Reading this book is better than having sex!

Oh come on…you know that can't be true…but now that I have your undivided attention, here is what a few people really do think about this book.

Outstanding! This is a fun book and an easy read, as well as being very informative. You have written an excellent book that will be a great teaching tool for years to come. I truly hope the public will pick up this book, devour the information, and then apply it in their daily lives. They would be so amazed and blessed with the results!

Judy Gedney, BS, MS
Professor of Biomechanics at Western Illinois University for 38 years
Co-founder of both The World, and The American, Drug-Free Powerlifting Federations
Competing powerlifter at the world championship level

I don't think anyone has presented such a case before and I truly believe it is the "right" answer for a huge percentage of our population. This book takes a great position so that the many people with already busy schedules can do something really positive about their body fat, nutrition, and overall health, and also be convinced that they can succeed. Great dietary information, including a simple enough explanation of exactly how it all works.

I completely love the way you have boiled the key information down to a very useable length as well as how you have used a very straightforward, "no BS allowed" delivery. People need to see how all the BS floating around is only there to take their money, not to help them reach their goals. Your humor throughout is also wonderfully direct, just like the information.

Neil Schmitt, BS, MBA
Multiple All-American
Former University of Iowa gymnastics coach
Former Marketing Executive for Hewlett Packard

Up till now, the problem with books on exercise and nutrition has been that you had to practically be a doctor to understand them, or they were so boring that you fell asleep trying to get through them. Bobby's book has definitely solved both of these problems. It's a terrific book.

Rob Haans
Certified Fitness Instructor
World Jiu-Jitsu Champion

Bobby is truly a guru for people who are interested in their total health but don't know where to start. This book is the perfect vehicle for helping so many more people than he could ever manage to help in person. It really sorts through the garbage and truly tries to educate people. Bobby never ceases to amaze me and I am overwhelmed with this product. I especially appreciate the chapter on gym etiquette!

Lucy Koviak, BS, MS
Former gymnast, former girlfriend (40+ years ago), and life-long friend
High School teacher for the past 18 years

This is a very well-written book. The information is essential for living a long, happy, and healthy life. This book should be in every school library.

Etta Dickson, BS, MS
Elementary School teacher for 25 years…having begun teaching at age 45
Yes…this is my mom who asked for some light dumbbells for her recent 93rd birthday.

Socrates said: "The unexamined life is not worth living by any man." The examination is considerably clearer now with Bobby's fine book.

Gene Murphy, BS, MS
38 years in education as a coach, teacher, Middle School and Jr. High School principal
Coached championship teams in football, basketball, track, gymnastics, diving, and golf
Multiple NAIA All-American in springboard diving
Member of the 1963 NAIA National Championship Golf Team
Winner of many long-drive (golf) championships (some at a body-weight of less than 140 lbs.) – longest drive in competition…376 yards…with the old wooden head, steel shaft clubs of those days.

This is a great book! It gives me specifics to go by rather than just wasting time at the gym. I changed my workouts to your recommendations and for the first five weeks I was gaining weight (muscle) but losing inches, especially around my waist. After that I began also slowly losing actual weight on the scale while continuing to build some muscle. I now do crunches the way you say and it really works.

After only five weeks on your program I was able to get off three blood pressure medications. My doctor could not believe that I was able to lower my BP that much, or that fast. Several friends (including a couple of doctors) want copies of your book when it comes out. I won't loan my copy out. Great book! Great workouts!

Jim Dickson
Retired TWA pilot…and yes…my older brother. If even he listens to me, I must be doing something right.

The book is great. It gives a new and original look at so many facts that most people overlook. The basic facts on diet and exercise are to the point and very realistic. It puts the responsibility of one's health directly on the individual – no excuses. The statistics regarding death in hospitals and overuse of drugs are fantastic.

Sam Bailie, BS, MS, & Avelyn Bailie, BS
Former gymnastics coaches at the University of Arizona
Former gymnastic coach at the University of Iowa (Sam)
Owners of Bailie & Assoc, Inc., developers of products for gymnastics
Owned and operated several very successful gymnastics training centers in both Florida and Arizona
Sam is also on the Board of Directors of the International Gymnastics Hall of Fame.

With the information contained in this well-written book you can make many positive changes in your life… and rather rapid changes at that. If you truly have the desire and the drive, you can work wonders with your body. I encourage all to read and heed the information in this book. It is valuable and will definitely enhance your life in many positive ways.

Dr. Ken Copeland, Ed.D.
Was a national caliber springboard diver at a weight of 250 lbs.
Ken has varied his bodyweight from a high of 330 lbs. to a low of 168 lbs.

CTTC™

CUT THRU THE CRAP©

of

FITNESS

and

FAT-LOSS NUTRITION

A no-nonsense personal prescription for
Exercise, Nutrition and a Healthy, Fulfilling Lifestyle

Efficient, effective, and practical techniques for producing maximum results
with a minimum amount of exercise!

Robert E. Dickson, BS, MS, CPFT

CTTC Health Publishing/USA

CTTC
health publishing

Cover design by Anoushka, (the late) Sandy Froeming, Karen McChrystal

ISBN 978-0-9797225-0-9

Printed in the United States of America

THIS BOOK IS DEDICATED TO THE LOVING MEMORY OF SANDY FROEMING

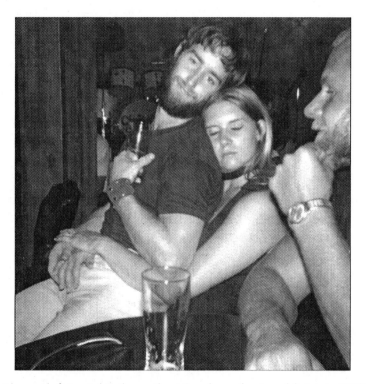

Above, left to right, the author, Sandy, author's publicist, in 1972

MOTHER TO A GENERATION OF GYMNASTS

A MOM TO PLANTS, PEOPLE, AND EVERYTHING IN BETWEEN

SHE LOVED AND CARED FOR ALL OF THEM EQUALLY

How to Read This Book

In order to completely comprehend the information, principles and concepts contained in this book, you should read it from the beginning straight through to the end.

I did not put any useless "filler" in this book. The information is important, relevant, and follows a logical progression from the beginning to the end of the book. Even the Preface, Foreword, Introduction and Acknowledgments (which many people never bother reading) contain information which is crucial to whether you will understand and accept the ideas within this book…or not.

If you skip parts of this book by first going to a chapter which you think will be most specific to your needs or interests, you will not be able to totally comprehend or evaluate what I am saying in that chapter. You will not be able to understand or appreciate how it logically "connects" with the information in the other chapters. Sadly, you will then miss one of the major concepts of this book, i.e., that these are NOT individual subjects but rather that each is critically involved in forming the "whole." A lack of understanding of this concept is what causes most people to fail, not only in their exercise and/or body fat loss programs, but also in life itself.

If your curiosity still demands to know more about what this book contains before you read it (or buy it), then go to Chapter 20: "22 Popular Myths and Fairy Tales." This chapter will give you a very good idea of the book's subject matter as well as how the information is presented. I wrote this chapter expressly for people who are tempted to begin reading at the back of a book.

Of course, this advice is optional. As I state again and again in this book, the choice to accept, reject or neglect any advice is ultimately yours and yours alone. In any case…

ENJOY!

CONTENTS

PREFACE

WHY DO WE NEED YET ANOTHER BOOK ON EXERCISE?

The short answer is: I simply can't continue to watch so many well-meaning exercisers waste so much of their valuable time and effort…with little or no results to show for it…and not do something to help. I sincerely hope that this book will change that situation for some people.

This is a straightforward and brutally honest exercise and nutrition book for genuinely serious men and women of all ages, all sizes and all abilities…but especially for those who love to eat and hate to exercise. I also include a good dose of fundamental lifestyle advice that is essential to anyone's health and well-being as well as to being successful at anything in life.

Between Extremes

There are many very good exercise and nutrition books on the market. I have many, many of them, and much of the advice you will read in this book has been gleaned from these other fine publications as well as from my more than four decades of personal experience helping other people to build more attractive, stronger, healthier bodies. The problem is, most of these books have been written for highly motivated, elite level athletes or bodybuilders at one end of the spectrum, or for people who are not genuinely serious about attaining a high level of fitness and health (the dreamers), on the other end of the spectrum. This is one reason why, even with these hundreds of books, magazines, videos, and DVDs on the market, most exercisers still know next to nothing about efficient, effective, result-producing **Quality Exercise**. For many years I have wanted to write a book which would help the many people who fall in between these two extremes. This is it.

The actual (non-adapted) **CTTC** Workouts are written for relatively healthy men and women who are already somewhat experienced at both cardiovascular (aerobic) exercise **and** exercising with weights. However, Chapter #11 tells you how the **CTTC** Workouts can easily be adapted to all levels of fitness, and to suit any personal exercise goals…regardless of your age or present physical condition (as long as you have no special or life-threatening medical problems).

This exercise program is the most logical, practical, time-saving, efficient and effective way to create a truly strong, healthy and shapely body. It is also a program that you can easily continue, with minor adaptations, for the rest of your life…which is how long a Quality Exercise program should last. You don't stop cleaning your teeth at sometime during your life, do you (even when they are not your own anymore)? An exercise program should be the same. A Quality Exercise program should form an integral part of your lifestyle.

Time Management

One of the main problems with so many exercise programs (even the good ones) is that they demand too much of your valuable time. Most people just don't have time to run 1-2 hours, 5-6 days a week and exercise with weights 4 -6 hours a week. Even if you do at this point in time, think about doing this for the next 20, 30, 40 years, and so on. You have to be a real fanatic to do something like this, and most of us are simply not exercise fanatics. We have real lives.

The **CTTC** Exercise Program is an excellent solution for the "time problem" that many professionals and other busy people have. Doctors, nurses and other health professionals, lawyers, business people, police, firefighters, and many others need to be healthy and in superior physical and mental condition in order to function optimally in their jobs. However, they have very little free time to exercise. The **CTTC** Exercise Program is **the** answer for anyone who wants to look good, feel great, function optimally, and be really healthy…but is always short of time.

Yes, it can be done and you do not have to give up everything else in your life in order to do it. In fact, by following the **CTTC** Exercise and Nutrition Programs, you will have more time to enjoy friends, family, and life…not less.

Above Average

These **CTTC** Exercise and Nutrition Programs are designed for men and women for whom average is not good enough…people who want to strive for something better!

When followed properly and conscientiously, this **CTTC** Exercise and Nutrition Program will help you to develop a superior level of health, and enable you to maintain that level…with a very small investment of your valuable time.

What **CTTC** Is Not

This is **not** another bodybuilding book, full of boring technical and scientific information explaining how to become a massive and muscular macho male…or massive and muscular macha female…by lifting tons of iron for 2-3 hours a day, five or six days a week. You will not find intricate charts and diagrams of complicated exercise plans which are impossible for us mere mortals to figure out…much less carry out.

Not a Wish Book

CTTC is also **not** another wish-book which promises that you can create a fabulous body in no-time by lifting and swinging your arms and legs around in the air for five or ten minutes a couple of times a week, without ever breaking a sweat or even breathing hard. There are no intelligence-insulting eat-as-much-as-you-want-of-anything-you-want-and-still-lose-body fat diets here either. You will not find

100 pages of food charts or useless recipes which use expensive ingredients, or which take hours to prepare. There are more than enough of these books already on the market.

CTTC does not contain super-strict, tortuous diets that you need to follow for months on end and, instead of having to wear out a pair of running shoes every week in order to lose your excess body fat, CTTC utilizes an innovative combination of exercises which, for many people, will require no more than 3 hours of Quality Exercise per week.

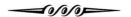

Logical, Practical, Informative

What you **will** find is pages and pages of practical, useful information that you can easily adapt to suit your own personal needs. Explanations are kept simple, logical, and relevant. They are intended to make you think about what you are doing and why you are doing it.

> A sensible understanding of exercise is a prerequisite to being successful at exercise.

Understanding exercise makes it possible for you to recognize what will work for you and what will not, thereby allowing you to make the right exercise choices. In turn, the right exercise choices will enable you to achieve a very high level of health and fitness and, at the same time, sculpt a stronger, firmer, and shapelier body…with the least amount of time and exercise possible!

Principles

The Principles of Quality Exercise and Nutrition presented in this book are so logical and practical that they can be applied to **any** exercise or nutrition program to enhance its effectiveness, and to increase your results.

Labor of Love

It is my goal to present this information, both old and new, in such a logical and entertaining way that it will make the material much more interesting and much easier to understand than it has been up to now. I hope to encourage some people to begin exercising, and to help the people who already exercise to reach their health and fitness goals much faster and more efficiently. If I can successfully do this, even on a small scale, then this book will have been more than worth all the time and effort it has taken to write it. If not, then it has still been a labor of love for me. That's what I like…win-win situations.

Repeating Myself

I repeat things often in *Cut Thru The Crap*. This is not my short-term memory loss at work. I do this because these things are important and I hope that...by repeating them often enough...they will begin to stick in your mind. I also use **bold** to emphasize words that I feel need emphasizing.

I am fully aware that these are considered to be appalling literary no-no's. However, **not** bestowing enough importance on these ideas, principles, and actions is causing thousands of otherwise serious exercisers to fail to reach their exercise goals and...for me...that is a much more serious no-no. Besides, I have not accomplished all that I have in life by always following someone else's rules. If I followed the rules, this would just be another in the myriad of pretty-picture exercise books, rehashing the same old information...once again...and that is sooooo not me!

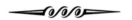

Too Much Information

The science of exercise and the field of building and maintaining optimal health are becoming more important at an ever-accelerating rate as health systems fall apart and health insurance premiums continue to skyrocket. For this reason, new research and information are also becoming available at a pace that makes it almost impossible to keep up. There has been more well-designed research conducted on the effects of exercise on healthy people in the last 15-20 years than has been done in the 50 years before that. The same is true for nutrition and the use of nutritional supplements for building and maintaining optimal health.

Unfortunately, much of this information is still being ignored by many in both the medical and the fitness communities.

Why...What...How Much...When

If you are a person leading an average life of working or attending school, paying bills, spending time with your significant other, kids, pets, hobbies, etc., then you certainly don't have time to sift through all this information yourself. Fortunately, others do and I would like to contribute to this worthy cause.

For those of us who have been passionately involved with health and fitness for the last 20-50 years or more, much of this information is not really new at all, but now we have scientific confirmation for what we already knew from experience long ago. The major difference is that now we know why, what, how much, and when, much more precisely than we did before.

Promises, Promises, Promises

As dinosaurs in the business, we have seen every fad diet, every piece of "miracle equipment," and every "revolutionary exercise system" come and go, only to see them return years later after people have forgotten that they didn't work the first time around. Usually they come back with pretty new names and fantastic advertising campaigns, but the results remain the same. After making people's wallets a lot lighter, they disappear once again to patiently await a new generation of victims.

Run Away, Run Away

You should run from anyone or any exercise program that promises you a "full-body workout with incredible results" in only five, ten, or fifteen minutes a day, once or twice a week...usually without ever having to break a sweat. Promising changes to your whole body by exercising only one part of it (usually your butt or stomach muscles), is another terrific way to scam you out of your hard-earned money. If I were clever, I would also write one of these "magic exercise programs." Unfortunately for my bank account, I still have too much integrity to do that...even though many of my friends would probably argue that point.

The same advice goes for weight-loss schemes which promise that you can eat as much of anything you want and still lose body fat. Nutritional supplements which promise "unbelievable results" should, in fact, not be believed. These should be no-brainers but, to the contrary, they have become multi-billion dollar businesses. They are selling hopes and dreams...NOT solutions to your problems.

Foolproof Test

I will give you an absolutely foolproof test to know if a system that makes these kinds of promises actually works or not...and here it is:

The person who comes up with a way to build a strong, healthy, and shapely body without having to exercise intensely...or to lose excess body fat while eating as much of anything you want...will become the richest person on the face of the earth...INSTANTLY! Within a week of this miracle system becoming known, the inventor's bank account will make that of Microsoft's Bill Gates look miniscule. I haven't seen that happen, so I guess the system isn't available yet...in spite of what the infomercials proclaim. When it is, I guarantee you that I will be one of the first ones to buy it...at any cost.

Warning

If all these products really worked, obesity would not be our national problem. The problem would be people completely disappearing!

These products would have to carry warnings on their labels like: "**WARNING:** If you use this miracle weight-loss product (or diet), in combination with any other miracle weight-loss products (or diets), such as, but not limited to: pills, patches, rubber or plastic clothing, teas, bracelets, miracle-working fitness equipment, fat-eating foods, massage machines, creams, belts, wraps, herbs, anything that shakes or vibrates, necklaces, tiny electric stimulators, magic stones, powders, magnets…and so on…you will run the risk of losing so much weight, so fast, that you could completely disappear before you realize it."

Lottery Tickets

Wake up people! You would be better off spending that money on lottery tickets. At least your chance of winning the lottery isn't completely ZERO!

A Better Way

Fitness and aerobics activities are unique in one aspect. They are usually accepted and blindly followed, regardless of whether they produce results or not!

Imagine that you were paying for golf lessons, but after several weeks your score was still 180 for 18 holes or, after weeks of tennis lessons, you still couldn't even hit the ball. At some point you would stop and say to yourself, "Self, something is wrong here." For some reason, this usually doesn't happen with fitness or aerobics (exercise). Most people either quit completely, or they continue on blindly. The idea that there may be **a better way** never seems to enter their minds!

I often return to gyms after several months, or even after a couple of years, only to find that more than half of the people who were there before have quit. Most of the ones remaining are still following the same "resultless" programs they were following the last time I saw them and they still look the same as before…or sometimes even worse. It is a very strange phenomenon which defies logic.

Results Count

Apparently, a lot of people seem to think that the goal of exercise is to punish their bodies for hours at a time, several days a week, in spite of minimal…or a total lack of…results.

> ✳   Your exercise goal should be to produce maximum results with the minimum amount of exercise possible.
>
> RESULTS are what count…not how MUCH exercise you do!

Diminishing Returns

Another factor that is rarely, if ever, considered, is the point of diminishing returns. This is the point in a successful exercise program where your results no longer keep up with your efforts. When I have reached a point where I would have to increase the intensity or duration of my exercise by 15-20% or more, in order to improve my results by only 5%, then I will choose to remain at the present level. The minimal improvement in results does not warrant so much extra time and effort, unless you are an elite athlete. I prefer to spend that extra time doing more productive things…like enjoying life.

Enough Is Enough

The better the condition you get into…the harder it is to get into even better condition. You have to decide at what realistic level you will be personally satisfied. **Your** health and **your** opinion are the only things that should really count here.

And if you hate to exercise…like I do… why would you ever want do more exercise than is necessary to attain, and then maintain, your personal health and physical goals anyway?

Smarter Is Better

A few systems of exercise and nutrition have withstood the test of time because they **do** work. Thanks to quality research, these same systems have become better and more precise over the years. Today we have a much better understanding of the genetic, hormonal and physiological influences on our bodies. We can now apply this knowledge to these systems which have always worked, to achieve even better results, more quickly. It's no longer a matter of working **harder** for better results, but working **smarter** for better results.

I'm Convinced

These are some of the things that convinced me that this book is necessary and this is also why I chose a title that would very clearly explain that the purpose of this book is to literally *Cut Thru The Crap of Fitness and Fat-Loss Nutrition.*

Better Is Better

As you will see, the **CTTC** Exercise and Nutrition Program integrates information synergistically, enabling you to:

1. Develop the muscle you need to create a shapely (ladies) or athletic (guys) body.

2. Burn your excess body fat away to reveal the shapely (or athletic) body underneath.

3. Keep your excess body fat off once it is gone or…even better…prevent gaining excess body fat in the first place.

4. Increase your strength.

5. Improve your cardiovascular fitness.

6. Increase your energy levels.

7. Improve your flexibility.

8. Enhance your health.

9. Strengthen your immune system.

10. Improve your quality of life.

You Can Have it All

The great thing about the **CTTC** Exercise Program is that you can accomplish all these things in the same workout. You can't be much more efficient than that. And I am not talking about busting your butt for 2-3 hours a day, 5-6 days a week. The **CTTC** Exercise Program is comprised of three short, but satisfyingly intense, workouts per week.

All Also Includes…

In addition to the physical advantages the **CTTC** Exercise Program will provide, it will also help you to:

1. Develop more self-esteem, so that you feel better about yourself.

2. Develop a better self-image, which will make your journey through life flow much easier.

3. Develop more self-discipline, which will make it easier to get what you want out of life.

4. Develop more self-confidence, which will make all aspects of your life better.

5. Enjoy life more.

More is not better…*better* is better!

FOREWORD

By Charles Froeming

When it comes to your fitness and exercise program – do you want to achieve maximum results in minimum time? Are you interested in learning how to achieve your personal goals for health, strength, endurance, appearance, or performance – and do it in the most efficient way, and in the least amount of time? If so, you have come to the right place because this book is about honesty. It is about the author being honest with you and it is about you being honest with yourself.

You see many books that are written for the sole purpose of selling books. The information is "packaged," and usually also ghost-written, to tell you what you want to hear instead of what you need to know. You won't find that to be the case in *Cut Thru The Crap*. The author, my friend Bob Dickson, tells it like it is. What you have in your hands is a lifetime of experience gained through meticulous trial and error. What you have is a shortcut to success that comes from years of study and hard-learned lessons about what works and what doesn't work.

It all starts by being honest with yourself. It is about clearly defining where you are now and where you want to be. It is about setting goals and measuring the progress along the way. It is about "feeling good" – feeling good about being in control, feeling good about who you are, feeling good about where you are going, and feeling good about what you can achieve in this life. None of us are getting out of this game of life alive…so why not make the most of the time you have? The best way to do that is by staying healthy, by staying fit, by discovering who the "real you" is, and by learning how to really enjoy life.

In this industrialized, computerized, remote control world, finding time to exercise can be a real challenge. We sometimes forget how important exercise is to our overall health and well-being and, thereby, to our happiness. This book is perfect for everyone who ever said, "I just don't have the time to exercise," because with this program you can't afford not to exercise – the positive results are just too compelling.

This book is written by a person who loves life, loves to have fun, loves to party, and who actually hates to exercise. I ought to know: Bob and I almost killed ourselves on a mission to outdo each other in the field of partyology. Is that a word? We have spent half our lives recovering from the other half of our lives. What is remarkable is what Bob was able to achieve despite his tendency to sway a bit from his training regimens. He constantly amazed teammates and friends with his ability to get ready for major gymnastic competitions, seemingly overnight. We knew that Bob knew something special; we just didn't know how much he knew…until now.

Bob is also an inspiring leader of people, helping them to reach deep down and pull out the best they have inside themselves. In fact, he is a leader in everything he does. He was using weights to improve both his health and his sports performances decades before it was accepted by the mainstream. He was already using special diets and nutritional supplements in the 1960's. During this time he also utilized meditation, visualization and yoga to enhance his sports performances, and was teaching them to others as well.

Exercise – My Dad used to watch me exercise all the time. He was always a bit confused as to why I would work that hard without being paid for it. As a high-level competitive gymnast, I had a focused goal in mind. What is yours? Do you even have one? Read this book and apply what you learn…and you will know, with confidence, that you are moving in the direction you want to go, with a program that can truly become part of your life…for the rest of your life!

Thank you, Bob, for sharing this important information with the world, and for sharing your humor and your life with Sandy and me. It has been a great run. She is watching over us and is very proud of what you have accomplished with this book.

   ~ Charles "Charlie" Froeming, B.S., M.A.

Chapter 1

INTRODUCTION

THE "CUT THRU THE CRAP" EXERCISE AND NUTRITION PROGRAMS

CTTC is a brutally honest guide to creating a stronger, shapelier, and healthier body…in the shortest amount of time…and with the least amount of exercise possible.

My hope is that this book will not only motivate you to use Quality Exercise and nutrition to improve your body and enhance your health, but that it will also inspire you to better your "self."

This book will not only put you in control of your weight…it could also put you in control of your life.

IT CAN DEFINITELY CHANGE YOUR LIFE FOR THE BETTER!

> I have never been able to understand why people who would never accept living in a house that is broken down and falling apart, allow their spirits and minds to live in one. – R.E. Dickson

Different

I think you will find this to be a little different from your normal, run-of-the-mill exercise book. I sincerely hope that the way I present the information in this book will open exercisers' minds to what they are actually doing…or at least shock them into thinking about what they are actually doing.

If this book can convince only a few exercisers to stop blindly following advice, and to begin thinking and analyzing what they are actually doing, then I will have done the job I set out to do. These readers will then become better, healthier, more successful exercisers…with more attractive bodies to show for it.

Words

One of the things that makes this book different is the way that I use words. Words are very powerful. They cause actual physiological changes in both our bodies and our minds. For this reason, I do not sugar-coat my words, my opinions, or my advice. If I happen to offend your sensibilities in the process, that's OK too. At least I will have gotten some kind of reaction out of you.

Think

I introduce several personal definitions in this book which I feel are necessary to eliminate the confusion caused by years of incorrect interpretation of certain words related to the fields of exercise, nutrition, and health. I do this because one of the main purposes of this book is to make you **think** about what you are hearing, reading, believing and doing when it comes to exercise, nutrition, body fat and your health.

Over-weight

For instance, are people over-**weight** or are they over-**fat**? Over-**weight** is such a benign word. It is almost cute, which is why it does not ring the alarm bells in us that it should…as soon as it should. The truth is, over-**weight** is like friendly-fire. They are both innocent sounding words, which is why people prefer to use them. However, with the one you are still dead, and with the other you are still fat. Is someone more dead if he gets killed by enemy-fire? Will you be less fat if we call it over-**weight**? Are you over-**fat**? What exactly is over-**weight**? Where does over-**weight** stop and over-**fat** begin?

Tell the Truth Now

When talking to yourself, always tell the truth. Don't hide the truth behind nicer sounding words. That is lying to yourself and it will only hurt you in the long run.

If you can't even bring yourself to call a problem by its real name, you certainly won't be able to bring yourself to seriously do something about it.

It Begins So Innocently

First we have baby-fat. That turns into pudgy. Then we become pleasingly plump. Next, we are just a little overweight…which is still OK, right? Then we become too heavy, which is also not too bad. The next step is just plain overweight, where we first start to consider the possibility that something may, in fact, be wrong. Eventually all these misnomers lead us…little lie by little lie…to a place we never wanted to be, and can no longer deny. We are just plain FAT. Oh, you don't like that word? How about obese? Doesn't sound enough like a disease that you can have no personal control over whatsoever? How about Lardosis? Now that has a nice medical ring to it, doesn't it?

What Happened?

After deciding on the politically correct name of your choice, the questions begin. "How did this ever happen to me?" It happened to you because, by continually lying to yourself (denial), you allowed it to happen. That's OK. We all lie to ourselves at sometime or another. I have done it as well.

The real question should be: After having finally decided to call the problem by its real name, what are you willing to do about it?

The same thing can happen with your health. You have it and then...whoosh...all of a sudden it's gone and you are asking the same question again, "How did this ever happen to me?" However, regaining your health is much more difficult than losing body fat, which is why I do not separate the two in this book. If your exercise/body fat loss program does not also contribute significantly to your health...and continue to do so...I do not consider it to be a "quality" exercise program.

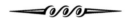

Quality Exercise?

In Chapter #2, I am sure you will be surprised to hear what I do not consider to be Quality Exercise. Most people only think they are exercising, which is why their results are usually so disappointing. **A sensible understanding of exercise is a prerequisite to being successful at exercise.** If you do not understand what exercise really is, you cannot make good exercise choices. Without good exercise choices, you will fail to achieve your exercise and health goals.

In order not to contribute even more to this confusion, I attempt to use the word exercise only when I am talking about my specific definition of Quality Exercise. I also try to not use words like training, working out, or lifting weights...to name a few...when I am referring to Quality Exercise. This way, you can have no doubts as to what I am talking about in this book.

I repeat: A Quality Exercise and nutrition program should do all of the following...and continue to do so:

- Increase your lean body mass (muscle)...or maintain it at a level at which you are personally satisfied.
- Decrease your body fat...or maintain it at a level at which you are healthy and personally satisfied.
- Improve your cardiovascular condition...or maintain it at a level where you remain completely functional.
- Increase your strength...or maintain it at a level where you remain completely functional.
- Improve your flexibility...or maintain it at a level where you remain completely mobile.
- Increase your energy levels...or maintain them at levels at which you can function optimally.

- Enhance your health…and keep you as healthy as possible.
- Strengthen your immune system…and keep it strong.
- Improve your quality of life.

If it does not do all these things…and continue doing them…it is not a Quality Exercise program.

All Mixed Up

You will find references to fat-loss, exercise, aerobics, and physical and mental health everywhere in this book…not only in the specific chapters regarding these subjects. This is not only to emphasize their importance, but also because they are inseparable. You cannot intelligently discuss one of these subjects without involving all of them to some degree. This goes against modern "magic bullet" thinking, where you have to consider…or do…only one thing in order to achieve a certain outcome. However, "magic bullet" solutions rate right up there with "politically correct" thinking in my mind and, from what I can see, neither one of these works very well.

I consider being politically correct to be, in most cases, an insidious form of lying. For instance, I myself am not "motivationally challenged." I am plain lazy…pure and simple. I admit it, I accept it, and I manage my life with that fact in mind. If you base your life on bullsh.t, that is exactly what you will eventually wind up with.

Honesty clarifies problems, which then makes them much easier to solve.

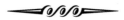

The Information Gap

When I first started exercising in the 1950s, there was very little information on exercise available. Thankfully, that is no longer a problem. The problem now is that there is too much information. There is so much really good information out there and, at the same time, so much really bad information, "old wives' tales," and just plain crap about health and exercise, which stubbornly refuse to go away. It is very confusing and **most people don't have the experience or the knowledge necessary to separate the good from the bad.**

It takes even more experience and knowledge to separate good from better…and better from best. There are several good programs, techniques and systems of Quality Exercise, but they are not all equally suitable to help you to reach your personal exercise goals. This can be really confusing. This book will provide you with the facts, information and ideas you need to make better exercise choices. Even if you choose not to follow the **CTTC** Exercise and Nutrition Programs (which I think would be a BIG mistake), the ideas and information in this book can be applied to any exercise, body fat loss, or nutrition program, as well as any program designed to increase health.

Not a Pretty Picture

If you are looking for a book with lots of pretty pictures…this is not it. This book is, however, crammed so full of important, practical, and useful information that you will definitely want to (and need to) read it over and over again.

Not a Textbook

Keeping in spirit with the title, I want this book to be an easy read, so I do not attempt to educate you about anatomy, kinesiology, physiology, or any other ology. If you are interested in learning more about these subjects, there are dozens of books that will do that much better than this one does. This is not a medical or a scientific textbook. It is a thoughtful, practical, doable guide for helping you to achieve your personal goals in the areas of fitness, body fat loss, control of body fat, mental and physical health and creating a shapelier and/or more athletic body.

Many other books have also been written with these things in mind. However, most of them address only one or two of these subjects, which still leaves you with missing parts to a puzzle. *Cut Thru The Crap* combines all these subjects into one super efficient and time-saving twelve-week program.

Most exercise books are written for a single group of people. There are exercise books written specifically for young people, older people, in-between people, not-really-serious exercisers, serious exercisers in every type of sport, aerobic exercisers, anaerobic exercisers, exercisers using weights, bodybuilders and so on. If you don't happen to fit into the one specific category that the book addresses, much of the information can be useless for achieving your specific exercise goals.

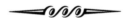

Principles

The vast amounts of information you will encounter in this book can be applied to virtually any type of exercise you could ever choose to do, because the information is based on **Principles of Quality Exercise**. After reading this book, you will understand what will work…and what will not work…to achieve your personal exercise goals, and, even more importantly, you will understand why!

Holistic

Cut Thru The Crap uses a holistic/integrated approach. The length and frequency of the **CTTC** Workouts, the duration of the three phases (four weeks each), the combination of traditional and Cardio-aerobics, the choices of exercises, the order of the exercises, the changes in exercises, the exercise positions, the number of sets and reps, the length of the rest periods, the grip positions, the exercise intensities…and so on…make **CTTC** an extremely efficient, complete, well-rounded, Quality Exercise program. The Quality Exercise program has been carefully integrated with a quality nutrition program not only to improve your outer beauty, but also to strengthen your inner beauty and increase your health.

Fight Fat

This book places a great deal of emphasis on losing body fat and keeping it off…permanently, simply because most people's main concern is controlling their body fat (nearly 70% of Americans are over-fat).

I'm not going to **show** you how to lose **weight**. Instead, I'm going to **teach** you how to lose your **excess body fat**.

CTTC is the most logical, practical, timesaving, efficient, effective and healthiest way to lose excess body fat, and keep it off…permanently! You did not put your excess body fat on in a couple of weeks and you will not take it off in a couple of weeks. Get that thought out of your head right now. It is possible to lose body fat a little more quickly than with the **CTTC** programs, but only if you are very highly motivated, extremely self-disciplined, and are able to devote much more time to both your exercise and your nutrition than is necessary with the **CTTC** Exercise and Nutrition Programs.

Unless you could have written this book yourself, you would also need the services of an excellent personal trainer. After all that, you will still need a program such as **CTTC** in order to keep the body fat off permanently, so you might as well save yourself a lot of time, money and physical torture by giving the **CTTC** Exercise and Nutrition Programs a fair chance right from the beginning.

The **CTTC** Exercise and Nutrition Program is an intelligent and effective alternative to today's inefficient dieting and exercise madness. Try it…you'll like it!

Personalizing

If your goal is to add solid bodyweight and build a more muscular, athletic body, this **CTTC** program can be easily adapted to these goals as well.

You will learn how you can easily make small changes in the **CTTC** Exercise Program to better suit your personal situation, problems, and goals. This makes **CTTC** an ideal exercise program for the vast majority of people…both men and women, young and old…who are genuinely serious about creating a stronger, healthier, shapelier body…and improving their overall quality of life as well.

Hear me

I wrote *Cut Thru The Crap* as if I were personally instructing and talking to you on a one-on-one basis. I do attempt to inject a little humor, some sarcasm, and I even make up some words when I think it will help to make my point…or if it will make you really think about what I am saying.

I don't want you to just read what I wrote…I want you to hear what I am saying!

Who needs this program?

- If you do no exercise at all…you definitely need this program.

- If aerobics is your only form of exercise…you definitely need this program.

- If you only exercise with weights…you definitely need this program.

- If you are not satisfied with the results you are getting from your present exercise program… you definitely need this program.

- If your present exercise program is taking up too much of your valuable time…you definitely need this program.

- If you catch the flu (or colds) more than once every several years, or scratches and small cuts become easily infected, or heal too slowly, the **CTTC** Exercise and Nutrition Programs will definitely help to strengthen your immune system and make you healthier.

In other words, if you want to have a stronger, healthier, shapelier body and all the benefits in life that come with it, the **CTTC** Exercise and Nutrition Programs can help you to reach these goals quickly and efficiently. The **CTTC** Programs can be easily adapted to accommodate all ages, different ability levels, different goals, and different levels of motivation.

- If you are new to exercise, you now have the chance to bypass most of the mistakes the rest of us have had to make over many, many years of trial and error. The **CTTC** Exercise and Nutrition Programs will save you years of wasted time and effort in your quest to attain your exercise goals and build a strong foundation for future health and happiness.

- If you have been exercising for eight weeks or longer, and are not satisfied with your results, the **CTTC** Exercise and Nutrition Programs offer a better solution.

- If you only do aerobics and/or callisthenic type exercises, the **CTTC** Exercise and Nutrition Programs will put you on the right track to creating a truly strong, healthy and shapely body… not just a skinny one.

- If you are already a successful exerciser, the **CTTC** Exercise and Nutrition Programs can become welcome additions to your arsenal of other successful programs.

- If you are just bored doing the same programs over and over, the **CTTC** Exercise and Nutrition Programs can renew your interest, and put enthusiasm back into your exercising.

Give It a Chance

I hope you will decide to give the **CTTC** Exercise and Nutrition Programs a fair chance to do their intended jobs and I wish you success in life, great mental and physical health, and lots of enjoyment of your stronger, healthier, shapelier body.

Never forget to enjoy life … you only have one shot at it!

Chapter 2

WHAT EVER HAPPENED TO THE "T" IN EXER(T)CISE?

This is in reference to the myriad of exercise programs and equipment, past and present, which promise amazing results without anyone ever having to exer(t) themselves. For someone who is morbidly obese, or is recovering from an illness or injury, just walking to the end of the block and back could be strenuous enough to be considered exercise. However, if you are not in one of these two categories and an "exercise" program in which you move your arms in little circles and lift your legs up and down, etc., gives you sore muscles and makes you actually feel like you have really "exerted" yourself, then you are just plain physically unhealthy. Acknowledge it…and then do something about it!

Just Moving Is NOT Exercise

Of course, nearly anything is better than nothing…but is that honestly the quality of life that will really satisfy you?

Do not let yourself be conned into believing that these kinds of programs can build truly strong, healthy, shapely bodies. There is a German word I like to use when describing these kinds of physical "activities." "Krankengymnastik" means exercise for sick people. The Dutch do not even have a word for exercise. They call more strenuous exercise "sporting" and anything less than that is referred to as "beweging," which means, literally, moving. Dutch doctors then say that people need to "move" more to be healthy and prevent obesity, so most Dutch people think that just moving is the same thing as exercise. They say, "But I do "beweg." I clean the house, I do some gardening, I wash the car, I go for a stroll with the dog for ten minutes every day," and so on.

A stroll is not exercise. It is standing still…speeded up a little! Taking strolls as your only form of exercise is certainly better than nothing…but it is still Krankengymnastik.

Tell Them What They Want to Hear

How many out-of-shape, unmotivated people would ever join a gym if they were told from the beginning that they would have to work really hard in order to attain their fitness and body fat-loss dreams? The truth…not many! Exercise equipment advertised on TV has to promise "miracle results" with only a few minutes of "fun and easy" exercise a day, in order to sell their products.

A Personal Favorite

My favorite one at the moment promises unbelievable results from exercising only one muscle (abdominals, of course) for only one minute a day. They don't say anything about any other exercise, so I guess you don't need any, and they don't say anything about nutrition, so I guess you can also eat anything you want…and as much of it as you want. All I know is that they show some 300 - 400 pound people who, after exercising for only one minute a day with this "miracle machine," became 115 lb. models after only a few weeks of this "fun and easy" exercise.

Not only that, but their stretch marks and cellulite completely disappeared, they have no loose skin, and even their makeup and hairstyles got better. The "miracle machine" somehow gave each of them a great tan as well.

With something as wonderful as this on the market, I don't understand why there are any over-fat people left on this earth at all! One minute a day…right. Before I continue, let me go get a "Hi, I am an idiot" stamp on my forehead.

Masochists

A doctor telling his unhealthy patients just how much they will really need to exercise in order to regain their health is just begging for a second opinion. Let's face it, there is a very limited number of exercise masochists, and there are not enough of them to financially support all the commercial gyms and sell all the exercise equipment out there…so they have to stretch the truth a little…or a lot.

How … Not What   *INTENSITY IS KEY*

Unless you are obese, or recovering from an injury or illness, taking a walk is also not exercise. It is a slow form of transportation. Power-walking **is** exercise. Once again, **it's not** *what* **you do, but** *how* **you do it that makes the difference.** Don't compare a soap opera with an Academy Award winning movie. They are both entertainment on film, but you can't seriously say that they are both the same "quality" of entertainment.

How Much Is Really Enough?

If you want to enjoy a high degree of health benefits from exercise, research tells us that you need to expend a minimum of about 1500 calories per week doing both Quality Exercise and exercise activities. It is not a coincidence that the CTTC Exercise Program, when followed correctly, will expend approximately 500 calories per workout, or 1500 calories per week, based on a 150-pound man. Smaller persons and women will expend a little less and larger persons will expend a little more.

The health benefits of Quality Exercise continue to increase up to approximately 3,500 calories per week. Above that, "the law of diminishing returns" begins to kick in, which means that, from that point on, you will be getting **minimal** results for all your extra effort.

One long-term study of 785 men and women who had lost at least thirty pounds, and kept it off for five years or more, showed that they burned an average of 2800 calories per week through exercise.

Therefore, for the most efficient results, your exercise program should fall somewhere between 1500 and 3,500 calories per week, depending on your personal circumstances. So why do more exercise than is necessary to reach, and thereafter maintain, your personal health and fitness goals? Or do you just have lots of extra time that you can afford to waste?

The three **CTTC** Workouts will expend about 1500 calories per week, which covers your **minimum** weekly exercise requirements for higher health benefits. This will cost about **three hours** of your valuable time. Or you could walk for **ten hours per week** for the same 1500 calories, but with many fewer positive results to show for it. It is your choice.

I like to add a safety margin of another 500 calories per week for a total of 2000 calories per week. This means that you only need to burn another 500 calories (with exercise activities) during the other four days of the week in order to reach a goal of 2000 calories per week. That is an average of only 125 calories a day, which should make it very difficult to make excuses not to do this.

Just thirty minutes of either power-walking or riding your bicycle at about 70% of your MHR (maximum heart rate; MHR will be explained in the following chapter) will burn about 150 calories. Tennis, squash, racquetball, golf (walking, not riding), swimming, all kinds of skiing/boarding, and other enjoyable exercise activities are also productive ways to increase your weekly caloric expenditure.

Of course your personal circumstances will determine how much exercise above the minimum of 1500 calories you will need to do, if any.

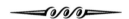

What Is Quality Exercise?

> The purpose of Quality Exercise is not to run a certain distance, or to lift a certain amount of weight. The purpose is to create a specific stimulation in your body which will then produce a specific and desired result.

The difference between Quality Exercise and an "exercise activity" is the same as the difference between studying a book in order to reach a specific goal (pass a test, earn a diploma, etc.), and reading a book just for pleasure.

> Quality Exercise is very structured and very exact exercise, designed to achieve a very specific goal.

An **exercise activity** is doing some type of exercise, physical game, or sport, just for the fun of it, with health benefits being secondary to the enjoyment of the activity.

Another Foolproof Test

So that you can have no doubts as to whether you are truly exercising or just "moving," I will give you a foolproof test to determine whether an activity qualifies as Quality Exercise or not. My test for Quality Exercise is very simple. It consists of only three questions:

1. Can you objectively measure the activity?

2. Can you control the movements of the activity?

3. Can you measure and control the intensity level of the activity?

If you can NOT answer yes to all three of these questions, then I consider it to be an "exercise activity," not Quality Exercise.

If you cannot accurately measure what you are doing, or cannot control the movements and intensity, you cannot accurately evaluate your results. **Without accurate results, you cannot design an effective exercise plan with a specific, desired outcome.**

1. **Measurement:** If you cannot, or do not, objectively measure the activity, you cannot know exactly what is happening to your body. If you don't know exactly how far you ran last time, exactly how long it took you to run it, and exactly what your heart rate was while you were running, you cannot know exactly how "hard" you ran. You also cannot plan to run "harder," or "less hard," next time because you have no objective measurements to work with.

   If you do not use actual weights for your strength exercises, you cannot know exactly how much resistance you used last time, this time, or how much you need to use next time. If you try to rely on elastic cords, or something similar – did you stretch the elastic ½ pound more than last time, or was it 1 pound less? You just can't know. These types of resistance exercise are just not precise enough!

2. **Control:** Being able to control the movements of the activity is another necessity in my test for Quality Exercise. Power-walking, jogging, some other types of aerobics and exercising with weights are all examples of controlled movement exercise. In basketball, tennis, racquetball and many other physical activities, your movements cannot be controlled, so they remain "exercise activities," according to my test.

Compare these first two factors to studying a book. If you begin at the beginning of the book (control) and study one consecutive chapter every day (measurement), your results will be much different than if you arbitrarily open the book to a random page each time, and only study for as long as you feel like it. Come to think of it, that may be why it took me so long to graduate from high-school…and college.

3.   **Intensity:** Now that we can we can accurately measure the activity and control the movements of the activity, we can control the intensity of the activity as well. The first thing distance runners do when they cross the finish line is to check their stopwatches. If they don't know their exact times, they can't compare them to their previous times to know exactly how they did, or where they are in their training programs. If they ran the same distance faster than before, then they exercised more intensely. If they ran the same distance slower, they exercised less intensely.

   Callisthenic type activities do not pass my test. Did you circle your arms or lift your legs more often, or more intensely this time than last time? How much more? Taking an aerobics class is also not Quality Exercise by my test…unless you constantly measure and control your heart rate!

   Playing basketball or tennis is taking part in an "exercise activity." Did you play tennis more intensely today than you did last time? Maybe you did, and maybe you didn't. You can't know for sure because you cannot accurately measure a tennis game or a basketball game, and you cannot control their movements either. These are great "exercise activities," but they are inefficient tools for reaching a specific exercise goal.

If you choose your types of exercise according to my test, you will reach your exercise goals much more quickly and much more efficiently than if you try to do it haphazardly with "exercise activities." After you reach your exercise goals, you will enjoy your exercise activities even more.

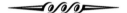

Weights and Quality Exercise

Of course, these three **Principals of Quality Exercise** apply to exercising with weights as well. Many people just move the weights instead of exercising with the weights. There is a big difference!

Elite athletes **train** with weights to improve some specific aspect of their performance. Weightlifters and powerlifters want to **lift** as much weight as possible. These are measurable activities with controlled movements, a high intensity level, and they are designed to achieve a pre-determined goal. However, we are also interested in our fitness and health, which are not specific goals for these two particular groups of athletes. They are only concerned with improving performance. Since we are concerned with **exercising** with weights, the time factor becomes much more important.

People who do one set of a resistance exercise which doesn't even make them breathe hard, then "rest" for two or three minutes (or more) before beginning the next set, are only moving the weights

up and down. They are not exercising and they will enjoy none of the benefits of Quality Exercise because the intensity factor is completely missing!

If you exercise with the same amount of weight, but complete your workout in less time than usual, or you exercise for the same amount of time, but use more weight, then you have increased intensity. It is measurable and it is able to be controlled. Now you only have to make sure that you are exerting yourself enough to be truly exercising. Once again, if you are not breathing hard when you exercise with weights, then you are not exerting yourself enough.

Exertion

Normally my wife Anoushka always travels with me. However, one time I had to take a short business trip and she decided to stay home. A friend of ours, who was a competitive bodybuilder at the time, jokingly said that Anoushka could "train" with him for that week. She agreed, but said that they would "train" using her exercise program, which she and I had designed together … and her training tempo. Our friend laughingly agreed, thinking he had a week of easy "girly" workouts in his future. He lasted about fifteen minutes into the first workout before he had to run to the bathroom to "lose his lunch." He had **trained** with weights, but he had never **exercised** with weights, so he had no muscular endurance and he had really lousy cardiovascular conditioning as well. Needless to say, Anoushka **exercised** by herself for the rest of the week.

I often see joggers, even over-fat ones, whose technique is so smooth and efficient that I probably burn more energy watching TV than they do jogging. If your goals are to lose excess body fat, increase your health, improve your fitness, build a shapely or athletic body, or any combination of these, you will have to **exert** yourself. If you do not, you are only wishing and hoping…not exercising to reach a goal.

Only when you fully understand the importance of these three factors, which are so necessary to Quality Exercise, can you intelligently choose an exercise program that is both efficient and effective. In other words, one that not only works in the beginning, but also one that will continue to work because it can be adjusted and fine-tuned…indefinitely. The **CTTC** Exercise Program has been designed with this in mind.

How Many Calories?

You can also very easily approximate how many calories your resistance exercise is burning. You burn about one calorie for each 100 pounds that you lift. For example, if you bench press 100 pounds ten times, you will have burned approximately ten calories (and I am being generous here). Do five sets of these bench presses and you will have burned about fifty calories. So if you are curious, you can add up the poundage from your entire weight workout, divide that sum by 100, and you will know approximately how many calories you have used during that workout. And you thought you would never have an opportunity to use that math you had to learn in school. Well, here is your chance. Done? Now look how many calories are in that candy bar you are thinking about eating. Is it really going to be worth it after all that hard work?

—◦/◦/◦—

Goals

OK, now you have the right tools: the **CTTC** Exercise and Nutrition Programs. So what else makes so many well-intentioned people fail to reach their exercise goals? There you have the answer: goals. Too many people have no goals at all or they have unrealistic goals, which is just as destructive. This is a major cause of failure and unhappiness for many people, not only in their exercise programs, but also in their daily lives!

> A desire without a plan is a wish, not a goal.

Every action begins as a thought but, **without realistic goals, you will never succeed.** You need realistic goals in order to know where you are going, in health, fitness, and in life!

First we need to define what a goal is, and then how to set realistic, attainable goals. **A desire without a plan is a wish, not a goal,** and you cannot make a commitment to a wish. Guys who want to get "BIG," ladies who want to just "tone up," and anyone who wants to lose "weight" are not setting goals and making commitments. They are wishing and dreaming. What they actually want is, respectively, to develop more muscle, to create a shapelier body, and to lose excess body fat.

If you are forty-five years old and think you can look eighteen again, or you haven't exercised in years (or ever) and think you can get into really great shape in a few short weeks, then you are living in a dream world and you will FAIL – definitely, totally, and miserably. Set real, attainable goals for yourself, and relish the joy of success instead of suffering the constant misery of failure.

Short, Medium, Long

You can have a realistic, attainable, long-term goal of graduating from school. However, your medium-term goal has to be that of successfully completing the current semester. The only way to insure successful completion of the current semester is to successfully complete your short-term goals of doing your best today, the rest of this week, and the rest of this month. Then you need to complete these same short-term goals again next month, and so on. Just hoping and dreaming about graduation isn't going to get the job done. Believe me. I tried it, and my university "education" was the happiest eight years of my life.

So once you have defined your long-term goal(s), you need to make more specific medium and short-term goals. These should be designed to program yourself for continued success. **Hoping** to lose thirty pounds of excess body fat in one month is programming yourself for failure. **Planning** to lose five pounds this month is an entirely attainable medium-term goal, so you will be programming yourself to succeed. Continued success assures that you will stick with your commitments and, after all, a mere five pounds a month is thirty pounds in only six months. Do you have any idea how much volume there is in thirty pounds of body fat? It is an enormous amount and unless you are extremely obese, the loss of thirty pounds of body fat will not only completely change the shape of your body, but also your mind-set. That is not a small result.

Short-term goals are the small steps to your future successes and they can be as simple as deciding not to miss any workouts this week…or not to miss your workout today.

As you get into better shape, you will still need goals, but they will need to become more and more specific to match your progress. You should never be completely satisfied, because then you will have no more short-term goals. Maintaining your well-earned hardbody should then be your long-term goal but, to stay motivated, it always helps to keep striving to improve something. Maybe you want to develop just a little more definition in your abdominals, or to fill in that area between your shoulder blades, or improve the shape of your calves just a bit. There will always be something to improve on and, when you do, it will once again earn you personal satisfaction, motivate you, and increase your self-esteem, self-confidence and self-discipline. That's a darn good payoff for a **minor** improvement.

It's About You

Set goals that you want to achieve for yourself, not for another person. Don't set a goal just to impress someone else, although that can be a perfectly valid short-term goal when used as a motivational tool. For instance, you can use an upcoming reunion to boost your enthusiasm and keep yourself better focused and disciplined for that period of time.

Time Limits

This brings up another thing that people often fail to do, and that is to put a definite time limit on their goals.

In order to win…you have to know where the finish line is!

When I was in my late thirties, I set a long-term goal of being able to squat, deadlift, and incline bench press 220 pounds each on my fortieth birthday. Being a former gymnast and professional acrobat, I am quite strong when throwing my own body around, but I have never been particularly powerful when it comes to pushing iron. The "big boys" will laugh at these weights, but they were darned heavy for my meager 140 pounds and it took me long enough to build up to them. Besides, I was doing this as a personal challenge to myself, knowing that, **when** I accomplished it (not **if** I accomplished it), I would be in excellent all-around condition and ready to start a new decade of my life. The amount of weight was completely irrelevant. It was simply a means of peaking my exercise interest once again by setting a realistic goal with a definite time period attached to it. After I reached this goal, I set another long-term goal, which required a completely different exercise plan to achieve, but which also had a definite time limit.

"…till death do us part" is another good example of setting a specific goal with a definite time limit.

Inspiration

Use whatever works to keep you on the road to your medium and long-term goals. Both external and internal inspiration are necessary. Use pictures of persons who inspire you. Use old photos of yourself if you were ever in good shape. Read inspiring books and magazines. Most importantly, **program your internal thoughts to be positive and inspiring**. After all, you are doing this for yourself, so make sure "self" is on your side.

Visualization

First, develop a realistic picture in your mind of exactly what you want to achieve with your exercise program. You have to know **exactly** what you want. **If you can't perceive it, you can't achieve it.**

Next, **constantly visualize achieving these goals**, especially while you are exercising or just resting quietly. The more you do this, the more it becomes ingrained in your brain, and the stronger you will become mentally. You will be making positive thinking and goal achievement a normal part of your being which, in turn, will positively influence every other aspect of your life as well.

Would you have ever thought that exercising could put you more in control of your life? I hope you are beginning to see that exercise is more than huffing and puffing and sweating…or just moving various body parts around.

Make It Real

Write your goals down. Writing them down makes them real instead of just being abstract ideas floating around somewhere in your head. If you put them on paper, they will constantly confront you. This is a very important step in transforming your goals from intangible ideas into concrete motivational materials.

Baaaaa, Baaaaa

Don't let the latest fad, whether it be for clothing, a tattoo, a hairstyle or a certain type of body, determine your goals for you. You have a certain basic type of body. Analyze the positive and negative aspects of your body. We all have both and **acknowledging your personal weaknesses will make you a stronger person.** Then form a vision of the best possible body you could create from the raw materials you have been given. **Determine your goals for yourself.**

I do not have the type of body I would have liked to have been born with either. I am 5'6" and small-boned. I will never be a 200-pound muscular monster, an NBA, NFL or an NHL player. However, I can be a darn fine 145-150 pounds and I have been very successful as a gymnast and professional acrobat, where my body type was a definite advantage.

I may admire Arnold Whatzizname for his determination and his achievement of personal goals, but for my physical inspiration, I look to other successful people who have raw materials more similar to mine. There are plenty of them worthy of your admiration if you only take the time to look around. Trying to imitate some idol or other image is not a realistic goal, especially if he/she is nothing like you. It is only wishing and dreaming. You will be programming yourself for failure and unhappiness, instead of success and satisfaction.

Don't be one of the sheep...be the sheepherder!

Be your own person. Some people say that my legs are too small and my arms are too big. That does not bother me. I do not personally like big legs and yes, my arms are big for the rest of my body. So what? It does not compromise my health in any way. It is simply a matter of taste. I like it and if other people have a problem with that, then they have the problem, not me. Once again, I do this for myself, not for them. **Think for yourself and believe in yourself.** Build more self-esteem, more self-confidence, and a better self-image...for yourself.

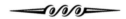

Those who fail to plan are planning to fail

So, other than having no goals, the wrong goals or unrealistic goals, what else causes people to fail in their exercise programs...or at anything else in life for that matter? The second major reason for any failure is having no plan, the wrong plan, or an unrealistic plan.

To build a beautiful, strong house, you first need a specific vision, and then a good blueprint. To design and sew a dress that fits correctly, you first need a specific vision, and then a good pattern. To create a strong, healthy and shapely body, you first need a specific vision, and then a good exercise and nutrition plan. Having no specific plan will definitely stop you from achieving your goals.

It's Not Rocket Science

Let's see if we understand this now. If you don't know exactly what you want (specific vision), you can't develop a precise goal(s). Without a precise goal(s), you can't design the correct plan(s) in order to successfully achieve the desired result(s). This doesn't sound like rocket science to me.

> Specific vision + precise goal + good plan = SUCCESS!

Designing the Plan

OK, what kind of mistakes can be made when designing an exercise plan? The following can cause you to fail in your exercise program, or to achieve less-than-optimum results:

- Choosing the wrong type(s) of exercise
- Wrong choice of exercises
- Wrong order of exercises
- Exercising too much
- Not exercising enough
- Exercising too hard
- Not exercising hard enough
- Exercising too often
- Not exercising often enough
- Trying to use too much weight
- Not using enough weight
- Using too many sets for a specific body part
- Not using enough sets for a specific body part
- Resting too long between sets
- Not resting long enough between sets
- Keeping the muscle under tension for too long
- Not keeping the muscle under tension for long enough
- Not using the correct repetition tempos
- Using incorrect exercise form
- Changing workout programs too often
- Not changing workout programs often enough
- Not considering the safety factor
- Unhealthy nutrition
- Inadequate nutrition
- Not getting enough quality sleep at night
- Not knowing how to manipulate your hormones, enzymes, etc., with exercise
- Not knowing how to manipulate your hormones, enzymes, etc., with nutrition

- Not knowing how to manipulate your hormones, enzymes, etc., with nutritional ✓ supplementation
- Not keeping exercise journals, nutrition journals, photos and records of body measurements

Too Complicated

Oops! It suddenly becomes complicated again, doesn't it? Do you have the time and the interest to go through all the study, research, and trial and error it takes to design an efficient and successful exercise plan for yourself? Probably not, and this is exactly why you need help from someone who is not only very knowledgeable in all the above factors, but who can also analyze exercises and correctly combine them into efficient and effective exercise programs. The same is true for nutrition programs.

As you can now see, this is not a simple task, and not everyone is capable of doing this. Diplomas, certifications and experience are important, but they offer no guarantees.

The **CTTC** Exercise and Nutrition Programs take all these factors into consideration. I carefully analyzed all aspects, and then designed three different workouts…each four weeks long. This twelve-week program will be extremely effective for almost everyone. It may be too intense for very unhealthy people (even at the beginners' level), and not sport-specific or intense enough for some elite athletes. However, for the rest of us who fall somewhere in between these two extremes, the **CTTC** Exercise and Nutrition Programs, when followed correctly, with commitment and determination, will create a stronger, healthier and shapelier body than you ever dreamed possible…and all with a minimal investment of your precious time.

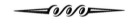

Results

How do you know if an exercise or nutrition program is any good or not? Three words: results, results, and results! If you have conscientiously followed an exercise and/or nutrition program for eight weeks or more, and have negligible results to show for all your efforts, then something is very wrong. Keep in mind that less than eight weeks does not give any program a fair chance of success.

Insane Exercisers

My favorite definition of insanity comes from Albert Einstein, who said: **"Insanity is doing the same thing over and over again…but expecting different results."** Don't be an insane exerciser. THINK!

- Is your exercise program time-efficient?
- Is it producing the (realistic) results that you want?

Success

When has an exercise or nutrition program been successful? Answer: When **you** are satisfied with your results. Success is what **you** say it is…not what someone else says it is. We don't all have the same goals. Your honest opinion should always be at the top of your list. I do want to emphasize that I am talking about your **honest** opinion (evaluation) here. Other people's opinions should only serve as reference points and reality checks.

However, **you can usually judge the value of your successes by what you had to give up in order to achieve them.** Easily obtained successes usually don't amount to much in the long run.

The **CTTC** Workouts adjust automatically to your improvements in strength and conditioning, which means that you can continue to follow the twelve-week program almost indefinitely. At a later date I will also offer other **CTTC** programs which will cater to more specific problems and goals. However, they will all be based on this **CTTC** Exercise and Nutrition Program…so get off your butt and get going on this one…NOW!

"Try" is usually meant as a negative word.

Stop trying…start doing.

Chapter 3

AEROBICS: RUNNING NOWHERE FAST

> Every progressive spirit is opposed by a thousand mediocre minds, self-appointed to guard the past.

This chapter is going to upset a lot of people. Why? Because what most people believe about aerobics is dead wrong. The way aerobics has traditionally been done is **not** the best way to lose excess body fat and it is also not the best way to keep excess body fat off after you have lost it. In fact, you can actually perform aerobics in a manner that will cause your body to hang onto the body fat it has and, in the long run, even cause you to gain body fat more easily. Let's look at some traditional advice about aerobics.

What Is Aerobics Anyway?

When most people refer to aerobics, they are generally talking about doing some kind of extended, low-to-medium intensity exercise, for the purpose of losing and/or controlling their body fat.

Cardiovascular conditioning is a close relative to traditional fat-burning aerobics, but they are not necessarily the same. The purpose of cardiovascular exercise is to strengthen your heart and circulatory system. However, it is possible to do aerobics without improving your cardiovascular conditioning at all.

The terms aerobic and anaerobic refer to how energy is produced within the body's cells. Aerobic refers to energy produced with oxygen and anaerobic refers to energy produced without oxygen. The word anaerobic is a bit confusing to many people because all exercise requires oxygen. It is called breathing. The difference is actually just a matter of when and where the oxygen is used by the cells. Most experts will say that exercising with weights is anaerobic. These people have definitely never done multiple sets of twenty rep breathing squats with short rest periods between the sets.

Keep It Simple

I like to simplify the definition of aerobics by saying that any type of movement which involves most of the body, lasts longer than a few minutes, and makes you breathe hard, is aerobic. Yes…even that…but it has to last longer than just a few minutes. Sorry guys.

So using my definition, almost any exercise is aerobic to some extent. For someone recovering from an illness or injury, just getting out of bed and struggling to the bathroom and back can be aerobic.

Anyone who has ever had their lower back go out on them knows exactly what I am talking about here. It is painful and extremely exhausting.

The effects or results received from any type of exercise are determined, not only by **which** exercise you do, but also by **how** you do it, and **when** you do it. **How** you do it is by far the most important of these three factors.

Cardio

Cardiovascular conditioning has three main requirements, and differs only slightly from traditional fat-burning aerobics. A cardiovascular activity should traditionally be done for at least fifteen minutes and it should be done for a minimum of three times a week. The third requirement is that your target heart rate be above 70% of your maximum heart rate (MHR).

Traditional fat-burning aerobics still often recommends that you exercise at least three times a week for a minimum of thirty minutes at a THR (target heart rate) of 60% - 70% of your MHR (maximum heart rate). However, for cardiovascular conditioning, your THR requirement **begins** at 70% of your MHR (assuming that you are relatively healthy and already in reasonably good cardiovascular condition).

Using these numbers, if you increase the intensity of your fat-burning aerobics by only a few percent, you will not only still be burning fat, but will also be improving your cardiovascular fitness at the same time. As you can see, the differences in **how** you do it can be minor while the difference in results can be major. Two for one. Better efficiency. That is why this concept has been incorporated into the **CTTC** Exercise Program.

Do the Math

First you have to know what your Maximum Heart Rate (MHR) is. You determine your MHR by subtracting your age from 220. Multiplying this number by 60, or 70, or 85 will give you 60%, 70%, or 85% of your MHR. This is your Target Heart Rate (THR).

Traditional aerobic advice also still often says that exercising at 60-70% of your MHR, for a minimum of thirty minutes, several times per week, is the best way to lose excess body fat because a target heart rate (THR) of 60-70% of your maximum heart rate (MHR) burns a higher **percentage** of fat than exercising at a higher heart rate. This is only partially true!

While it is true that it burns a higher **percentage** of fat, what they neglect to tell you is that it also burns **fewer** total calories, **fewer** actual calories from body fat, and the after-exercise fat-burning process **is less** than when exercising at a higher heart rate.

More Math

A light aerobic activity burns approximately 200 calories per hour at 60-65% of your MHR. We will say that of these 200 calories, 60% are from fat and 40% are from carbohydrates. 60% of 200 calories is 120 calories burned from fat. A more intense aerobic activity at 80-85% of your MHR will burn approximately 550 calories per hour. We will say that of these 550 calories, only 40% come from fat. 40% of 550 calories is 220 (fat) calories. Even according to the math I learned in school (which wasn't much), 220 is more than 120. Do you still not get it?

Something You Will Understand

Let's put this in monetary terms then. Everybody understands money. Which would you rather have, 60% of $200, or 40% of $550? By exercising at a higher intensity, you not only burn more total calories, but you also burn more calories from fat, burn more after-exercise calories from body- fat, and you improve your cardiovascular fitness…all at the same time. You are now exercising more efficiently and you are getting a much bigger bang (results) for your exercise buck (time and effort).

Sleep Yourself Thin

If the **percentage** of fat burned were the most important factor, you would be able to sleep your body fat off because your body uses a very high **percentage** of fat for energy during sleep. Unfortunately, the amount of calories burned during sleep is so low that, even if they were 100% fat calories, the effect on your body fat would still be negligible.

This negligible effect on body fat also holds true, in many cases, for low to medium intensity aerobics, especially if the aerobics is not done in combination with a Quality Exercise program which also incorporates the use of weights.

Depressing Fact

If you were to exercise at your highest **percentage** of fat-burning (low to medium intensity aerobics), it would take you about **sixteen hours of constant exercise** to burn just one pound of body fat. And if that sounds extremely inefficient…that's because it is.

Non-Fat Exercise

It is also true that at 60-70% of your MHR you have to exercise for about twenty minutes before you begin to burn much body fat at all, because your body has to use most of its available carbohydrates first. So you are spending the first one-third of your one hour-long fat-burning exercise class…**not** burning body fat. Once again, my rudimentary math skills tell me that this is not very efficient. There must be something more productive that you could do with these twenty minutes. There is, and I will tell you what that is a bit later.

Misunderstanding

So why do these ideas persist if they are so misleading? There are several reasons, but the main one is that many trainers and medical professionals still don't really understand how different types of exercise actually affect different body types as a whole, and the loss of excess body fat in particular. And even if they do understand, many times they don't know how to put this knowledge to work efficiently.

For instance, exercising at 60-70% of your MHR to lose body fat can be absolutely correct:

- If you are not obese.

- If your cardiovascular condition is already quite good.

- If you are doing this aerobics in order to help you lose a relatively small amount of body fat.

- If you are doing this aerobics **in addition to** a Quality Cardio-aerobics exercise plan. Cardio-aerobics is included in the CTTC Exercise Program and will be explained later in this chapter.

- If you are doing this aerobics **in addition to** a Quality Exercise program which also uses weights.

This level of aerobics can then help you to more effectively lose those notorious "last 5-10 pounds," or to make up for a little overindulgence during a vacation or holiday. Otherwise, exercising at this level of intensity is a massive waste of time unless you happen to be doing it as an exercise activity…just for fun. Then, you will at least be enjoying yourself.

How Much Is Enough?

Unless you have special problems, one hour of **combining** exercise in the traditional aerobic heart rate zone and the cardiovascular heart rate zone, three times per week, should be the **maximum** amount of aerobic exercise that you should need to do for your health and to keep your body fat under control. I will explain later why this hour should **not** consist exclusively of traditional aerobic exercise.

In fact, if you are quite healthy and do not have a problem keeping your body fat under control, then you only need to be concerned with cardiovascular fitness for health purposes. You can take care of this by exercising at 85% of your MHR, or above, for only fifteen to twenty minutes, three times a week. **That is only forty-five to sixty minutes of aerobic exercise per week**, not including warm-ups and cool-downs. Any more than this is a waste of time and energy, unless you are an elite athlete.

Any further improvement in cardiovascular fitness will be very small in relation to the amount of extra work you will have to do to achieve it. This is another example of how exercising intelligently will result in your exercising less…not more!

Coincidentally, exercising at 80-85% of your MHR for fifteen minutes, three times a week, is also the most efficient means of elevating your metabolism with aerobic exercise…**not** doing low-medium intensity aerobics for hours at a time.

For most shorter, smaller people who do not need to lose more than ten pounds of body fat, and for most taller, larger people who do not need to lose more than twenty pounds of body fat, the body fat burning effects of the **CTTC** Exercise Program, in conjunction with the **CTTC** Nutrition Program, should be more than enough to take control of your body fat problem. For the others, occasional extra, low-to-medium intensity aerobics and/or exercise activities may be necessary until you reach your fat-loss goal.

More Is Not Better

Excessive aerobics will cause a survival response in your body. This will result in you body doing three things:

1. Your body will gain body fat more easily.
2. Your body will use less body fat for energy.
3. Your body will hang on to the excess body fat it already has.

This is very similar to how your body responds to low calorie diets. I could be wrong, but I seriously doubt that this is the response people are expecting from their many, long aerobic sessions.

Now we come to the biggest drawback to excess aerobics as it relates to losing body fat. After a certain point, excess aerobics will also start to burn lean body mass. In other words, you will start to lose muscle.

Since everyone is a little different, there is no hard and fast rule for determining exactly where this certain point begins. However, if you are doing forty-five minutes of aerobics above 70-75% of your MHR, five times a week, you are probably getting very close to this point. If you are doing more than this, you are almost certainly doing too much. If you are doing this much aerobics and are still not losing body fat, the problem lies with the rest of your exercise program (weights), or your nutrition program, or both. The solution is **not** to do even more aerobics.

Burn That Muscle

The longer and more often that you exercise aerobically above this point, the more lean body mass you will lose, especially if your nutrition is bad, or if you are on a low-calorie diet, and/or if you are also exercising with weights.

Cannibals

Higher intensity aerobics, combined with a low-calorie diet will result in almost half of your energy coming from the breakdown (cannibalization) of your own muscle tissue, instead of from your excess body fat. This will definitely slow down your metabolism instead of raising it, and that is exactly the opposite of what you want to be doing. With less muscle and a slower metabolism, you can flush your dreams of a shapelier (fat-free) body down the toilet. This is especially true if your nutrition…both before and after exercise…is not 100% in order. I will address this in the chapter on nutrition.

Aerobics and Immunity

Excessive aerobic exercise also depresses the immune system, which explains why many distance runners and aerobic instructors get sick so often. When followed correctly, The **CTTC** Exercise and Nutrition Programs do not allow this to happen.

Sooner or Longer?

Look at the bodies of 100- and 200-meter sprinters compared to long distance runners. The sprinters are going all out for only ten to twenty-five seconds, while the distance runners are running at a much lower intensity for more than two hours, in the case of the marathoners. As the distance of the race increases, the lean body mass of the runners decreases.

The sprinters – both men and women – have powerful-looking upper and lower bodies…perhaps too powerful-looking for some people, but that is a matter of taste. The fact is, they have firm, full muscles which give shape to all parts of their bodies…and they have butts you could crack an egg on. No sagging here.

The marathoners, on the other hand, have small, wiry legs and very little upper body musculature. Some even look emaciated, with sunken cheeks and drawn faces. Yet most people would be very surprised to know that the actual percentage of body fat is lower in some sprinters than it is in many distance runners.

What Kind of Body Do You Admire?

Now some of you are going to say, "Yes, but I don't like either one of those body types." How about gymnasts then? Their training is also short, but intense. A strength move such as a "cross" on the still rings only has to be held for a couple of seconds and the most aerobic discipline in gymnastics (the floor exercise) only lasts fifty-seventy seconds. Yet gymnasts, both men and women, are some of the strongest and leanest athletes in the sports world. I also think most people would agree that many gymnasts, both men and women, have very shapely, aesthetic bodies. Of course, I am talking about the more mature young ladies here, not the pixies who still have little girls' bodies.

Muscle = Shape

For you ladies who think that female gymnasts are still too muscular, take a look at the rhythmic gymnasts with the hoops, ribbons, etc., who, even though they are extremely thin. are still shapely and strong. Other than skin, bones and internal organs, their weight is comprised of about 85-90% healthy, supple, form-giving muscle…yet no one has ever mistaken one of them for being a female bodybuilder. The fact remains that muscle **builds** shape and body fat **destroys** shape so, even if you lose all your body fat, you will still not have a nice body shape unless you have enough healthy, form-giving muscle underneath your lost body fat.

You ladies also need to realize that most muscular looking women do not look that way because they have especially large muscles, but because their body fat is usually under 15%. This low level of body fat makes their muscles **appear** larger, even if they are not. If you are an averagely over-fat American woman (35% body fat), you would have to lose more than half of your total body fat before you could even begin to look "too muscular." The average aerobics instructor has about 18% body fat, so I really don't think that most women need to worry about this too much.

Skinny Ain't Where It's At

These rhythmic gymnasts are much different from what I refer to as "skinny fat girls." I am referring to those very thin girls (and women) who have almost no muscle and, therefore, no shape to their bodies. Their arms form one straight line from shoulder to wrist, and their legs from hips to ankles. On some of them, their elbows and knees are the largest parts of their arms and legs. If you squeeze their arm, it feels like a thin sack of pudding. There is no firmness anywhere on their bodies because what little muscle they do have is also unhealthy. "Skinny fat girls" definitely do not qualify as "hardbodies." They are walking clothes hangers. But then again, this is also a matter of personal taste, so each to his own, as long as you remain healthy.

More Than One Way

The point is, you should be aware of the fact that the traditionally accepted way of doing aerobics is not the only way (and certainly not the most efficient way) to lose excess body fat and keep it off, or to create the kind of shape you probably want your body to have. Having been a gymnast myself for twenty years, I can assure you that gymnasts do not reach such low levels of body fat by doing hours of aerobics every day.

So if you also think, as many still do, that traditional fat-loss aerobics is the only way to achieve your fat-loss goals, then your chances of success will be greatly diminished and your struggle will be long and unnecessarily difficult.

Right Kind, Right Pace, Right Place

Although at this point it may seem so, it is not my intention to trash all aerobics. Aerobics most definitely has a place in every exercise program. But in order to reach your fat-loss, fitness, and health goals as quickly and as efficiently as possible, you have to be doing the right kind of aerobic exercise, at the right pace and at the right place in your exercise program.

You Need It

Properly done, aerobics will improve your muscles' ability to use fat for energy by increasing the number and size of the "fat furnaces" (mitochondria, for those of you who care) in the muscle fibers themselves. Aerobics also causes an increase in the fat burning enzymes in the working muscles. Aerobics increases the blood flow, and thereby the oxygen supply, to the working muscles. This is also necessary for increased and efficient fat burning.

In short, aerobics, when done properly, will teach your muscles to use more fat for energy **all the time**…not just while you are exercising. Now isn't that a much better way to lose excess body fat than just indiscriminately burning calories?

There have been well-designed studies done which show that multiple, short bouts of aerobic exercise can actually burn more body fat than one longer session of the same total amount of time. This is because the amount of body fat that you actually burn **during** aerobic exercise is minimal. Yes, you read that right.

Happy Fact

The good news is that with any type of exercise that you do, more than two-thirds of the increased fat-burning takes place **after** you have finished exercising…**not** during it.

This happens because the exercise has not only temporarily raised your metabolism so that you burn more total calories, but has also increased the amount of those calories burned which come from fat. This is why multiple, short bouts of aerobic exercise…spread out over your day…will work better than one longer session of approximately the same total exercise time. How often, how long, and how intense will depend on your personal circumstances, but when it comes to aerobics, **frequency is more important than duration.**

New Terms

To avoid confusion, let's call the traditional, low-intensity form of this exercise simply **T-aerobics** and we will call the more intense form **Cardio-aerobics**.

Cardio-Aerobics Does It Better

Most people still think that doing traditional aerobic exercise is also the best way to keep your metabolism elevated and increase fat burning. Sorry to destroy another one of your sacred aerobic beliefs, but it just ain't so.

Amazing Fact

Studies have shown that traditional aerobic exercise elevates metabolism for only one to six hours, depending on the intensity. Metabolism remains elevated for much longer after Cardio-aerobics… while **Quality Exercise using weights can raise metabolism for up to eighteen hours.**

Once again, **an intelligent combination** of these three different kinds of exercise will result in better, faster, and longer lasting results than using any of them alone. That is why the **CTTC** Exercise Program uses the best possible combination of these three different types of exercise.

Less Work = Less Fat

One well-designed study showed that a group of Cardio-aerobic exercisers expended less than half the amount of energy over a five-month period than a group of T-aerobic exercisers did, but the Cardio-aerobic exercisers lost significantly more body fat than the T-aerobic exercisers. Burning more body fat **with less work** certainly sounds like a good thing to me!

Cardio-aerobics keeps your after-exercise metabolic rate raised much longer than T-aerobics does, so you will also burn more total calories…and more fat calories…in the hours after you finish exercising. Burning body fat **without exercising** also sounds like a good thing to me!

Cardio-aerobics also improves insulin sensitivity better than T-aerobics does. In the next chapter you will see how incredibly important this is for keeping your body fat under control.

Winning Situation

Cardio-aerobics not only does these things better than T-aerobics, but it also improves your cardiovascular fitness and helps to maintain your muscle mass, all at the same time. This makes Cardio-aerobics a win-win-win situation. Cardio-aerobics is so good and so efficient that we even use it to keep our Chihuahua in top condition. That was not a joke. We really do use Cardio-aerobics to exercise our dog.

Build a Fat-Guzzler

By now you should be beginning to understand why muscle is indispensable for losing body fat, keeping the body fat off, and creating the shapely "hardbody" you want. Muscle is the only thing in your body that burns fat when you are at rest. This is one reason that the sprinters and the gymnasts can get away with doing little or no T-aerobics and still have such low levels of body fat. They have more muscle ... and that muscle is constantly burning fat.

If you want a car that burns very little gasoline (energy), you buy one with a small engine. The bigger the engine, the more of a gas-guzzler (energy burner) you have, even when it is just idling. More muscle equals a bigger engine equals a fat-guzzler.

Muscle is your body's engine. You should not see muscle as your enemy, but as the best weapon (fat-guzzler) you can have against your real enemy, which is excess body fat.

First Things First

This is why, if you want to lose excess body fat and keep it off, you need to concentrate FIRST on building a reasonable amount of lean body mass (muscle), instead of just mindlessly burning calories with aerobics. Remember, the more muscle you have, the more fat calories you will also burn with your aerobics.

Eat More...Weigh the Same...Be Smaller

The more muscle you have, **the more you will have to eat to maintain your bodyweight**. Each pound of muscle needs approximately twenty-five calories per day just to maintain itself, even without exercise. And here again lies the secret of the sprinters and gymnasts versus the distance runners... more muscle!

If a muscular sprinter has forty pounds more muscle than a skinny marathoner, then he will burn 1000 calories more...every day...while doing absolutely nothing (25 calories x 40 pounds = 1000 calories). The marathoner has to run those 1000 calories off, or eat 1000 calories less, to keep from gaining body fat! Which of these two scenarios sounds better to you?

So if you lose ten pounds of body fat and gain ten pounds of muscle, you will weigh exactly the same on your scale, but you will be smaller (one pound of fat has about four times the volume of one pound of muscle). You will also be firmer and shapelier...AND you will have to eat about 250 calories a day **more** just to maintain this same weight.

Let's see now...smaller, firmer, shapelier, AND you will have to eat **more** in order to keep from losing more body fat. Who would ever want to be in that situation? Wouldn't you prefer to continually do hours and hours of aerobics and eat less and less in order to control your body fat? Not me! No thanks!

More Muscle = Less Body Fat

Another well-designed study was done comparing the body fat loss results of different kinds of exercise. Diet alone was compared with diet combined with aerobics, and both of these were compared to diet combined with aerobics **and** exercising with weights.

As anyone would suspect, the diet and aerobic group lost much more body fat than the group that relied on diet alone. However, the group that also exercised with weights lost the same amount of **weight** (as seen on the scale) as the diet and aerobic group…**but lost twice as much body fat** as the diet and aerobic group. In other words, they gained some muscle and lost **double** the amount of body fat. Please read that again.

So don't just try to lose weight. Replace some of your body fat weight with lean (muscle) weight. This way, **you will eventually be able to eat more and exercise less** and still keep your body fat level under control. Your body will also become more firm and shapely…as if any of you are interested in that.

Those Twenty Minutes

Unless you have special problems, the **CTTC** Exercise Program should take care of all of your fat-burning and cardiovascular/aerobic needs. The **CTTC** warm-up raises your heart rate through the T-aerobics level to the Cardio-aerobic level right at the beginning of the workout. When done properly, the weight workout will keep your heart rate in the T-aerobic range, or higher, for the entire weight workout.

By the end of the weight workout, you will have lowered your blood sugars significantly, making fat much more available as an energy source. This is basically what happens during those first twenty minutes of a fat-burning aerobic session, except that the **CTTC** Exercise Program uses those twenty minutes to also build muscle tissue, instead of only mindlessly burning calories. Two for one. Better efficiency again with **CTTC**.

Hormones

The quality **CTTC** Weight Workouts also do something else that T-aerobics cannot do. They cause certain hormonal changes in your body which are needed in order to switch over to a better and more effective fat-burning mode. This puts your body in an optimal body fat burning situation before the last part of the **CTTC** Workouts – the Cardio-aerobics.

The **CTTC** Workouts end with ten minutes of Cardio-aerobics. This insures that you will have exercised in both aerobic ranges for a total of at least forty-five minutes each time you complete a **CTTC** Workout…three times a week. The time you save can be used to enjoy life more.

Special Problems

If you are too over-fat…or obese…you will need to do more fat-burning exercise than this until you have reached your fat-loss goals. This extra exercise could be done from Monday to Friday, or only on Tuesday and Thursday – the days you do not follow the **CTTC** Exercise Program, depending on your personal circumstances.

The **CTTC** Workouts are not extra exercise. They must be done as consistently as possible. I do not recommend seriously exercising on the weekends, except in very special instances. Weekends should be reserved for enjoyable "exercise activities," enjoying life, family, and friends, and recovering from your **CTTC** Workouts. If you follow the **CTTC** Exercise Program correctly, you will need this recovery time.

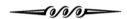

The Best Time

The absolute best time to do extra aerobic exercise (or any exercise for that matter) is first thing in the morning, before you eat anything. You can definitely burn much more body fat by exercising at this time of the day. Some say that you can burn up to three times more body fat at this time, or that of the calories you burn first thing in the morning, 70% come from fat, whereas only 40% come from fat if you exercise at another time during the day. But these are just interesting numbers. All you really need to know is that this is the best time…period.

The reason for this is that your body has had no food all night, so your blood sugar levels are lower than at other times during the day. This puts your body and hormones in a much better fat-burning mode than at any other time of the day.

Secondly, after you exercise, your breakfast calories will go to replenishing the muscles you just exercised, instead of immediately being turned into body fat.

The third advantage is that exercising before breakfast kick-starts your metabolism from a sleep mode to a fat-burning mode as early in the day as possible.

Earlier in this chapter, you read that Quality Exercise can elevate your metabolism for up to eighteen hours. If you exercise in the morning (or at least early in the day), your metabolism will remain elevated all day long. If you exercise later in the day, or in the evening, your metabolism will only remain elevated until you go to sleep. Then it will drop like a rock until you get up the next morning. This is another reason why exercising first thing in the morning is so important if you are attempting to lose excess body fat. **It is absolutely essential if you are obese!**

Second Best

The second best time for this extra aerobic exercise (or any exercise for that matter), is whenever you can work it into your schedule. I do not recommend doing this extra aerobic exercise for longer than thirty minutes at a time, unless you just really enjoy doing it. Then you can exercise for up to forty-five minutes. After forty-five minutes, the advantages of this extra aerobic exercise begin rapidly diminishing.

Obesity Aerobics

If you are obese, you should do some aerobic exercise in the morning, and do your **CTTC** Workout later in the day (for a second fat-burning session), three days a week. As I explained earlier, the **CTTC** Workouts mimic the early morning situation as best as possible by finishing with Cardio-aerobics after exercising with the weights has put your body into a similar state of low blood sugar. Of course, if you are obese you must do extra aerobic exercise at other times too, including before breakfast on the two days in between the three **CTTC** Workouts during the week or, in other words, five days a week.

Variety Is the Spice of…

Be sure to change your Cardio-aerobic exercises occasionally so that your body cannot adapt to any one type of aerobic exercise. If you don't, your body will become very efficient at that particular type of aerobic exercise and it will begin to use less energy. Remember the efficient joggers in the preceding chapter?

In other words, your body will burn less and less body fat as it becomes more and more efficient at any one type of exercise…or you will continually have to increase the intensity of the exercise in order to attain the same results. Occasionally changing exercises will help to prevent this. I usually use a limit of about six weeks of doing any one particular Cardio-aerobic exercise. After six weeks, change exercises. You can also change more often. You can change every week if you wish. You can even change every time you exercise. I recommend doing the same for T-aerobic exercise. If it is possible to change aerobic classes every four-six weeks, do so.

Aerobic Stresses

Many forms of aerobics are very stressful on the ankles, knees, hips, lower back and neck, so keep this in mind when choosing aerobic exercises and exercise activities for yourself, especially if you are obese or if you have previously injured any of these body parts.

Coordinated Grace

One positive point about T-aerobics is hardly ever mentioned. Aerobic dance and other types of T-aerobics are wonderful for improving coordination and learning to move more gracefully. Most people, both men and women, could use a lot more of both of these two qualities.

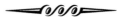

Obesity Is Different

What is obesity? Clinical obesity begins already at 20% body fat for men and 28% body fat for women. Chronic obesity begins at 28% body fat for men and 32% body fat for women.

Obese people need to **physiologically re-educate their bodies** in order to change their metabolisms from a fat-storing mode to a fat-burning mode. In other words, their bodies have to re-learn how to effectively use body fat for energy. This is the real reason they need to do low-intensity aerobic exercise, not to just mindlessly burn calories. This is where we run into a serious problem with the MHR (maximum heart rate) and the THR (target heart rate).

MHR and THR for the Obese

MHR and THR were originally developed to increase cardiovascular fitness, not as guidelines for losing excess body fat. However, if you understand MHR and THR, they can still be very useful for monitoring exercise intensity and for losing excess body fat.

A THR of 60-70% of MHR will supposedly put you just below the level of intensity where your body changes from using mostly fat for energy to using mostly carbohydrates for energy. This is sometimes called the aerobic/anaerobic threshold. However, the aerobic/anaerobic threshold has nothing to do with age (subtract your age from 220, then multiply by .7 to get a THR of 70%). The aerobic/anaerobic threshold is determined by your level of cardiovascular fitness, not your age.

Huffing and Puffing

This means that for someone who has a very high level of cardiovascular conditioning (such as marathoners), the aerobic/anaerobic threshold may be 75% or even 80% of MHR, but the aerobic/anaerobic threshold of someone who has very little cardiovascular conditioning (an obese person, for instance) will be much lower. This is why the old-fashioned advice, "During aerobics, exert yourself until you are breathing hard…but not so hard that you can't carry on a conversation," will actually work better for obese persons than a predetermined THR will.

A Step Further

However, I advise obese persons to drop it even a step further. Exert yourself to the point of breathing hard, and then ease up just a little. This is because the point where you begin to huff and puff is the point where your system begins to shift over from using fat for energy to using carbohydrates for energy. You want to stay just under this point in order to re-educate your metabolism most efficiently. This is one reason that brisk walking is so effective for obese people…and why **it is absolutely essential for obese people to also do this kind of aerobics.**

Too Intense

For most obese people, 60-70% of MHR is too intense. Because of their low level of cardiovascular fitness, most obese people will be breathing much too hard at 60-70%, which means that they will be burning too low a percentage of fats to efficiently re-program their bodies to better use body fat for energy. They need to exercise at a THR of about 40-50% of MHR in order to re-program their bodies as quickly as possible. As their cardiovascular condition improves, their THR will automatically increase so, for best results, they should always coordinate their THR with the breathing advice in the previous paragraph.

To summarize, at 60-70% of MHR, most obese people will be exercising too intensely to efficiently re-program their bodies to effectively use body fat for energy. However, I do also recommend short bouts of exercise at higher levels of intensity, simply because cardiovascular health should be an important part of any exercise program. The **CTTC** warm-ups and the Cardio-aerobics at the end of the **CTTC** Workouts will take care of this nicely, and the build-up to this intensity level for obese exercisers is done very slowly…just to be on the safe side.

Back to School

Another difference for obese people is the frequency and duration of the aerobics that they need to do. Doing aerobics five or six days a week for thirty to sixty minutes each time is not necessarily the best way.

Remember, you are endeavoring to re-program your fat-burning systems. That is a learning situation. If you need to learn some specific task, what works better, practicing that task for thirty minutes once a day…or practicing that task for ten minutes in the morning, ten minutes in the afternoon, and ten minutes again in the evening?

Stimulating your body to react to exercise two, three, or more times a day will outweigh by far the calorie burning results of a single thirty- to sixty-minute aerobic session.

Results

One well-designed study compared the exercise results of fifty women. In the first part of the study, they exercised (brisk walking) one time a day for thirty minutes, five days a week. Later, they switched to exercising (brisk walking again) three times a day for only ten minutes each time, five days a week. The three times ten minutes a day plan **resulted in better reduction of body fat** (determined by loss of inches around the ladies' waists) than the one time, thirty minutes did.

Lose the Excuses

There are other advantages to this system. Since you don't need to find one thirty-minute block of time in your busy day, you lose the excuse, "I just can't find time." For ten minutes of aerobics at this level of intensity, you don't even need to change clothes...except for possibly your shoes.

You can even combine this type of aerobics with your daily schedule. Is your children's school close by? Walk them to and/or from school. You can get in some quality time with your kids and you will also be instilling healthy exercise habits in them so they don't wind up with an excess body fat problem later in life. Don't think of this as exercise. Think of it as an act of love towards your children. That just might be the motivation you need. If not, then find another source of motivation that does work. I can't do it for you.

Do you need milk or bread, and is there is a grocery store within a ten minute walk or bicycle ride from your house? Go for it. Don't want to carry that heavy carton of milk back from the store? Get a basket for your bicycle, or a backpack if you are walking.

A brisk ten-minute walk before and/or after dinner can become a very pleasant and relaxing part of your day instead of just being "another ten minutes of boring exercise." My wife and I always try to take our dog for a fifteen- to thirty-minute walk before or after dinner and, since we have a Chihuahua, believe me, our speed never gets above the brisk level.

Those Twenty Minutes...Again

I can hear some of you already. "But you said earlier that it takes about twenty minutes of exercise before your body even begins to use much body fat for energy, so what good is a ten-minute walk?"

Wrong! What I said was that it takes about twenty minutes...if you are exercising at more than 60% of your MHR...before your body begins to use a high percentage of fat for energy. Walking is so low on the intensity level that your body will begin using a high percentage of fat for energy almost immediately, thereby helping to re-program your fat-burning systems each time you do it. However, make sure that you stay just under the huffing and puffing level of exertion.

Metabolism…Again

Another advantage of breaking up your low-intensity aerobics into shorter sessions is that it will ensure that you keep active during the entire day and, with each short session, you will elevate your metabolism a little bit…all day long.

Pick a Number

Don't misinterpret what I am saying. 3 x 10 minutes is just an example. 3 x 15 minutes, or 3 x 20 minutes, or 1 x 10, 1 x 20 and 1 x 15, or 6 x 10 minutes would be even better, but the point here (as with all exercise advice) is that it has to be doable.

If you just don't have 3 x 30 minutes during the day, then it is useless for me to say that this is what you **have** to do. What is important for you to know is that 1 x 30…or 45…or 60 minutes of aerobics is **not** the only way to achieve good results. If you only have ten minutes right now…then at least get that ten minutes in. Maybe later you will find another ten minutes…or maybe more…but you will have at least done ten minutes, which is infinitely better than having done nothing at all.

How Often?

And yes, **obese persons need to do this type of aerobics as often as possible,** and as many days per week as possible, until they have reached their desired body fat level…and maybe even after that. Sorry, but this book is not about lying to you to give you false hope and make you feel better. It's about giving you the truth about exercise and nutrition, as I know it. What you do with this information is entirely up to you.

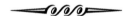

Enjoyable Aerobic Activities

So where do enjoyable aerobic activities fit into the **CTTC** Exercise Program?

For people who are not over-fat, or who only have a few pounds of excess body fat to lose…anywhere except on the three **CTTC** Workout days…if possible. On **CTTC** Workout days, extra aerobic activities could interfere with your recovery from the **CTTC** Workouts, depending on the length and intensity of the exercise activity. On the other days you can do aerobic activities that you enjoy, just for the enjoyment.

Remember, according to my definition, every activity is aerobic. Only the intensity varies. Walking your dog is aerobic. The size and age of your dog will determine how fast (intense) your walk will be. If you really enjoy jogging, then jog with your dog. If you really enjoy taking T-aerobics classes, then do it. Just don't look at it as something you **have** to do.

Don't look at exercise activities as being part of your exercise program. **Make exercise activities part of enjoying life.**

Play golf, tennis, squash, basketball, racquetball or handball. Go hiking, bicycling, skateboarding, rollerblading, water skiing, snow skiing, cross-country skiing, snowboarding, canoeing, kayaking, scuba-diving, snorkeling, or just plain swimming. I consider the martial arts to be some of the very best exercise activities because they also develop so many positive mental characteristics.

A well-designed exercise program will improve your performance in any sport or recreational activity, thereby making them even more enjoyable. In turn, sports and exercise activities will enhance your exercise program, thereby making it more productive…another win-win situation.

Family Affair

Plan more exercise activities with your spouse and the rest of your family. When you get home from work, take a brisk walk around the block with your spouse, or your dog (or both), to unwind, instead of sitting down right away and having a beer or watching TV. Make it a family activity. Have your kids join you. You can use this time to ask them about their day and you will be instilling healthy exercise habits in them as well. You can always have the drink when you get back from your walk…if you still want it…or need it.

It doesn't matter so much **what** you do, or **when** you do it, **as long as it is something that you enjoy,** and that gets you off your butt and away from the TV, computer or whatever else keeps you more sedentary than you should be. It has to be enjoyable or you won't do it regularly…or continue doing it. Not everybody looks forward to running two or three miles at 5:00 every morning…rain, snow, or shine. I know I certainly can't do it for any extended length of time…and I have great self-discipline.

On Your Own

You should have some enjoyable exercise activities that you can do alone or with only one other person. The more people you need for an activity, the greater the chance is that you are not going to continue to do it.

For the same reason, the activity should not require elaborate preparation. Remember, we are looking for exercise activities that will become part of your daily lifestyle, just like brushing your teeth. If you try to force yourself to do something that is boring, unpleasant or feels too much like work, you will not do it for long. That makes the activity worthless for our purposes. Keep in mind that even pleasurable activities can become monotonous, so they may also need to be changed once in a while.

I am not talking about doing **one** specific exercise activity for the rest of your life. I am talking about doing **some** exercise activities for the rest of your life. **Learn to play again!**

A Little Can Be a Lot

Exercise activities can also be more strenuous. Some people actually enjoy jogging miles at a time. For them it is relaxing and a way of relieving daily stress. Great! Go for it. But if you don't enjoy jogging…don't jog. Find something else that you do enjoy, or at least that you don't hate so much. If you do an exercise activity that burns only 200 calories on each of the four days you are not working out with the **CTTC** Exercise Program, you will still burn more than 41,000 extra calories a year. If you normally eat 2,000 calories a day, you will have burned more than twenty days' worth of food by doing something you enjoy…for a few minutes a day…four days a week.

> You should exercise like a sprinter; but building and maintaining a strong, healthy and shapely body is a marathon.

Some Good News…And Some Bad News

The bad news is that the building part requires some hard work…and a little time. The good news is that when the building part is done, maintaining your strong, healthy and shapely body is much easier.

Restoring a classic car or a piece of antique furniture also requires a lot of work in the beginning, but when finished, or re-finished, as the case may be, they only require occasional maintenance to keep them in great condition. As you progress on the **CTTC** Exercise Program, your body will become more efficient at burning body fat and at maintaining your lean body mass (muscle). **You will need to exercise less, not more, and you will be able to eat more food, not less!**

For the college-oriented among you, look at it this way. Say you need 140 hours of credits to graduate. If you study hard your freshman and sophomore years and build up seventy hours of a 4.0 grade-point, you could coast through your last two years of college and still graduate with a decent grade-point. The opposite is also true. It is almost impossible to significantly raise a lot of hours of bad grade-point. Now guess how I know that.

This is also true with your health and fitness. If you build a good base of health and fitness at an early stage in your life, then it is very easy to maintain that level. The longer you wait, the more difficult it becomes. Maintaining is always easier, and always requires less time, than building, rebuilding or repairing.

Having said all that, I do want to emphasize the fact that it is never too late to start! After all, I eventually did manage to graduate.

Sticking to It

This is precisely why you will be able to stick with this **CTTC** program long-term. You don't have to dread a lifetime of having to do more and more exercise and eat less and less, just to stay in the same place. I certainly would never have continued to exercise for more than three decades (since the end of my competitive sport career) if all I had to look forward to was hours and hours of some kind of boring exercise…day after day…for the rest of my life. That is just not my idea of enjoying life.

My Way

Using myself as an example, the ten-minute warm-up and the ten minutes of Cardio-aerobics built into the three **CTTC** Workouts per week are more than enough to keep my body fat under control. I even skip the ten minutes of Cardio-aerobics once in a while on my leg workout day, because the breathing squats and/or leg presses are enough for my personal needs. I address adapting the **CTTC** Workouts to fit your personal needs in Chapter 11.

Adapting

The gym where we mostly exercise is not far from where we live so, when the weather is not too bad and we have enough time, my wife and I bicycle to the gym, using a warm-up intensity. When we get to the gym we can immediately begin the weight portion of our workouts because we are already warmed up and in our exercise clothing. We only need to change our shoes. After the weight workout, we bicycle back home at Cardio-aerobic intensity (partially), which takes us fifteen to twenty minutes (depending on the wind). That is our Cardio-aerobics for that day. When we get home, we stretch and drink our **After CTTC Workout Recovery Shakes** (Chapter 12). On these days, we shower at home, in case you were wondering.

After so many years of exercising, our weight workouts are very short and specific, so this whole scenario from leaving home until returning home, takes us about one hour and fifteen minutes. You can't get much more efficient than that. Well, actually we can. If we drive to the gym and do our normal **CTTC** Workouts, we can be back home in just over an hour.

Three Hours

Think about that for a minute. What I am telling you here is that **we exercise for an average of only three hours per week**. If I can not only maintain, but still even improve my sixty-year-old body with only three hours of Quality Exercise per week, then you can certainly make major improvements by following the **CTTC** Exercise and Nutrition Programs.

Two Hours

/ LORI

If I am not exercising to lose excess body fat, I will do a five-minute warm-up, exercise for twenty-five to thirty minutes with weights, and then I will do five minutes of Cardio-aerobics…three times per week. If you don't count my ten-minute cool-down and stretching, then **this is only two hours of exercise…per week!**

Now…thinking logically…someone who spends two hours per day…five days per week in the gym should look five times better than I do and should be in five times better condition than I am, regardless of any age difference. Well they aren't, which should make you ask, "Why aren't they?" The answer: inefficiency.

I Could Be Wrong

It all sounds crazy doesn't it? But if you had been in the hundreds of gyms I have been in all over the world, and seen so many people doing T-aerobics…year after year…with little or no apparent improvement, you would also start to wonder. I often see T-aerobic instructors who give class after class, day after day…and are still over-fat, or have big butts…or both…so something isn't working for them either.

I can hear some of you saying to yourself right now, "This guy doesn't know what he is talking about. Most of the people I know who have lost a lot of excess body fat did it using T-aerobics."

Probably true, but don't forget that most of the exercisers who have **failed** to lose their excess body fat, or **failed** to keep it off, were also depending on T-aerobics to do the job, and this is a much larger group, no pun intended.

I am not saying that it can't be done using T-aerobics alone. I am saying that using **only** T-aerobics is inefficient and one-sided. The **CTTC** Exercise Program is healthier, much more efficient, produces better and longer lasting results and is much more complete than T-aerobics alone. That's all.

If It Ain't Broken…

However, if what you are already doing is working for you…and you are satisfied with your results… simply forget everything I have said about the subject. I never argue with success. But if it isn't working for you, give the **CTTC** Exercise and Nutrition Programs a shot at it. What have you got to lose…some excess body fat?

Confused?

I admit it. This chapter is confusing…even to me…so let's summarize the basics for getting the best possible results from your aerobic exercise.

Not
my
body

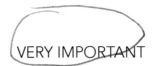

VERY IMPORTANT

Only after having slowly progressed to doing the complete twelve-week **CTTC** Exercise Program (as detailed in Chapter 11) should you begin adding **extra** aerobics, as described below, to your program. This includes obese exercisers. Otherwise you will be attempting to do too much, too soon, and you will burn out. Your body is not yet ready for that much exercise.

After completing the twelve-week **CTTC** Exercise Program for the first time without any adaptations, some exercisers will not even need to add extra aerobics anymore.

AEROBICS FOR REAL RESULTS

To Lose 1-10 Pounds of Excess Body Fat: ✓

- Follow the twelve-week **CTTC** Exercise and Nutrition Program as it is.

- Add some enjoyable exercise activities on some…or all…of the remaining four days of the week.

- Continue until you have lost the desired amount of body fat, then adjust your nutrition to maintain that level of body fat.

- Continue the **CTTC** Exercise and Nutrition Programs.

To Lose 10-20 Pounds of Excess Body Fat: 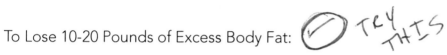 TRY THIS

- Follow the twelve-week **CTTC** Exercise and Nutrition Program as it is.

- Add 30-45 minutes of T-aerobics (preferably before breakfast) at approximately 60-70% of your MHR on the two days of the week which fall between the three **CTTC** Workouts. Remember to exert yourself until you are breathing hard, but not so hard that you can't carry on a conversation.

- Add some enjoyable exercise activities on the weekend.

- Continue until you have lost the desired amount of body fat, then adjust your aerobics **and** your nutrition to maintain that level of body fat.

- Continue the **CTTC** Exercise and Nutrition Programs.

To Lose 20-40 Pounds of Excess Body Fat:

- Follow the twelve-week **CTTC** Exercise and Nutrition Program as it is.

- Add 30-45 minutes of T-aerobics (preferably before breakfast) at approximately 60-70% of your MHR on Monday through Friday (five days a week). Remember to exert yourself until you are breathing hard, but not so hard that you can't carry on a conversation.

- Add some enjoyable exercise activities on the weekend.

- Continue until you have lost the desired amount of body fat, then adjust your aerobics **and** your nutrition to maintain that level of body fat.

- Continue the **CTTC** Exercise and Nutrition Programs.

To Lose More Than Forty Pounds of Excess Body Fat:

- Follow the twelve-week **CTTC** Exercise and Nutrition Program as it is.

- After completing the Cardio-aerobics at the end of the **CTTC** Workouts, add 10-30 minutes of T-aerobics, at approximately 40-50% of your MHR, between the Cardio-aerobics and the cool down. Remember to exert yourself to the point of breathing hard, and then ease up just a little.

- Add 15-45 minutes of T-aerobics before breakfast, at approximately 40-50% of your MHR, on Monday through Friday (five days a week). Remember to exert yourself to the point of breathing hard, and then ease up just a little.

- Endeavor to get in another two or three (or more) 10-30 minute sessions of T-aerobics during the day. Make these a part of your daily activities.

- Add some enjoyable exercise activities on some days of the week, and absolutely on the weekend.

- Continue until you have lost the desired amount of body fat, then adjust your aerobics **and** your nutrition to maintain that level of body fat.

- Continue the **CTTC** Exercise and Nutrition Programs.

Don't Just Move Your Fat...Remove it!
Run Along now!

LORI

To Gain Lean Body Mass (Too Skinny)

- Follow the twelve-week **CTTC** Exercise and Nutrition Programs, adjusted for people who are attempting to gain healthy lean body mass (explained at the end of Chapter 11).

- Stop doing all types of aerobics, **except for the CTTC Workout # 1 warm-up,** but cut this warmup down to five minutes. Also use this warm-up for **CTTC** Workouts # 2 and #3. Do no other form of aerobics, and very few exercise activities, until you are close to your desired weight. Then begin slowly adding the **CTTC** Workout # 1 Cardio-aerobics.

- Slowly increase your Cardio-aerobics until you stop gaining muscular weight, then ease the Cardio-aerobics back a notch until you begin gaining muscular weight again.

- Repeat the above step occasionally until you have achieved your desired lean body weight, then adjust your aerobics, your exercise activities **and** your nutrition to maintain your desired lean body weight.

- Continue the **CTTC** Exercise and Nutrition Programs.

Chapter 4

WHY WOULD ANYONE IN HIS RIGHT MIND WANT TO LOSE "WEIGHT"?

You read about it in magazines. You see it on book covers. It is a constant theme on TV and people are always talking about it: What is it? Losing **weight**! But why would anyone want to lose **weight**? Do you want to lose some bone mass because dense, healthy bones weigh too much? Or do you want to lose some of those horrible muscles which give shape to beautiful legs, arms, shoulders, mid-sections, rear-sections and so on. Muscle **weighs** a lot, you know. Alternatively, you could consider donating some organs to be taken out now, instead of waiting until you no longer need them. Be sure to choose the heavier organs so that you will **weigh** less when they are gone.

Oh yes, I nearly forgot water. Our bodies consist of more than 70% water so, theoretically, you could lose 70% of your **weight** just by never ingesting any more fluids. You would lose **weight** alright. You would also be very dead and you would look like a fat, dried prune because muscle tissue is 70% water while body fat contains about the same amount of water as your bones do – only about 20%. Theoretically then, your muscles would shrink by 70% while your fat would shrink by just 20%. But hey, we are only concerned with losing **weight** here, right?

What You Really Mean

You see now how really ridiculous this sounds, but words are powerful and they do affect our thinking processes, so I prefer to use the politically incorrect word: **FAT**. That is actually what we are talking about losing, isn't it? **FAT**! To be even more specific, we are talking about **excess BODY FAT**, aren't we?

When I was at my heaviest muscular weight, I weighed 176 pounds at 5 foot 6 inches tall. According to the BMI (Body Mass Index), I was borderline obese. However, my body fat was actually under 10%, which is the level of a well-trained athlete. This is the problem with the BMI. It only deals with **weight**, not body fat. So, according to the BMI, I know lots of athletes who are over-**weight**, but they are certainly not over-**FAT**.

I do, however, know lots of people who are within their BMI limits, but who are still over-**FAT**. If a person **weighs** only 100 pounds, but 30% of the 100 pounds is **fat**, then that person is over-**FAT**. Over-**FAT** describes exactly what we are actually talking about, so that is the term I will use from here on. If this term offends you, then you have not yet fully accepted your problem and you are probably not yet ready to seriously do anything to solve it. That is your decision to make…and make no mistake about it, it is a conscious decision that you will have to make in order to solve your excess body fat problems.

By the way, I have also been over-**FAT** at only 165 pounds but with more than 25% body fat. That was one of the times I stupidly let my body fat get out of control.

Here Are Some Facts About BODY FAT

But I Weigh the Same!

So **weight** means nothing. Adults lose from one-half to one pound of muscle per year after about the age of twenty-five, if they do not exercise to maintain muscle mass. Scales don't know if they are measuring lean weight or fat. They can only give you a number. So if you are forty-five years old and weigh the same as you did when you were twenty-five, don't pat yourself on the back too hard. If you don't exercise…and especially Quality Exercise with weights…you probably have fifteen to twenty-five pounds more body fat than you did at age twenty-five, even though you may still **weigh** the same.

The average woman loses about ten pounds of muscle and gains about twenty-five pounds of **FAT** during these twenty years. The average man doesn't do any better. This means that you will have to continually eat less and less as you get older, just to keep from gaining **weight**. You will, however, continue to lose muscle and gain body fat. Are you still wondering why most people get flabby as they get older, even if they have not gained any **weight**?

The Golden Years

Of course, as you eat less you will ingest fewer and fewer nutrients. If you still listen to the majority of doctors and nutritionists, you will also not be taking a good multi-vitamin/mineral supplement, so your bones will keep getting weaker and weaker, as will your immune system. Ah, I see brittle bones and bad health in your future, and I am not even clairvoyant. Welcome to middle-age, and later, your Golden Years…over-fat and underhealthy!

At the moment, 75% of retirees in America are over-fat and life expectancy is predicted to go down by five years in the near future, because of obesity. **It is the first time ever that life expectancy has fallen in America.** In other words, this is the first time in history where children have a lower life expectancy than their parents. Not a pretty picture, is it? Don't you think it's finally time to get more involved, Mom? Dad?

Bigger Yes…But Better

I have just seen the newest figures from the Centers for Disease Control (CDC), which show that in 1960 the average American man was 5' 8" tall and weighed 166 pounds. In 2004 the average man is only one inch taller, but weighs 191 pounds. In 1960 the average American woman was 5' 3" tall and weighed 140 pounds (already much too over-fat, even then). In 2004 the average woman is also only one inch taller, but weighs a whopping 164 pounds…almost what a 4" taller man weighed in 1960. This is a gain of twenty-five pounds since 1960 for the average man and woman. This also means that half of American men and women weigh even more than this.

The cost of obesity to the American healthcare system has increased from $3.6 billion in 1987, to $36 billion in 2002. And you wonder why people can't afford healthcare anymore?

Enough Is Enough

The average American male has about 25% body fat and the average American female has about 35% body fat…or so I have read. Looking around, I would put the figures much higher than these, but the numbers don't really matter. What matters is that obesity, which already starts at 20% body fat for men and 28% body fat for women, has now overtaken smoking to become the number one cause of preventable death in America. Clinical obesity begins at 20% for men and chronic obesity begins at 32% for women, which means that the **average** American man is already clinically obese and the **average** American woman is already chronically obese.

How Little

"But you **need** some body fat." True…but no one ever tells you exactly how **little** body fat you actually **need** to be healthy, do they? Men only **need** about 3% body fat and women only **need** about 6% body fat to stay healthy. That is all you really **need**. That means that a 200-pound man or a 100-pound woman only **needs** six pounds of body fat to stay healthy. Now you know. Oops…there goes another rationalization out the window.

How Much

OK…so how much body fat can we **allow** ourselves and still be healthy? Experience tells me that 15-18% body fat for men and 20- 25% body fat for women are absolutely reasonable and attainable goals for the majority of people. After all, this is just below where clinical obesity begins. Well-conditioned athletes have body fat levels which are about half of these figures, so I am not being overly fanatic with these percentages. Not so long ago, these were considered "normal" levels of body fat. Now they are considered (by some) as "ideal" levels. How times change.

Are You Really Over-fat?

I can't tell you if you are over-fat or not. It is your body and you have to be happy with it. I will, however, offer another simple, foolproof test for you here. Strip down to your underwear, stand in front of a full-length mirror, and be really honest with yourself. Simply ask yourself if you look as good as you could…or should…look, and be honest…no excuses, and no denial.

If you want to be even more critical of yourself, take the pinch test. Pinch yourself just below your navel, on the sides of your waist, and at the small of your back. You decide then whether you are pinching too much excess body fat between your thumb and finger…or not. If you decide that it is too much, start doing something about it…now! Of course, if you can grab handfuls of flab, your answer is obvious!

You can pinch-test other places too, but excess body fat on the waist area, and especially the stomach, is much more dangerous to your health than excess body fat on other areas of the body. Fat thighs are more of a cosmetic concern than a risk factor for your health.

Am I Really Over-fat?

These two tests are much more accurate than electronic body fat meters, mathematical body fat formulas, the Body Mass Index, other people's opinions, or any other type of body fat measurements. I don't let devices tell me if I am over-fat or not. I decide if I am over-fat…or not. I look in the mirror, pinch test myself, and my answer is a simple YES or NO. The little lie of "I'm just a tiny bit over-fat" is not an option for me. I am either over-fat…or not over-fat. This attitude keeps me honest with myself, and then I am much less likely to let my body fat get out of control…again.

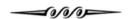

Begin at the Beginning

Unfortunately, instead of exercise being instilled in young people as something positive and enjoyable, it is often used as a form of punishment. "Drop and give me twenty," or, "The **losing** team has to run laps." These are great incentives to make exercise a pleasant and integral part of their future lifestyles, aren't they? Exercise equals punishment and only losers exercise. Dumb, dumb, dumb!

It is part of every parent's responsibility to instill healthy exercise habits in their children from a young age. You can't wait until they are over-fat teenagers. That is like allowing them to only watch TV and play computer games and then, when they are sixteen and flunking classes at school, suddenly trying to interest them in reading good books. Good luck!

Fortunately, it doesn't have to happen like this. Let's begin at the beginning. If young people would be properly introduced to intelligent, effective, Quality Exercise and exercise activities before the whole destructive cycle begins, they would have far fewer mental, emotional and physical problems. Besides getting a head start on preventing over-fatness and eating disorders, they would be building a strong, solid foundation for a lifetime of health and happiness. Young girls would be building strong bones, which would greatly minimize the effects of bone loss later in their lives, instead of permanently dieting away their bone mass before they are even out of their teens.

Learn and Earn

Youth is the time to start developing self-esteem, self-confidence, self-discipline, a good self-image, a healthy body-image, realistic and attainable goals and the correct priorities in life. Please notice that

I continually use the words **develop** and **self**. These qualities do not just happen. They have to be worked at, practiced and developed. No one is going to walk up one day and simply give them to you. Each person has to learn and **earn** them by him/her self. An intelligent, well-designed exercise program will go a long way in helping to develop these qualities in anyone, young or old.

Be a Winner

Not everyone can be a star in sports, on stage, or in the movies…but everyone can be a winner when they compete against themselves!

> True success is not measured by being superior to someone else, but by being superior to your former self.

To Error Is Human

It is difficult enough to develop all these qualities without having major roadblocks in your way, but if your parents allowed you to become over-fat before you were old enough to take responsibility for yourself, you started with a definite disadvantage. If you became over-fat later in life, then accept that it was your responsibility and that you blew it. It doesn't matter now how it happened. What matters now is what you are prepared to do about it.

> An error only becomes a mistake if you don't do anything to correct it.

Good

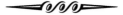

Stupid Diets Always Fail

Now let's examine why all weight-loss programs and most fat-loss programs fail.

Weight-loss programs fail because they are based on the fact that most people will be temporarily satisfied by just losing **weight**, instead of by losing excess body FAT.

This is extremely easy to do. You just have to follow a zero carbohydrate diet for a few days and you will "magically" lose several pounds of **weight**. Our bodies can store up to 500 or 600 grams of carbohydrates, mostly in muscle tissue. Each gram of carbohydrate binds four grams of water to itself, so we are talking about four to five pounds of **weight** right there. Unfortunately, none of this **weight** is body fat, so as soon as you eat or drink your usual amounts of carbohydrates again, you gain the water **weight** back, plus some more body fat to go with it.

Remember, body fat is only 20% water while muscle tissue is 70% water, so losing water **weight** only makes your muscles look smaller and your body fat look bigger in comparison. Not a very positive result.

Losing Muscle

Most **weight**-loss diets also cause you to lose actual muscle tissue, which you will not gain back unless you exercise correctly with weights. If you follow a stupid diet and also don't exercise correctly with weights, only about 35-50% of the **weight** you lose will be from body fat. The other 50-65% of the **weight** you lose will be muscle. Less muscle means a lower metabolism, fewer calories that your body can burn, and more body FAT. You are doing the exact opposite of what you want to be doing…again.

One pound of fat has 3,500 calories, while one pound of muscle has only 600 calories. It doesn't take a mathematical genius to figure out what will happen if you lose **weight** incorrectly. Bye, bye muscle (and with it, your metabolism), and hello more body FAT.

Losing Body Fat

These kinds of **weight**-loss diets not only cause you to lose muscle, but can also leave you with loose skin and loose, hanging rolls of body fat. Is that really the body shape you are going for?

Cut Those Calories

Many fat-loss diets are also one-sided. Most are still based only on cutting calories, which can not only slow your metabolism, but also, once again, cause you to lose muscle tissue. Low calorie diets also suppress your thyroid hormones. You know, the ones many people still blame for their gains in body fat.

The Perfect Recipe

Combine a metabolism-slowing, muscle-reducing diet with a calorie-burning, muscle-losing exercise program (excess aerobics, for instance) and you will have the perfect recipe for **gaining** body fat! It may not happen while you are doing it, but the second you stop either the diet, or the exercise…or both…you will gain all the weight back…plus some. **Some** of the weight you lose while on the diet will be muscle, but **all** the weight you gain back will be from excess body FAT. And no, you were not just imagining it – you actually can gain back weeks of lost body fat in a matter of days.

These are the real reasons that low-calorie diets only have a 5% success rate.

One More Time

These negative results will be the same if you diet like this, or if you exercise improperly. It will just happen more quickly if you exercise improperly and follow a stupid diet as well. Each time you try this approach it will be more difficult. You will have to eat less or exercise more…or both…to get any results. And each time, the rebound will be stronger. You will get fatter, and fatter. Finally you get to the point where you just give up altogether and that is when you really start packing on the pounds.

Eventually, your system becomes so programmed and so efficient at storing excess body fat that bariatric surgery (gastric bypass) may seem to be your only hope. Gastric bypass surgeries have increased by 600% in recent years and other weight-loss surgeries are up by 400%, so you will certainly not be alone.

Talented Fat

Do you recognize the pattern here, if not from yourself, then from someone else? Many people who seem to be able to gain body fat even though they eat very little, have actually developed this dubious talent over many years of following stupid diets…and the wrong kind of exercise…if they exercised at all.

Bad Taste

The reason these systems do not work is that they are based on how many calories go into your mouth and how many calories you can burn by endlessly torturing your body with (mostly) aerobic exercise. This is absolutely not the right way to go about losing excess body fat. Even if these systems would work, I can't think of a more inefficient and unpleasant method of trying to keep your body fat under control. They would sentence you to being hungry (from the lack of food) and tired (from the excess exercise) for the rest of your thin life. That certainly leaves a bad taste in my mouth.

With Me It's Genetic

Now let's examine one of my all-time favorites: "Yes, but with me it is genetic. One (or both) of my parents is (are) fat."
And your point is? If one (or both) of your parents is not very intelligent, do you just give up and not go to school because you may have to study a little harder than the students whose parents are more intelligent? If one (or both) of your parents is an alcoholic, does it mean that you might as well start drinking now because you are genetically destined to become an alcoholic anyway. Of course not! THINK!

You can **choose** to take another path. Of course you will have to be more careful, and much more attentive to your problem than people who do not have a genetic predisposition, but it can be done. **You** are the controlling factor.

You, You, You

Please note that I did not say that it **can be** controlled, which infers that someone else has the responsibility. I said **you** can control it. No one else can do it for you. They can support you, gladly, but they cannot do the work for you. That is entirely up to you.

Genetics does determine which of the three basic body-types you inherit. Naturally thin (ectomorph), naturally muscular (mesomorph), and naturally heavy (endomorph) are the three basic body types. Most people are a mixture of two of these. You can be basically thin but leaning towards muscular, or basically muscular but leaning towards heavy, or just basically thin…or basically heavy.

Doomed

However, your inherited body-type does not doom you. It only predisposes you. Being basically heavy doesn't sentence you to becoming over-fat. Bad nutrition and lack of exercise, or the wrong choice of exercise and stupid diets will do that, no matter which body type you have inherited!

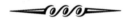

Child Abuse

What about parents who do not address the problem of their children's body fat getting out of control? I personally consider this to be a serious form of unrecognized child abuse. These parents are contributing to the bullying, social and emotional problems, unhappiness and bad health of their children. By the time the kids are old enough to realize that something is not right, they have already been saddled with lifelong problems – physical, mental, and emotional. Gee…thanks Mom…Thanks Pop! I'll be sure to mention both of you to my therapist.

Isn't He Cute

Some experts say that you are born with all the fat cells that you will ever have. However, I am not alone in believing that fat cells can be added after birth by overfeeding babies, young children, teenagers and even adults, especially if they are being overfed with unhealthy food choices. This is why "plump," "pudgy," or "chubby" babies should not be considered to be cute. They should be considered to be over-fat and immediate steps should be taken to make sure that their cute "baby-fat" doesn't get completely out of control. And please people…I know that healthy babies are not born skinny, but when their little eyes are nearly shut from folds of fat, you have the beginnings of a major problem. You know what I am talking about here. Fat babies are not cute, healthy babies. They are over-fat!

More than 10% of American pre-school children (two to five years old) are now over-fat. In the last twenty years, obesity has **doubled** in grade-school children and has **tripled** in teens. This is simply unacceptable!

Kiddy Onset Diabetes

At the moment, there are more than 400,000 children in America diagnosed with Type II diabetes and the number is rapidly growing. It used to be called adult onset diabetes, but they certainly can't call it that anymore since twelve-year-olds are now developing this disease…and the age just keeps dropping. In the most susceptible groups (African-Americans and Latinos), children as young as three and four years old are now being diagnosed with the preventable Type II diabetes. Now read the paragraph about "cute baby-fat" again.

Something is drastically wrong here! This is totally unacceptable, and simply changing the name of the disease doesn't solve anything either. 90% of all newly diagnosed cases of diabetes are of the preventable Type II, so the adults aren't doing very well here either. Type II diabetes is now the fastest growing disease in America, having doubled in only one decade.

Excessive

If parents give their kids excessive amounts of alcohol (some cultures allow a small glass of wine with dinner), it is considered child abuse. If parents give their kids excessive amounts of (legal, but unnecessary) drugs, it is considered child abuse. If parents give their kids cigarettes, it is considered child abuse. If parents provide their kids with excessive amounts of unhealthy foods…what do you want to call it?

Setting Examples

Don't get me wrong. I am not saying that parents can control their kids' eating habits twenty-four hours a day, but they should have a great deal of control at home, and they should be setting much better examples themselves. You can't tell your children to exercise and to eat healthy if you don't. You will have no credibility with them whatsoever.

Education

It is the same as educating them at home about alcohol, drugs (not only illegal drugs), and…dare I say it…yes, I dare…sex! As parents, you can't simply shove responsibility for things this important onto someone else (teachers, doctors, etc.) and expect a satisfactory outcome. I am talking here about parents who do nothing, or very little, about the problem of their over-fat children. After a certain age, the problem does become partly the responsibility of the young person, but by then the foundation has already been laid.

You Can Only Teach What You Know

Parents share the responsibility for educating their kids about health-building nutrition. It is part of preparing your children for success in life. Learning what they need to know in order to be able to teach their children about nutrition wouldn't do most parents any harm either. **But how can you teach your children about something you yourself know very little about?** Learn about health, nutrition and exercise yourself...and then teach your children about them. **In order to teach, you must first be willing to learn!**

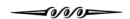

The Real Deal

OK, if cutting and/or mindlessly burning calories is not the way to go, then what does work? Pay very close attention to what I am about to tell you now. This is the real deal for taking control of your body fat and for permanent body fat loss, which is probably the main reason many of you picked up this book in the first place.

The real reason that stupid diets fail is that the people who dream them up do not really understand how the human body truly reacts to food, and how the human body actually uses body fat for fuel.

Your Choice...Again

Once again, **how can you expect to be successful at something you don't even understand?** Is it more logical to rely on hit-and-miss, trial-and-error and old wives' tales, or on scientifically proven principles?

Remember...it is your body...and it is your choice.

> ### The Only Way
>
> Building healthy, shapely muscle, and controlling your
> fat-burning/fat-storing enzymes and hormones is the ONLY efficient,
> effective, successful, and permanent solution to controlling your body fat.

Enzymes and hormones tell your body what to do with the food and liquids that it takes in, i.e., use them to build muscle, or to store carbohydrates in the muscles for quick energy…or to turn them into body fat. Enzymes and hormones tell your body to either store fat or to burn fat.

Apart from building muscle, **what** you eat and **when** you eat it will determine whether you become over-fat in the first place, or not. It will also determine whether you will successfully lose body fat and keep it off, or not. If you are eating health-building foods, **how much you eat is secondary to this**. These are the reasons that some people "hardly eat anything" and still gain body fat. They are eating the wrong things at the wrong times and their hormonal systems are completely out of whack.

Eat

You can and should eat as much health-building, nutritious food as you want, as long as you do not throw your enzymes and hormones into a fat-storage mode. Eating less is actually counterproductive to controlling your body fat, if done for long periods of time.

Of course this goes against the age-old advice of "a calorie in, a calorie out…all calories are the same" but, based on results (a 5% success rate), that system hasn't seemed to work very well, has it? So let me finally put this one to bed with "the world is flat," "the sun revolves around the earth," and "the check is in the mail."

NO MORE

Calories, Calories, Calories

Of course calories do matter to a certain extent. If they did not, stomach reduction surgery would not work. However, the quality of the food you eat, the size of your portions, and the length of time between your meals are much more important factors than simply counting calories.

After being on a low-calorie diet, your body will replace the body fat it has lost before anything else! The diet has programmed all your hormones and enzymes to do this. Does this sound familiar?

All calories are not the same. I will absolutely guarantee you that if you eat a diet of 40% fats, 40% carbohydrates, and 20% proteins, you will look and feel much differently than if you eat a diet of 40% proteins, 40% carbohydrates, and 20% fats…even though the total calories of both diets are exactly the same. I will also guarantee you that you will not like the difference that you will see with the higher fat, lower protein diet.

A fat calorie causes a different reaction in your body than a protein calorie does, and a carbohydrate calorie causes a different reaction in your body than either of the other two. Some calories can become body fat much more easily than other calories. For instance:

- Calories from unhealthy fats can be more easily **stored** as body fat than any other type of calories.

- Calories from **simple** carbohydrates can be more easily **converted** to body fat than any other type of calories.

- Calories from alcohol are not only easily **converted** to body fat, but will also **inhibit** your body's ability to use your excess body fat for energy — a double whammy!

A Perfect Formula

Combine these three "foods" and you will have the perfect formula for adding excess body fat. Combine them often enough and in large enough quantities and you will not only have a major body fat problem, but you can kiss your health goodbye as well…guaranteed!

Quality Counts

I will also absolutely guarantee you that if you eat a diet of 40% low-quality proteins, 40% simple carbohydrates, and 20% unhealthy fats, you will look and feel much differently than if you eat a diet of 40% high-quality proteins, 40% complex carbohydrates, and 20% healthy fats, even though the total calories of both diets are exactly the same. I will also guarantee you that you will not like this difference either.

High-quality proteins cause a different reaction in your body than lower quality proteins. Healthy essential fatty acids cause a much different reaction than unhealthy saturated fats and trans-fatty acids. A fibrous carbohydrate causes a different reaction than a starchy carbohydrate, and simple carbohydrates are also different.

For instance, eating too many simple carbohydrates…too often…will not only raise your insulin levels (bad) but will also destroy your body's ability to metabolize (burn) fats. These are the real reasons simple carbohydrates will make you over-fat and keep you over-fat…not just the empty calories they contain.

> If you really want to stimulate your hunger and elevate your production of excess body fat, then eat and drink lots of simple carbohydrates…often!

These are the things that should be determining what you eat and drink, and this is why just cutting calories doesn't work. Your body needs nutrient dense, high-quality nutrition, i.e., lean protein foods, bulky, filling, complex carbohydrates, and healthy fats…not concentrated, nutritionally empty, unhealthy calories. I will discuss these matters more in the chapter on nutrition, Chapter 12.

You can actually **gain** body fat on 1500 calories a day…or **lose** body fat on 2500 calories a day, depending on how you manipulate your hormones with the choices you make. For instance, if you eat

1500 calories of unhealthy foods spread out over only two meals, much of it could wind up as excess body fat. However, if you spread 2500 healthy calories fairly evenly over five or six meals, this will not happen, especially if you are also exercising correctly.

Enzymes And Hormones

So which enzymes and hormones are we talking about here? I mentioned enzymes in the chapter on aerobics. They work in close connection with hormones and will generally rise or fall with them. The major hormones we are concerned with are growth hormone, insulin, glucagon, testosterone, and cortisol.

Your levels of growth hormone, testosterone, and cortisol are determined by BOTH exercise and diet.

Your body's production of insulin and glucagon are determined ENTIRELY by your diet.

Exercise And Nutrition…Duh!

This is exactly why even a Quality body fat loss Nutrition plan will not work optimally unless it is combined with a Quality body fat loss Exercise program…and even a Quality body fat loss Exercise program will not work optimally unless it is combined with a Quality body fat loss Nutrition plan.

Quality Exercise produces the hormonal responses needed to insure a gain of muscle (or to prevent a loss of muscle) while optimizing and accelerating the loss of excess body fat. In addition, you need a Quality Nutrition program to control your levels of insulin and glucagon.

Just the Facts

Sorry to burst your excuse bubble once again, but those are the cold hard facts. Now you have to decide what you are going to do with them. Your local gym and fast food restaurants are eagerly awaiting your answer.

Break Point

Earlier in this chapter I said that clinical obesity begins at 20% for men and 28% for women. Then I told you that the average American male already has 25% and the average American female already has 35% body fat levels. That means that half of the U.S. population has even higher body fat levels than this!

Now you need to understand that a curious thing happens at around 20-25% body fat for men and 25-30% body fat for women.

At these levels of body fat, your body begins to release less growth hormone and (for the guys) produce less testosterone. And the more over-fat you become, the less your insulin works.

The origin of the word hormone is Greek and means "to put into motion." If you have too little of these hormones, no fat-burning can be put into motion. Without these hormones working at normal levels, your metabolism begins to slow down and your entire system begins shifting into a major fat-storage mode!

The result of this is that the more over-fat you become, the easier it is to become even more over-fat, and the more difficult it becomes to lose your excess body fat. Does this sound familiar?

Prevention Is the Best Prevention

Of course, never allowing yourself to get over-fat in the first place is the best solution. The good news is that preventing over-fatness, curing over-fatness, and building health are all done in exactly the same basic way.

Hormone Control Ain't So Tough

Let's take a closer look at what we can **easily** do to gain better control over these hormones.

Growth Hormone

Growth hormone (GH) helps to build muscle, hinders the accumulation of body fat, and increases the use of fats for energy, while decreasing the use of carbohydrates for energy. GH strengthens bones, tendons, ligaments and other connective tissues, and even slows down the aging process. It does much more, but these are the things that we are concerned with here because they affect health and the loss of excess body fat. So what influences our body's production of growth hormone?

Increases Growth Hormone Release	Decreases Growth Hormone Release
• Infrequent, **higher rep**, large muscle exercise	• Overtraining
• Exercising intensely enough to cause a burning sensation in the working muscle(s)	• Intense exercise of longer than about one hour
• Keeping rest periods short between sets	• Extended low or medium intensity exercise (including aerobics) that lasts more than one hour at a time.
• Exercising intensely enough to be out of breath	• Overuse of forced reps and/or negative reps
• Exercising intensely enough to raise your body temperature slightly (cause sweating)	• Getting too little sleep
• Drinking an after-exercise recovery shake immediately after exercising	• Restless, shallow sleep
• Taking a 20-30 minute nap after drinking your recovery shake	• Excessive or chronic stress
• Not eating or drinking anything (except water) for one hour after drinking your recovery shake	• Cold or cool temperatures (outside or inside)
• Eating a high-protein, low-fat, medium carbohydrate meal about one hour after drinking your recovery shake	• Not having enough quality proteins in your diet
• Periodically changing exercise routines	• Eating meals too high in carbohydrates
• Short, high-intensity interval aerobics (Cardio-aerobics)	• Eating or drinking simple carbohydrates
• Heat, saunas and steam baths	• Eating or drinking carbohydrates immediately before, during, or immediately after exercise (except for the After CTTC Workout Recovery Shake, explained in Chapter 12)
• Deep, restful sleep	• Eating or drinking carbohydrates before sleeping
• Keeping stress under control	• Not eating a nutritious breakfast
• Eating small, nutritious meals every 3-4 hours	• Having an unhealthy diet
• Having enough high-quality proteins in your diet. The higher the quality of the protein, the higher the growth hormone response.	• Excess body fat
• Having enough essential fatty acids in your diet, especially the Omega 3s	• Alcohol
• Having low blood glucose levels	• Not keeping cortisol under control
• Maintaining a low level of body fat	
• Sensible exposure to sunshine	
• High-quality whey protein supplements	
• Creatine supplementation	
• Glutamine peptide supplementation	

Insulin

Insulin decreases the level of blood glucose (blood sugar) when it gets too high. It does this by pushing the blood sugar into the muscle cells to provide them with fuel for energy. When the muscle cells are full, any remaining blood sugar will activate your body fat storage systems (enzymes and hormones)…and will then be stored as body fat. The more muscle tissue you have, the more blood sugar (carbohydrates) you can store as muscular energy…rather than as excess body fat.

Quality Exercise increases the amount of blood sugar your muscles are able to absorb…even more! In other words, **the more muscle you have, and the better your exercise program is, the more carbohydrates you can eat without them being turned into excess body fat.**

In order to do this most effectively, you need to be in control of your insulin levels. If you can control your insulin, you can use it to build and maintain muscle tissue…and to lose body fat.

Insulin also has an influence on how your body metabolizes fats. If your insulin is out of control, it will make you over-fat. Body fat cannot be stored without insulin. High insulin levels also stimulate your appetite. **If you have elevated insulin levels, losing body fat will be virtually impossible.** So what influences your insulin levels?

Positive influences on insulin levels	Negative influences on insulin levels
• Eating small, nutritious meals every 3-4 hours	• Eating large, infrequent meals
• Combining small to medium amounts of complex carbohydrates with medium amounts of high-quality proteins and small amounts of healthy fats	• Consuming meals, snacks or drinks containing large amounts of carbohydrates
• Having enough fiber (25-35 grams) in your diet	• Consuming meals, snacks, or drinks containing only carbohydrates
• Having enough essential fatty acids in your diet, especially the Omega 3s	• Frequently consuming meals, snacks or drinks containing large amounts of simple carbohydrates
• Having enough vitamin E in your diet	• Having a diet high in saturated fats and trans-fatty acids
• Having enough vitamin C in your diet	• Having a diet low in fiber
• Having enough chromium in your diet	• Not eating a nutritious breakfast
• Drinking an after-exercise recovery shake immediately after exercising	• Caffeine (not only from drinking too much coffee, but from all sources of caffeine)
• Maintaining a low level of body fat	• Alcohol
• Chromium picolinate supplements	• Excess stress
• Vitamin E supplements	• Having a high level of body fat
• Vitamin C supplements	• Not keeping cortisol under control
• Alpha Lipoic Acid supplements	• Not exercising
• Having a high ratio of muscle to body fat	• Not taking a high-quality multi-vitamin/mineral supplement
• Exercising (influences insulin levels already in your system, not the production of insulin)	• Certain medications such as diuretics, beta blockers, anti-inflammatory drugs, antacids, female hormones, high blood pressure medications, and many others
	• Quitting smoking (one of the main reasons most people gain weight after they stop smoking…now you know why)

Glucagon

Glucagon does exactly the opposite of insulin. It releases glucose (sugar), stored in the cells to raise your blood sugar to a normal level when it gets too low. **Glucagon accelerates the breakdown of body fat and stimulates the use of body fat for energy…but only when your body is low on carbohydrates.** Glucagon burns body fat, but an increase in blood sugar will inhibit glucagon release. What can you do to maximize glucagon's effects on your excess body fat?

Increases Glucagon Release	Decreases Glucagon Release
• Quality Exercise • A diet higher in high-quality proteins • Drinking a high-quality protein (whey), very low carbohydrate shake, on an empty stomach, before doing your fat-burning exercise first thing in the morning • Drinking a high-quality protein (whey), very low carbohydrate shake, on an empty stomach, 45-60 minutes before doing your CTTC Workout • Drinking a high-quality protein, very low carbohydrate, shake, on an empty stomach, before going to sleep for the night, especially on CTTC Workout days	• Not exercising • A low protein diet • Inferior proteins in your diet • Eating or drinking carbohydrates before, during, or immediately after your fat-burning exercise • Eating or drinking carbohydrates immediately before, during, or immediately after your CTTC Workout (except for the **After CTTC Workout Recovery Shake**, explained in Chapter 12) • Eating or drinking carbohydrates before going to sleep for the night

Testosterone

Testosterone is the male hormone that allows men to develop large muscles. The lack of large amounts of this hormone in women's bodies is what prevents women from being able to build large muscles. Testosterone also helps to keep body fat levels low and increases protein synthesis. What increases or decreases testosterone?

Increases Testosterone	Decreases Testosterone
• Infrequent, **lower rep**, large muscle exercise • Heavy, intense exercise with weights • Short, high-intensity interval aerobics (Cardio-aerobics) • Longer rest periods between sets • Gaining muscle • Having enough essential fatty acids in your diet, especially the Omega 3s • Having a diet higher in monounsaturated fats (olive oil, for example) • Taking a high-quality multi-vitamin/mineral supplement • **Sensible** exposure to sunshine	• Intense exercise of longer than about one hour • Exercising too often • Excessive aerobic exercise • Not getting enough quality sleep • Extremely low-fat diets (less than 15-20% of total calories) • Low calorie diets • Trans-fatty acids in your diet • Having a high level of body fat • Not keeping cortisol under control • Drinking excessive alcohol (more than 1 drink per day if you are small, or 2 drinks per day if you are a larger person)

Metabolism

Of course, keeping your metabolism raised is also essential to an effective fat-loss program. Your basal metabolism accounts for 60-70% of the energy your body uses…every day…365 days a year. Now do you understand why your metabolism is so important for controlling your body fat? The longer you can keep your metabolism elevated, the more body fat you will burn…all day, every day…without doing anything. That sounds good to me, so what increases metabolism best and…just as important… what lowers it?

Elevates Metabolism	Depresses Metabolism
• Higher lean body weight (muscle)	• Having a higher level of body fat
• **Intensive** exercise with weights	• Not exercising with weights
• Raising body temperature by exercising	• Excessive aerobic exercise…again
• Physically demanding exercises such as high rep squats and leg presses	• Not eating for several hours & skipping meals Your body begins to think it is starving about 5-6 hours after its last meal, and your metabolism will start dropping
• Exercising at 80-85% of MHR for 15 minutes, 3 times per week	• Stupid diets…especially low-calorie diets
• Keeping active during the entire day	• Not eating enough high-quality protein
• Heat (weather, room temperature, saunas, steam baths)	• A diet high in saturated fats and trans-fatty acids
• Eating small, nutritious meals every 3-4 hours	• Eating too few complex carbohydrates (lowers thyroid hormone)
• A diet higher in high-quality proteins	• Frequently consuming meals, snacks, or drinks containing large amounts of **simple** carbohydrates
• Eating some high-quality protein at every meal. A high-protein meal will raise your metabolism by 30% for several hours (fats & carbohydrates raise metabolism by only about 4%)	• Sleeping for more than 8 or 9 hours at a time
• A diet higher in fibrous carbohydrates	• Not eating a nutritious breakfast
• Having enough essential fatty acids in your diet, especially the Omega 3's	• Eating less than your basal metabolism needs (diets too low in calories)
• Drinking an after exercise recovery shake	• Not keeping yourself hydrated
• Spicy foods	• Not keeping cortisol under control
• Drinking lots of pure, clean, **cool** water	
• **Sensible** exposure to sunshine	

Note: Basal metabolism is the amount of energy (calories) that your body uses when at rest in order to carry out all your necessary (basic) bodily functions, such as maintaining a constant body temperature, keeping your heart beating, breathing, digesting the food you eat, making enzymes and hormones, sending electrical impulses, maintaining brain function, etc…although, in my case, maintaining brain function has never been a major expenditure of energy.

Cortisol

Cortisol is a catabolic hormone produced by the body. Catabolic means that it breaks down body tissues. This breakdown can include muscle tissue. It can suppress your body's synthesis of new proteins, making it more difficult to build muscle. It can also hinder your body's ability to metabolize (burn) fats and carbohydrates. Cortisol, if not kept under control, will negatively affect your metabolism and slow down your thyroid function…thus making you over-fat.

Too much cortisol can also suppress your immune system, cause high blood pressure, elevate your cholesterol, increase calcium depletion, and accelerate aging and memory loss. A little cortisol is necessary, but an excess is definitely bad news.

Cotisol is sometimes used as a medicine to treat conditions such as asthma, certain allergies, some types of arthritis, and other inflammations. When used as a medicine it is called cortisone and you can easily see the side effects it has on many of these patients. These include rapid gains in body fat and severe bloating. Not a pretty picture.

Suppresses Cortisol	Increases Cortisol
• Eating small, nutritious meals every 3-4 hours	• Going several hours without eating
• Eating a nutritious breakfast. (Your cortisol levels are usually highest around 8:00 in the morning.)	• Low-calorie diets – cutting calories by 50% can raise cortisol levels by up to 40%.
• Drinking an after exercise recovery shake	• Unhealthy nutrition
• Eating some high-quality protein, or drinking a high-quality protein, very low carbohydrate, shake, on an empty stomach, before going to sleep for the night…especially on CTTC Workout days	• Sugar, caffeine, alcohol, nicotine, chocolate – 3 cups of coffee can elevate cortisol levels for several hours. Adding sugar to the coffee increases this effect even more.
• Keeping your growth hormone levels high	• Not eating a nutritious breakfast
• Keeping your insulin levels under control	• Not eating (or drinking) some high-quality protein before going to sleep
• A diet higher in monounsaturated fats (olive oil, for example)	• Restless and/or inadequate sleep
• Having enough essential fatty acids in your diet, especially the Omega 3s	• Long periods of mental or emotional stress
• Having a positive attitude	• Fear, anger, worry, anxiety, guilt, unhappiness
• Being happy and laughing often	• Not exercising at all
• Having optimistic, positive-thinking happy friends	• Excessive aerobic exercise…once again
• Keeping stress under control with meditation and/ or other relaxation (anti-stress) techniques	• Excessive exercise with weights
• Having regular sport massages	• Exercising intensely more than 2 days in a row
• Getting enough deep, restful sleep	• Intense exercise of longer than about one hour
• Vitamin C supplements	• Not drinking an after exercise recovery shake
• Glutamine peptide supplements	• Injuries and physical pain
• Alpha Lipoic Acid supplements	• Illness
	• Not taking a high-quality multi-vitamin/mineral supplement

Impossible

Now that we know how to control our enzymes and hormones, we come to the horrible realization that we cannot do this all the time. You simply cannot always eat four, or five, or six perfectly nutritious meals every day, or never miss an exercise session. It just isn't humanly possible…and life would be no fun and really boring if it were possible.

Enjoyment

I really enjoy a cold beer in the summer, a glass of wine with a meal, an occasional pizza, ice cream on a hot day, and French fries once in a while with a nice, juicy hamburger. When I go to a party or on a short vacation, absolutely the last thing I want to do is eat only "healthy" foods. In fact, even when I am busy dropping a few excess body fat pounds…again…I am really strict with myself only during the week. On the weekends I am careful with my choices and amounts of foods and beverages, but I still make sure to enjoy myself. However, if you are more than a few pounds over-fat, it would be an intelligent choice to put this off until you are quite close to your target body fat level.

This "weekend exception" not only helps me to stick to my fat-loss program but, as you will read in the following paragraphs, it is also actually necessary for a continued loss of body fat. This is where sticking points, set points and self-discipline come in.

Sticking Points

Sticking points are, unfortunately, a normal part of the fat-loss process. A sticking point is when you reach a point where you are no longer losing body fat. You are stuck. Most people try to break a sticking point by reducing calories even more and/or increasing exercise. An athlete may have to resort to this because of a competition deadline, but for the rest of us, the correct solution is to ease off a little.

Your body will not lose body fat at an even rate for a prolonged period of time. You will not lose one pound every week for ten weeks. You may lose one pound the first week, two pounds the second week, nothing the third week, then again two pounds the fourth week. Your body will occasionally stop to evaluate its situation. It is trying to find out if something dangerous…like starvation…is happening to it or not. Give it some time to adjust to the new weight.

Instead of cutting calories, eat a little bit more for a couple of days. The important thing at this point is to make sure that your weight does not go up more than a pound or so…no matter what.

Self-Discipline

This is where the people who have developed self-discipline succeed, and those who haven't fail. I don't care if it is your daughter's wedding, your son's bar mitzva, your anniversary or someone's birthday…you have to stick to your guns and keep your bodyweight in check during this time. You cannot eat foods that disrupt your fat-storage hormones and enzymes during this time. Of course you can treat yourself a little bit…but do it with healthy foods! Do not binge on unhealthy foods!

After a couple of days, your body will realize that it is not starving. The extra calories will help it to realize this. Then it will change its chemistry from a holding-on-to-body fat mode back to a body fat-losing mode. Now you can return to your fat-loss nutrition plan…and the process starts all over again. You continue this pattern until you have reached your goal. You can very definitely lose the ten pounds in ten weeks (or maybe in even less time), but body fat loss never happens in a straight line, so forget that idea…it will only depress you.

Less Takes Longer

You must also deal with the fact that the lower your body fat level becomes…the more difficult it becomes to lose more body fat. Someone who is 200 pounds over-fat can lose ten pounds of body fat in a very short time, without putting a great deal of effort into it. However, if you are only twenty pounds over-fat, it will take longer and will require much more effort and self-discipline on your part to lose ten pounds of excess body fat.

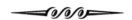

The Set Point

A set point is the weight which your body perceives to be its "normal" weight. Your body will fight you to keep from going under this weight and it will also fight you to keep from going over this weight. Unfortunately, it fights going under harder than it fights going over. Your personal set point is partially determined by your genetically inherited body type. If you are genetically predisposed to be heavier, you will never be able to re-adjust your set point to that of a very thin person…so keep your goals realistic.

Attempting to re-adjust your set point to an unrealistically low percentage of body fat is programming yourself for failure. You can, however, lower your set point to a level that will make it much easier to keep your body fat manageable for your body type. In fact, you **must** lower your set point in order to be successful in the long-term control of your body fat.

LORI

If you are thin and attempting to gain muscular weight, you will have to **raise** your set point in order to more easily maintain your hard-earned new muscle. The principle remains the same.

Acceptance

There is another problem with the set point. After you have reached your desired body fat level, your body must learn to accept that as its new "normal" weight. This also takes some time. How much time? I don't know. Everyone is a little different. I have to maintain my new weight for about three months before it gets really "set." From experience with other people, I don't believe it can be done in less than two or three months. To stay on the safe side, and insure success, I tell my clients to go with six months. You cannot go over this new weight limit for any reason whatsoever during these "setting" months, or your new set point may not become really "fixed."

If you let your weight pass this new set point before it becomes really "fixed," it will take off like a runaway train and you will be back at your old weight, but fatter, in no time. Don't let this happen!

I Thought It Was Gone for Good

This is another reason most people fail at keeping their excess body fat off after successfully losing it. They fail to maintain the new weight long enough to really fix their new set point. Once again, this takes a lot of self-discipline. You have to be motivated, you have to be committed, and you have to make this a priority in your life for a few months!

Pick a Time

If you need to lose much more than about ten pounds of body fat, you will probably have to re-adjust your set point more than once on the way down. Set a medium-term fat-loss goal for yourself, reach it, hold it for a while…and then go on to your next medium term fat-loss goal. As you can see, this is no quick fix. It will take time, so you also need to plan your time.

Please don't start this program just before going on vacation, or the day after consuming too much alcohol at a party. Don't start the **CTTC** Exercise Program, the **CTTC** Nutrition Program, stop drinking and stop smoking all at the same time. Don't start any of this if you are currently going through a marriage, a divorce, a death, a job loss or any other emotional roller coaster. If you do, you will be programming yourself for failure.

Trust me on this one. I once tried to stop smoking, stop drinking, stop eating junk-food, stop swearing and stop thinking about sex…all at once. It was the worst five minutes of my entire life. I'll never try that again!

Pick a period when you have a good chance of devoting enough time, energy and mental fortitude to the project. Get organized. Prepare yourself mentally. Have your whole game plan: goals, time frames, etc., written down on paper. That will make them more real to you. When everything is right…go for it. You will now be programmed to succeed…and you will.

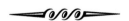

The Secret

Now you know how and why people become over-fat in the first place so you cannot use the "I didn't know…" excuse anymore. It is time to let you in on the absolute secret of never becoming over-fat. By ignoring this "secret," I stupidly allowed myself to become over-fat a couple of times in my life. Notice that I said "allowed myself." No excuses…no denial. No one forced me. They were my very own bad choices. Afterwards I had to fight my way back to being lean and healthy again so…yes…I know what that is like too. The secret is not in the set point because the set point is too easily broken. The real secret is the next step in the plan.

The Secret Is a "Line"

This means that when you reach your desired bodyweight, or when…for whatever reason…you can't continue with your fat-loss program for a period of time, you have to draw **a line** for yourself. This **line** is a weight somewhere above your desired bodyweight, or the bodyweight you are at when circumstances force you to temporarily put your fat-loss program on hold.

This **line** should be ten pounds (at most) above either of these two bodyweights if you are a shorter, smaller person and twenty pounds (at most) if you are a taller, larger person. Five pounds and ten pounds would be even better choices, but I will leave that up to you. That depends on your levels of commitment and self-discipline. The important thing is to pick **a line** that you can stick to…no matter what.

Give It a Rest

The reason this is necessary is that your life, like mine, probably doesn't flow in a constant, positive, upward direction. Your life has ups and downs, and so will your weight and physical condition. It is just not humanly possible for people with normal lives to always be in tip-top condition. Even professional athletes cycle their training because it is not possible, or even desirable, to maintain a very high level of fitness and a very low level of body fat all the time…unless that is just a natural state for you that you don't have to work at…and if that's the case, the rest of us hate you for it.

Inspiration

I actually use this fact to help keep myself inspired and motivated. After the summer, I ease up on my workouts a little. I don't push myself so hard with the weights or aerobics. I allow my body to rest and recover more during this period. I experiment with different exercises or machines and I even skip the Cardio-aerobics once in a while. To be perfectly honest, I also party a lot harder too. During this time, I do strive to keep my set point under control but…when I occasionally fail to do that…I reaffirm my commitment to myself to never, ever, under any circumstances…cross my **line**.

About the end of January I start my three-month plan to be in "beach shape" again by May. I maintain this "beach condition" throughout the summer and then I start the cycle all over again. This seasonal cycle bolsters my enthusiasm and helps to keep me committed to a lifetime of healthy exercise.

Lifetime Commitment

Here is the real deal with the **line**. You have to make a pact with yourself, a conscious decision, a written-in-stone commitment that you will never, for any reason, or under any circumstances whatsoever, allow yourself to cross your **line**.

When talking about the set point, I said that you have to stay under your set point weight for a few months to initially "fix" it. The **line** is different. You have to make an ironclad commitment to yourself to stay under this weight **for the rest of your life!** The **line** will provide you with a lifetime safety margin of those ten or twenty pounds (five or ten pounds would be better). That is leeway enough for you to be able to successfully keep your body fat under control for a lifetime…**if you make the decision to do it.**

The Payoff

If you never cross your **line**, you will always be able to make it back to your desired set point and healthier bodyweight without suffering major lifestyle changes, or having to torture yourself with extra exercise and food deprivation for months on end.

The other side of the coin is that every time you do cross your **line**, it will become less defined. If you cross your **line** often enough, it will disappear completely, putting you right back where you started – over-fat and out of control…again!

Self - Discipline

Once again we come back to self-discipline, because self-discipline is the only thing that will keep you from crossing your **line**. No one can do it for you. However, every time you come close to your **line**…without going over it…you will build a better self-image and more self-confidence. Each time you do this you will become mentally stronger and it will become easier and easier to never cross your **line**. This is how you can conquer over-fatness forever…and become master of your own body.

With a Little Non-Help From My Friends

Family and "friends" are often the ones who make the self-discipline so necessary. Unfortunately, a lot of people will want you to fail. Even worse, they will do anything and everything they can to make you fail.

You know the routine. They will offer you alcohol and/or cigarettes if you are trying to quite either of these. "Oh come on…just one won't hurt you. You have to live a little." They will do the same with exercise and food, providing you with all kinds of excuses to skip your exercise and constant temptations to eat things you know you should not. "Just eat one…it's a special occasion," or, "But I baked/bought them just for you."

Lives of Quiet Desperation

Why do they do this? Seeing other people fail probably makes them feel better about themselves. Losers hate winners. Unsuccessful people don't like to see others succeed. Who cares why? You are doing this for yourself, not for them…so use their negativity to make yourself stronger. Each time you say, "Thanks, but no thanks" to these people you will feel better about yourself, become mentally stronger, better disciplined and more determined than ever to achieve your goals.

Mental Muscle

These mental strengths, in turn, will carry over to all other aspects of your life. That definitely makes this another win-win situation…so go for it. Don't let these negative people bring you down. Once again, use their negativity to make yourself stronger.

> The only person who can stop you from succeeding…is YOU.

Reality Check

Remember, your goal is to never cross your **line**. In spite of all your sincere intentions, you may still allow this to happen sometime. I have already admitted to my couple of errors. However, **an error only becomes a mistake if you don't do anything to correct it.**

Feel a little guilty for allowing it to happen. A little guilt is good. It means you care. Then kick yourself in your butt and get busy correcting your small error before it becomes a huge (pun definitely intended) mistake. Make a conscious decision to never let your weight get out of control again…to never cross your **line** again.

De-Size

Another commitment that you absolutely have to make to yourself is to never again buy larger clothing. When your present clothes start getting tight…take a hint. Spend your time losing excess body fat and getting healthy, not shopping for a new, larger wardrobe to expand into.

In fact, you can reward yourself for losing your excess body fat by buying some smaller sized clothing instead of rewarding yourself with food. It's a much better choice and the enjoyment will last much longer. Each time you wear the new, smaller clothing, you will be re-enforcing your success and you will be even more motivated to continue achieving your goals.

Lying Again

NEVER buy pants, shorts, skirts, kilts, incontinence diapers, or anything else if it has an elastic waist. Elastic waistbands are just another way of lying to yourself. Don't do it.

Are you really confident and motivated? Start systematically giving away your present clothing as they become too large for your new body. Burn the bridges back to being over-fat again. Now there is a personal challenge…and it gives a whole new meaning to "coming out of the closet" too.

Too Complicated

This might all seem very complicated at this point, but if you compare the different lists in this chapter you will find that they have many things in common. **The Principles of Quality Exercise** have all been incorporated into the **CTTC** Workouts, so when and how to exercise is no longer a problem for you. Now you only need to adjust your eating habits in order to turn your body into a fat-burning machine.

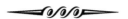

A Review

Let's review the nutritional do's and do not's for losing body fat...and keeping it off permanently.

Do	Do Not
• Eat small, nutritious meals every 3-4 hours (5-6 meals per day) • **Always** eat a nutritious breakfast • Combine small to medium amounts of complex carbohydrates with medium amounts of high-quality proteins and small amounts of healthy fats • Have enough **high-quality** proteins in your diet • Eat some **high-quality** protein at every meal • Eat a diet higher in fibrous carbohydrates • Have enough fiber (25-35 grams) in your diet • Have enough essential fatty acids in your diet, especially the Omega 3s • Take a high quality multi-vitamin/mineral supplement • Drink lots of pure, clean water every day	• Eat large, infrequent meals • Go several hours without eating • Consume meals, snacks, or drinks containing large amounts of carbohydrates • Consume meals, snacks, or drinks containing **only** carbohydrates • Frequently consume meals, snacks, or drinks containing large amounts of **simple** carbohydrates • Eat a diet high in saturated fats and trans-fatty acids • Use stupid diets, skip meals, or not eat enough calories • Eat or drink carbohydrates immediately before, during, or immediately after exercise (except for the **After CTTC Workout Recovery Shake**, explained in Chapter 12) • Eat or drink carbohydrates before going to sleep • Drink alcohol of any kind, in any amounts, as long as you are attempting to lose body fat • Let yourself become dehydrated

When we break it down like this, it doesn't seem so impossible. The necessary **basic** nutritional supplements, which are also uncomplicated, are covered in the chapter on nutrition, Chapter 12. That leaves us with just one more thing.

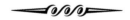

Diet Pills

What about diet pills? Wonderful...let's rely on some more drugs to solve another one of our problems. The quick fix again. Unless you can find a pill that also changes your bad lifestyle, unhealthy diet, and somehow forces you to exercise, you will only be treating a symptom (the fat) again instead of fixing the cause of the problem. Instead of just being an over-fat person, you can become an over-fat drug addict. Now, do you really think that would be a step in the right direction?

And let's not forget the recent fiasco with the weight-loss drug Fen-Phen, which seriously damaged heart valves in thousands of people before it was finally pulled off the market. You will read about "100% safe drugs…with no side effects"…in the chapter on health, Chapter 15.

Why resort to drugs when you can use your own body's biochemistry? It's cheaper. It's legal. It's a lot healthier than using drugs. The positive results gained from using your own body's biochemistry are both physical and mental…and they can be permanent.

Success

What do I think about diet pills? I think this:

Good

> Successful people are successful because they are willing to do things that unsuccessful people are NOT willing to do!

If you follow the **CTTC** Exercise and Nutrition Programs conscientiously and faithfully…you will not need diet pills. Do the work that needs to be done and stop wasting time looking for "magic" or "miracle" solutions to your problems…no matter what they may be.

Nutritional Fat-Loss Supplements

I will discuss specific nutritional supplements…also those which can assist in the loss of body fat…in a future publication and on the **CTTC** website, but first things first. You need to begin by doing what is in this book…then you can think about adding something extra. The only "fat-loss supplement" I will recommend here is 400 – 600 mcg of chromium picolinate daily. Chromium is hugely important for controlling insulin and **nobody** gets enough chromium from their food. This 400-600 mcg is including the amount that may already be in your multi-vitamin/mineral supplement. I repeat…it must be the chromium picolinate form.

If It's Between Your Ears

Some people have real mental and emotional problems with food and, if so, it is imperative that you also solve these problems if you ever want to successfully lose your excess body fat, and keep it off… permanently.

Dr. Phil

My only choice for addressing mental or emotional issues related to food is Dr. Phil McGraw's book, *The Ultimate Weight Solution.* Our thinking processes are very similar: we share many of the same thoughts on losing excess body fat, since much of it is just plain common sense and logic.

Dr. Phil also definitely "cuts thru the crap," so I can recommend his book without hesitation, and with absolute confidence. Cutting through the mental crap is exactly what you need if your problems with food go deeper than, "I just love to eat because it tastes so darn good." (This happens to be my personal difficulty…even if it does involve (mostly) nutritious, health-building foods.)

A Winning Combination

How do you know if you have an eating problem or not? Simple! Barring a medical condition, if you are seriously over-fat, you have a definite psychological problem involving food, so buy Dr. Phil's book, combine it with the **CTTC** Exercise and Nutrition Programs, and get started solving your excess body fat problem…now! In fact, you should buy his book and read it even if you don't think you need it. You will definitely learn something, and knowledge is power! Remember: Read…Study… Learn!

Low-Fat Success

Is the **CTTC** Exercise Program tough? Absolutely! It will probably be more demanding than anything many of you have ever done up to now…or it may be less demanding than what some of you have already been doing. In any case, the superior results will convince you that the **CTTC** Exercise Program is not only more effective, but also more complete and more time-saving than anything you have ever tried before.

Success…Again

Is it hard work? Absolutely…but always remember: **Successful people do what unsuccessful people are not willing to do!**

Be successful at building your health, losing your excess body fat and keeping it off…permanently!

Here's a Last Thought on the Subject:

Think less about your weight and more about your health! **If you take care of your health…your weight will take care of itself.** Why? Because properly taking care of your health automatically includes a Quality (fat-fighting) Exercise program as well as a health-building and practical (fat-fighting) nutrition plan.

FIGHT EXCESS BODY FAT...NOT WEIGHT!

Dr. Phil's *The Ultimate Weight Solution* is a great book. It will enlighten you to the psychological how's and why's of healthy weight loss. *Cut Thru The Crap* further illuminates the how's and why's of **specific** excess body fat loss and sculpting a stronger, healthier, and shapelier body.

In his book, Dr. Phil correctly emphasizes the importance of exercising with weights for body shaping and permanent weight loss. The **CTTC** Exercise Program provides you with **the exact tools** you need to successfully accomplish this.

The **CTTC** Nutrition Program does the same with your nutrition. It will take you a step further.

Two Heads Are Better Than One

Why should you use the **CTTC** Exercise and Nutrition Programs in combination with Dr. Phil's book? Dr. Phil is terrific at motivating un-motivated people. I have never been much good at that. My talent lies in helping motivated people to reach the level of fitness, wellness or athletic performance which they have chosen for themselves, whether that goal is simply to achieve a better state of health or to become a World Champion.

That is why these two books will complement each other so well. Dr. Phil's book will motivate you, get you started, and guide you to an above average level of health and fitness. You can continue the journey to even more optimal levels of wellness with the **CTTC** Exercise and Nutrition Programs...if that is your goal.

Forty Years

Dr. Phil likes to say that he has been doing this (psychology) for thirty years. Well I have been teaching **successful exercise and body fat loss** for more than forty years! Together, these two booksks will make an unbeatable team!

Chapter 5

THE CHAPTER THAT SHOULD NOT HAVE TO BE IN THIS BOOK

During my travels I have noticed that common courtesy (in many gyms) is no longer so common. Since gym etiquette is so important to having a positive exercise experience, I feel that, unfortunately, I need to include this chapter here before we get to the actual **CTTC** Workouts. Some of the things I have listed here will make most of you shake your heads in disbelief, but I assure you that they take place every day in gyms and locker rooms all over the world.

Following these reasonable rules will make exercising more pleasant for everyone…assuming that exercising can be pleasant. Remember…I hate to exercise.

Before You Exercise

- Clean your shoes at the front door. Dirt and mud belong outside, not in the locker room.

- Come to the gym clean. If you have had a hard, sweaty day, take a shower before training.

- Wear clean workout clothes. Can you believe that I actually have to include this one?

- Use deodorant…please…but use a subtle one, not an eye-burning, lung-choker.

- Unless you are a doctor, fire-fighter, hooker, or a member of some other emergency service, leave your cell-phone in your locker. If your calls were really that important, you would be rich and exercising in your fully-equipped home gym with an expensive personal trainer…not with us commoners. We should not have to wait for a piece of equipment because you want to sit on it and talk to your mommy, boyfriend/girlfriend…or whomever.

In the Gym

- Don't drag equipment across the floor. If you need to move it and it doesn't have wheels…pick it up.

- Put equipment back where it belongs when you are finished using it…even if that is not where you found it. It is distracting and aggravating to have to interrupt your exercise session in order to look for a piece of equipment that someone did not return to its proper place. Also, don't put the ten-pound dumbbells in the place marked for the twenty-five-pounders, etc. If you can't read and match the numbers, ask someone to help you.

- Don't leave loose weights (or any other equipment) lying around when you have finished an exercise. Someone else could break a toe, or slip and fall...breaking a lot more.

- Don't lay dumbbells or barbells on the exercise benches. At worst they can roll off and crush someone's foot...maybe even yours. At best they will eventually tear the covering on the bench. If you are too lazy to put them down on the floor and then pick them up again for your next set, then go exercise on the machines where you just have to move a pin.

  A professional bodybuilder recently self-amputated his big toe in just this way, so you can see that I am not just talking to unknowing novices in this chapter.

- Always use towels. If you sweat profusely, have a smaller one to wipe sweat off your face and hands, and a larger one to lay on the benches and machines when you are using them. Well-equipped gyms will also have disinfectant spray and paper towels to clean off equipment you have perspired on. When you are done, clean off the seat, backrest, handgrips and anywhere else your sweat has landed.

- Do not sit or hang around on the equipment if you are not using it. You should be exercising instead of hanging around anyway. Don't use benches or other equipment as a place to hang your towel, belt, gloves, etc...or as a chair.

- Do not do half of your sets on a piece of equipment, stop to have a ten-minute conversation with someone, and then finish your sets. Either finish the exercise first, or go somewhere else to have your conversation so others can use the equipment while you are busy flapping your lips.

- Use equipment for its designed purpose. For example, don't make others wait for the only cable crossover machine in the gym because you are using one side of it to do an exercise that you could just as well do on a single cable machine that no one is using.

- If someone asks if they can alternate with you on a piece of equipment...let them...especially if you are taking long rest periods (more than 60 - 90 seconds) between your sets. If it doesn't work out, you can always politely decline the next time that person asks...but give them a chance first. Having a gym membership does not mean that you bought the equipment.

- Do not try to talk to, or otherwise bother someone who is seriously exercising. If they have time, you can talk to them either before or after their workout. If you are correctly following the **CTTC** Exercise Program, you will not have the time or the breath to talk while you are exercising anyway.

- Unless you are employed as an instructor at the gym, don't give advice to the other members. The gym may have a certain system of teaching which their instructors are taught to follow. Your well-meaning advice, even if it is correct, just confuses the situation. If you want to give advice, get a job as an instructor or become a personal trainer.

- If you don't even know the anatomical names of the muscles, much less their origins, insertions, and kinesiological functions, and your only education comes from reading magazines and talking to "big guys"…you should be **seeking** advice…**not** giving it.

- Never, ever, make fun of anyone in the gym who is over-fat, skinny, handicapped, disfigured, or is in any way "different." Think of kids at school making fun of your child, or when you yourself were bullied. This is exactly the same thing. If you think it's hard to make yourself go to the gym, think how difficult it is for these people. They have taken a very difficult, positive step to improve themselves and to make their lives better. They deserve our respect and all the support we can give them. A friendly word can do wonders for them.

Just For the Ladies

- Don't douse yourself with a strong perfume before training. A hint of scent is alluring. More is air pollution…especially if you are next to someone who is huffing and puffing away in an aerobics class or on a treadmill, etc.

- If you come to the gym dressed like a walking demonstration for the maximum stretch capacities of spandex… or wearing lingerie…or to show off your new (or old) breast implants…that's great. But then don't give anyone the "Why are you looking at me? I am soooo offended" routine when they do look.

Just For the Guys

- Size is important…at least when it comes to workout bags. I can't imagine what some of you have in those footlocker size bags, but please don't put them on the benches people use to sit on…especially not in small locker rooms. Put them on the floor. Some of us with bad knees and/or bad backs need to sit down to safely put on, or remove, our shoes and socks. If there is not enough room to keep your oversized bag out of everyone else's way in the locker room… duh…get a smaller bag.

- Don't blow your nose…or clear your throat and spit…in the shower. It's dirty and unhygienic, and I can't believe that I actually have to mention this.

- When your soap/shampoo bottle is empty, don't leave it in the shower or on the locker room floor for someone else to clean up…unless your mommy or wife is the gym's cleaning lady. At least they are already used to picking up after you.

- While you are exercising, don't grunt and groan like a bull elephant having an orgasm. We all know that you are working really hard…and lifting really heavy weights…and we are all really impressed…really!

- If you are using 100 lbs on an exercise, don't load the barbell up with all the 5-pound plates in the gym so that there are no more left for others to use. It doesn't look cool…it just looks stupid.

- We all know that you can squat 800 pounds, bench press 500 pounds, curl 200 pounds, etc., so we don't need to be reminded of it after you have finished. It's OK to leave a couple of lighter plates on the bar but…once again…it can be dangerous for those with bad backs, knees or shoulders to have to take forty-five-pound plates off a barbell…and carry them to where YOU should have stacked them in the first place.

  Some exercisers will have to ask someone to help them…thereby unnecessarily interrupting two people's workouts…or they will just skip that exercise altogether. Neither of these is acceptable so…guys…have a little more respect for your fellow exercisers.

- Don't drop weight plates, barbells or dumbbells on the floor. We all know that you use big, heavy weights but, if they are too heavy to set down gently, don't pick them up in the first place. We are not impressed…just annoyed.

In a well-run gym, the management will warn people who break these kind of common-sense rules… once or twice…and then they will throw them out…to the delight of the rest of the members.

Or, if you prefer this kind of conduct, then join a hardcore gym where all this **is** considered acceptable behavior. I love those gyms too.

Show Some Respect!

Chapter 6

DON'T FORGET TO ACCESSORIZE

The 8 Essentials:

1. **A watch:** This is absolutely essential to the success of the **CTTC** Exercise Program. Unless there is a clock with a second hand that you can easily see from anywhere in the gym, you will need a watch with a second hand or a digital watch which shows seconds.

   The rest periods between sets in the workouts are of **monumental** importance, and estimating them is **not** good enough. Why are they so important?

   - Within ten seconds after finishing a set, the working muscle(s) recovers 50% of its initial strength.

   - In the next twenty-five seconds, it will recover an additional 30%, thereby regaining 80% of its initial strength.

   - At seventy seconds, the muscle has recovered 95% of its initial strength.

   - The last 5% of recuperation takes an **additional** 3-5 minutes. This last 5% is only important if you are training for pure strength, i.e., weightlifters and other strength athletes.

   For the purposes of this book…these extra 3-5 minutes are a complete waste of time.

   This should explain why the rest periods between sets in the **CTTC** Exercise Program are so short (mostly thirty to sixty seconds). Resting a muscle for longer than sixty to seventy seconds does not make any sense if your objective is to exhaust it with exercise. The **CTTC** rest periods that are longer than sixty seconds have more to do with your (lack of) cardiovascular conditioning than they do with muscle recovery.

2. **A pulse meter:** One of these is absolutely essential in order to be precise during aerobic exercise. If you don't know exactly what your body is doing, you cannot be in control of your results.

3. **A good lifting belt:** If you don't have a bad lower back yet, you need one of these. If you already have a bad lower back, you definitely need one of these.

   A good lifting belt is not only necessary at certain times when you are exercising with weights, but also any time you are doing heavy or awkward lifting such as moving house, rearranging the furniture, throwing your almost-too-big-for-it kids around…or any other situation which could be dangerous for your very vulnerable lower back. This is true for both men and women. Because these situations usually occur on the spur of the moment, I have belts everywhere. I have one in my workout bag; I have one at home where I can get at it immediately; and I have one in the car in case I need to change a tire or help someone push their car. My wife does the same.

There are many types of belts out there…some bad…some good…and some better. There are a couple of really important factors you need to consider when buying one.

First…the front of the belt should be only slightly narrower than the back of the belt. This will give even more support to your back by increasing the intra-abdominal pressure when your back needs it most. There is another advantage to wearing a belt like this. When you are doing certain exercises, such as squats, leg presses, bent over rowing, and overhead presses, this intra-abdominal pressure tends to push your stomach out when you apply force to the weights. Wearing a good lifting belt will prevent this by keeping you aware of your body's actions and it's positioning, i.e., by increasing your "body-awareness."

Secondly…if you are not tall, the distance between your hip bones (pelvis) and your bottom ribs is probably short. If so, you may need a belt that is cut down (narrower) on the sides and in front. Otherwise, the belt may be too wide there and cut into your pelvis and ribs. Not only is that uncomfortable, but you could even break a rib during certain movements. I also learned that one the hard way…the way I learn most things.

Other options, such as padding, choice of materials or type of closing, are up to you. I personally prefer a Velcro® closure because it is a very quick and easy method for tightening and loosening the belt. Quick and easy also means that you are much more likely to use the belt when you need it.

Note: Once you have learned to perform the exercises correctly, and your abdominals and lower back are strong enough, you should only use a lifting belt for the heavier sets in your exercise program. This will force your "core" muscles to work harder during the lighter sets, thereby making them stronger, better stabilizers. This will also further increase your "body-awareness."

4. **An elastic band:** You should use this for gently stretching (especially your shoulders) before, during, and after your workouts. With a little imagination, you can safely, effectively, and efficiently stretch every part of your body with the help of this simple, inexpensive piece of equipment. I personally use a six-foot length of surgical tubing for this purpose.

5. **Journals:** You will need to keep an accurate record of the weights you use…and your rest periods…for each of the sets…in each of the exercises. These will be different for each of the three **CTTC** Workout Programs and they will change as you get stronger and in better condition. You will need to refer back to your journal when you repeat the workouts, so keeping accurate records will save you a lot of time.

Speaking of time, you should always record that as well, so you will know if your workouts are speeding up, slowing down...or staying the same.

You should also definitely keep records of your body-weight, and whichever measurements (such as waist, hips, legs, etc.) are important to you, in another journal. This will provide you with an objective record of your progress.

Only weigh yourself once a week, always on the same day, always at the same time, always on an empty stomach, and always naked or only in your underwear.

I also very strongly suggest that you take front, back and side photos of yourself...at the beginning and end...each time you tackle the twelve-week CTTC Exercise Program. This will provide you with a subjective record of your progress and will be a source of further inspiration and positive reinforcement for you.

The photos should always be taken in the **same** place (if possible), from the exact **same** distance, with the **same** lighting, in the **same** type of clothing (two-piece bathing suit for the ladies and small shorts for the guys), and in the **same** positions, in order to provide an accurate record.

Most people don't like to take photos of themselves, especially when they are not in good shape. However, once the CTTC Exercise and Nutrition Programs change your body, you will regret not having taken "before" photos to compare the difference. Do it now so you will not regret it later.

6. **Shoes:** Good shoes are a must when you are seriously exercising.

When exercising with weights, you need sturdy shoes with relatively flat soles to give you a solid base and good balance, thereby helping to prevent turned ankles, twisted knees and other injuries. Sturdy shoes with a low, wide heel are also acceptable.

For any kind of serious cardiovascular activity, you need shoes that have been specially designed for aerobics, walking, hiking, jogging, running or whatever particular type of exercise you are doing. Believe me, the injuries and pain that good shoes will help to prevent make them well worth their price. If you are not clocking lots of miles every day, high-quality cross-trainers are a sensible and affordable choice.

7. **Clean, comfortable, non-restrictive exercise clothing** (which keeps you warm, when necessary): Anything beyond this is purely show-and-tell...but hey...as long as you enjoy it...go for broke. Have fun!

8. **A winning attitude and a willingness to work hard:** If I have to explain this one, then you need to read this book over again...from the beginning.

Three Optionals:

1. **Gloves:** I personally prefer the direct feel of the metal on my hands when I am exercising and without gloves I have to grip harder, thereby keeping my forearms strong without extra exercise. However, some people do prefer gloves. Gloves minimize calluses on your hands and enable some people to grip better, especially when they have sweaty hands. It's a personal choice.

2. **Sweat bands:** If you sweat profusely, head and wrist bands can be a big help. The wrist bands will help prevent sweat running down your arms onto your hands, which can be dangerous. They will also help to keep your wrists warm in cool gyms and cold weather.

    Headbands will help to keep hair and sweat out of your eyes while you are exercising. Being momentarily blinded or distracted during an exercise (or when running) can have catastrophic consequences.

3. **Neoprene** (rubber) **knee, elbow, and waist-bands:** If you have old, or new, injuries to these joints, certain arthritic conditions (ask your doctor first), stiff joints that are difficult to warm-up, or if you have to exercise in the cold, these bands can be an enormous help. They give minimal support, but they do increase blood flow to these areas and help to keep them warm.

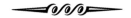

The Bottom Line

Your purpose is to exercise. Your exercise clothing should be:

First - Clean

Second - Functional

Third - Comfortable

Fourth - Fun

Fifth - Whatever turns you…or someone else on…so…go for it!

Have Fun!

Chapter 7

THE **CTTC** WORKOUTS: Scientific Fitness versus Science Fiction

Common Sense Is No Longer So Common

This is as good a place as any to put the "save my butt from lawsuits from idiots" clause so…for anyone out there who still proudly claims to be too ignorant to know that smoking cigarettes can cause lung cancer (among other things), or that regularly eating any meal which has 100 grams of fat and 2000 calories per serving could play a role in making you over-fat, or that Quality Exercise is necessary to be truly healthy…here we go.

If you really are that dumb, then you are a menace to yourself and others…and you should not be allowed to go anywhere unsupervised…or you could just stop living in denial. That might help.

DISCLAIMER:

Before actually doing, attempting to do, and possibly even thinking about doing ANYTHING recommended, not recommended, mentioned, not mentioned, or even insinuated in this book, whether of an exercise, body fat loss, nutritional, mental, emotional, or change of lifestyle nature…consult with and get the approval of the following: your doctor, mental health professional, priest, rabbi, clergyperson, local PTA, lawyer, city council, spouse, children, in-laws, distant family members, psychic, spirit guides and anyone else who would, could, or might be, in any conceivable way, negatively influenced, or offended by ANYTHING written, not written, misinterpreted or even inferred in this book. In other words:

- This book contains information and recommendations which, depending on your age, state of health (or un-health), and physical condition, could be hazardous, or even dangerous, to your health and well-being.

- Therefore, as with all exercise and/or nutrition programs, always get your doctor's approval before beginning the **CTTC** Exercise and/or Nutrition Programs.

- Anyone who uses any information in this book, for any reason whatsoever, does so at their own risk, and hereby accepts the fact that they, and they alone, assume all risks and all responsibilities for any injury or injuries, whether internal or external, physical, mental or emotional, which may befall them.

- By virtue of having read this book, the reader agrees not to initiate, or bring, any lawsuit or any other legal action whatsoever, against the author, his publicist, publisher or anyone else involved in the writing, publication, sale, or distribution of this book.

The Real Disclaimer

OK, this is what you **really** need to do…regardless of your age or your present physical condition:

- **Get a thorough physical examination**, explaining to your doctor that you are planning to begin an exercise program which is much more physically demanding than most other exercise programs. Make sure he/she understands this completely.

- **Insist that your doctor give you a maximal performance stress test.** This is necessary in order to see how your body, and especially your heart, reacts to intense physical exercise. This type of stress test can discover some existing, or potential problems which a normal physical examination may not.

- Make sure that your doctor monitors your pulse and blood pressure, both before and during your maximal performance stress test, as well as during the recovery period after your maximal performance stress test.

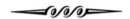

The Best Time

When is the best time to exercise? It would be best if you could exercise in the morning, for several reasons.

1. Many people's energy levels are highest then.

2. Some people even say it energizes them for the rest of the day by raising their metabolism above normal levels early in their day.

3. You will get it over with early and have the rest of the day to do other things.

4. You will have several meals left during the rest of the day to better recover from your exercise.

If you are over-fat and truly serious about losing your excess body fat as quickly as possible, then doing aerobics before you have breakfast is **essential**. If you are obese, it is absolutely **imperative**.

Second Best

The second best time to exercise is…whenever you can.

For a Great Workout

Here are eleven things that you need to remember every time you exercise with weights:

1. **Not too heavy.** Leave your ego in the locker room. Who cares how much weight you can lift? You are exercising…not weightlifting. I can't speak for you, but my muscles are illiterate. They can't read the numbers on the weights, so they don't know how much they are lifting. They only know if it feels heavy…or not…and if they are working hard…or not.

   How much you lift is not important. **How** you lift **is** important. I do some exercises for smaller muscles where I can make ten pounds feel like I am lifting fifty pounds.

2. **Not too light.** Exercising with weights that are too light to make your muscles work really hard is a complete waste of your time. Remember, if you are not breathing hard, you are not exercising.

3. **Always use good exercise technique** (exercise form). This insures that you will actually be exercising the intended muscle, or muscle group. Never use too much weight. You can't have good exercise form if all your focus is on just getting the weight to move. People cheat on exercise form to shift the work to stronger muscles and/or to include other muscle groups so they can lift more weight…usually to impress other people. Are you exercising for their benefit?

   This is fine if you want to be a weightlifter. But if your purpose is to exercise, leave your ego in the locker room and exercise with weights that you can handle with correct exercise form. This is an absolute necessity if you want the best results from your exercise program.

4. **Use a full range of motion on all exercises…unless specifically told otherwise.** This means exercising the targeted muscle from full extension to full contraction. This will give you the best results. It will also help to keep your muscles, connective tissues and joints healthy and flexible. Using a full range of motion means that you will have to use less weight than you otherwise could. This is another reason why you have to leave your ego in the locker room if you want to get the most out of your exercise program. Using partial movements will give you partial results.

5. **Use the correct exercise tempo for the CTTC Workout that you are using.** The different exercise tempos are there for very definite reasons. Do not ignore them.

6. **Concentrate while you are exercising.** Be aware of every movement you make. Feel the targeted muscles working as you go through the exercises. Each repetition is important. Block out all negative thoughts. Direct all your attention and energy to what you are doing. Don't use too much weight. You can't concentrate if all your focus is on just getting the weight to move. Through concentration, the actual physiological intensity in the working muscle(s) will be greater…using less weight…than it will be if you use a heavier weight but do not concentrate. Read that last sentence again.

7. **Don't look around, talk, or otherwise lose your focus while you are exercising.** Not only is this dangerous, but you will also be compromising your workout. I love to chat and joke in the gym, but I do it before and/or after my workout. During my workout…I am all business. If someone is talking to me and my rest period is over, I politely say, "Excuse me, but I have to do my next set now." They can continue talking to me, but I won't hear them because I will be totally concentrated on what I am doing.

8. **Visualize the goal you have for each exercise that you do.** Visualize the muscles working. See them taking on the shape you want them to have from doing each particular exercise. See your excess body fat melting away. Visualize your body as you want it to be. You cannot exercise with full intensity without using visualization.

9. **Use positive thinking.** Always think and talk about your goals positively. Remember, your emotions and state of mind cause actual physiological reactions in your body. If you believe that you can do something, you will be able to do it. If you truly believe that you will succeed, you will succeed. It is as simple as that.

   Every action begins with a thought. Positive thinking is all wrapped up with self-image, self-esteem, self-worth and self-confidence. These all work together. Building one will help build all the others. Believe in yourself and positive-think your way to success. Failure is for other people.

10. **Breathe!** Duh! But wait…this is not as dumb as it sounds. How you breathe during an exercise can make or break the exercise. It is not the same as breathing at other times. Remember…it is not **what** you do, but **how** you do it that makes all the difference. This goes for breathing too.

    I still often hear that you should breathe in through your nose and out through your mouth. If you are able to breathe this way, you are not exercising very intensely. Trying to forcefully breathe through your nose will cause your nostrils to partially close, thereby blocking the free flow of air into your lungs.

    The correct way to breathe when you are exercising intensely is to breathe in deeply, with your mouth open wide, so that there is no resistance to the air going in…and to breathe out forcefully through pursed lips. This will get the most amount of oxygen into your system, in the shortest amount of time. This type of breathing also necessitates fresh breath when you come to the gym…for obvious reasons.

    The above manner of breathing should also be used during the rest periods between sets of exercises. This will energize you and enable you to train harder and with more efficiency. It will also stimulate your metabolism and enhance the use of body fat during exercise. I will explain the exact breathing needed for each particular exercise in the chapters which describe each exercise in detail.

11. **Partners:** If you exercise with a partner and are using the same bench or exercise machine, try not to rest any longer than it takes him/her to complete his/her set. As soon as that person is finished, jump right in for your next set.

Ouch!

There are several things you can do to help prevent injuries when you exercise.

- **Always** warm up.
- Keep warm while you are exercising.
- Stretch lightly during your warm-up…more intensely between the sets of your exercises…and very thoroughly during your cool-down.
- Always use correct exercise form (exercise technique).
- Use full ranges of motion on all exercises, unless specifically told otherwise.
- Don't try to use too much weight.
- Always make sure both dumbbells are the same weight.
- Always make sure you have the same amount of weight on both sides of a barbell.
- Always make sure that the weights on barbells and dumbbells are secured in place.
- Always grasp bars, dumbbells, barbells and other equipment with your thumbs around the bar, unless specifically told otherwise.
- Always make sure that your hands are evenly spaced on barbells and other exercise bars.
- Always concentrate on what you are doing.
- Don't **over**-exercise (too much, too long, too often).
- Don't exercise if you are too tired from other things (work, being awake all night with a sick child, etc.).
- Keep a good balance of strength between opposing muscle groups.
- Practice health-building nutrition.
- Use proper nutritional supplementation.
- Start back slowly after any layoff of more than one week.

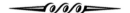

Recovery

One of the main reasons that people fail in their exercise programs is that all you ever hear them talk about is **how** they are exercising – how often, how long, which exercises, how much weight – and how exhausted they are afterwards. Nobody ever talks about **recovering from exercise,** and most exercisers do even less about it. Let me explain something here. Exercise is only a stimulus. If you do not fully recover from your last exercise session before you begin your next exercise session, you will be regressing…not progressing.

This is definitely not a good thing. Your expected results will appear very slowly…or never. Of course this is frustrating and depressing, so you will eventually give up and quit. Not a pretty picture…but it doesn't have to end this way. With a minimum amount of time and thought, you can insure that you fully recover from your exercise.

Rest

The **CTTC** Exercise Program provides you with one day of rest between workouts and two days of rest on the weekends. Under normal circumstances, this should be sufficient recovery time, especially if you are also faithfully following the **CTTC** Nutrition Program guidelines. However, there will be times when you are in no condition, either physically or mentally, to exercise. Cramming for final exams, overtime at work, being awake all night with a sick child, or simply being sick yourself, are all legitimate reasons to either cut your workout down drastically, or to drop it completely for that day…or days.

Intense exercise when you are sick, recovering from an illness, really tired or stressed out will not help you to reach your goals. It will, in fact, hold you back as well as delay your recovery from being sick, really tired, or stressed out.

Guilt

When you do have to miss one or two workouts for one of these reasons, do not attempt to make them up by exercising every day. Just begin exercising again wherever you left off and continue with the **CTTC** Exercise Program from there. Make sure that you don't try to do too much, too soon, thereby causing a relapse of the illness or fatigue. Be logical, reasonable, use common sense and learn to listen to your body.

It is OK to feel a little guilty about missing a workout. In fact, you should feel a little guilty. It shows that you care and that you are committed to your exercise program. That is a good thing. Just don't become fanatic about it. Rolling into the gym in a full-body cast the day after being in a car accident is not being committed. It is being stupid, just like exercising intensely when you are sick or exhausted. Your body doesn't need exercise then. It needs rest in order to fully recover.

Fatigue

What many exercisers don't realize is that, practically speaking, there are three basic types of fatigue. Two of these will stop your progress dead in its tracks. The first kind is the good kind. This is the local fatigue in the muscle(s) that you are exercising. Good. That is what you are attempting to do – work the targeted muscle(s) hard.

The second kind is **mental fatigue**. Students know what this is. You can only study intensely for so long before your brain starts to shut down. (My personal record is about ten minutes, which may be another reason it took me so long to graduate.) You have only been using your thinking processes, but your whole body feels tired. With some occupations you run the same risk. Mental and emotional stress can definitely put the brakes on your recovery processes.

If you can't concentrate on your workout because of mental exhaustion, you are wasting your time exercising. An obvious exception to this rule is if you are doing some type of "exercise activity" that actually reduces or gets rid of mental fatigue or stress. This is, of course, a good thing.

The third kind of fatigue is the worst kind. It is **a general fatigue of your entire system**. This is basically caused by beating your body into the ground long enough with overtraining, under-eating, having an unhealthy diet, not utilizing proper recovery techniques, mental exhaustion, stress, emotional exhaustion, illness, overwork…or a combination of these factors. When this occurs, you will have to stop doing everything that is not absolutely necessary to life itself, until your system has completely recovered. This is really a bad thing, so avoid this situation at all costs. Do everything possible to make sure that your recovery processes are working as efficiently as possible.

Back to Logic…Again

Quality Exercise is a logical process. All exercise uses muscles, so you must do the following:

1. **Stimulate the muscles** – exercise

2. **Feed the muscles** – health-building nutrition and proper supplementation

3. **Allow the muscles to fully recover between exercise sessions** – rest

Enhances Recovery Processes:

- Eating small, nutritious meals every 3-4 hours
- Drinking lots of pure, clean water
- Taking a good multi-vitamin/mineral supplement
- Extra vitamin E – when necessary (will be discussed in Chapter 12)
- Extra vitamin C – when necessary (will also be discussed in Chapter 12)
- Drinking a high-quality exercise recovery shake within thirty minutes after exercising (ditto, Chapter 12)
- Getting enough restful sleep
- Taking short naps during the day, if possible
- Having regular sport massages
- Taking saunas, steam baths, or just soaking in a hot tub, whenever possible
- Practicing some form of meditation, relaxation techniques and/or stress management

Too Much Fun

Remember that too many extra recreational or exercise activities will also cut into your recovery abilities, especially if they are of a strenuous nature. A simple way to know whether you are recovering completely from your exercise is to check your resting pulse rate (your pulse rate before you even get out of bed in the morning) for a few days in a row. If it is more than ten beats above normal for three or four days, you are probably overtraining, under-eating, not getting enough rest, stressed out, or a combination of these things. In any case, cut down or even stop all aerobics and most recreational exercise activities, and re-evaluate your nutrition while you are correcting the problem. Continue exercising with weights, if possible, but use less intensity until you are fully recovered.

Drugs...Again

What about steroids? Ah yes, back to the good old pharmaceutical solution again – relying on drugs for the quick fix (pun definitely intended) to all our problems. Hard work and self-discipline just don't fulfill most peoples' desires quickly enough anymore, do they? Instant gratification continues to be the theme of the day. And we wonder why people have so many self-esteem and self-image problems. Get off your butt and make some changes in your body that you can be proud of because you know that you made them happen through hard work and dedication, not some drug(s).

What do I think about steroids? I think successful people are successful because they are willing to do things that unsuccessful people are not willing to do.

> Successful people look for logical, practical, effective and efficient means of reaching their goals...not quick fixes!

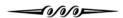

Chrome Is Pretty

You will notice that the **CTTC** Workouts revolve mostly around free weights instead of exercise machines. This is not because I am against exercise machines per se. There are some very good, well-designed exercise machines out there, but there is also a lot of pure crap on the market as well.

I forget who said it, but someone once compared exercise machines and free weights with clothing. He said that using exercise machines is like buying your clothes off the rack, while exercising with free weights is like having your clothes tailor made. This is a very good comparison.

Let's check out some of the advantages and disadvantages of both of these types of exercise, while keeping in mind that using the correct **Principles of Quality Exercise** is much more important than the choice of equipment you have.

Advantages of Free Weights	Advantages of Exercise Machines
• Free weights are more versatile.	• Machines are easier to use. ✓
• Free weights develop the secondary and small stabilizing muscles better. ✓	• With machines, you do not have to balance the weight.
• Free weights develop better overall strength. ✓	• With machines, you can change the weight by simply moving a pin.
• Free weights burn excess body fat more efficiently. ✓	• Some machines are more effective for isolating one particular muscle, or muscle group. ✓
• Free weights burn more total calories. ✓	• Some machines enable you to use a greater range of motion and a greater variety of angles, for certain exercises.
• Free weights allow you to do more work in a shorter amount of time.	• Some machines enable you to do exercises which otherwise might be too difficult, or even impossible, using free weights.
• Free weights develop balance and coordination.	• Some machines provide constant resistance, unaffected by gravity. ✓
• Free weights enable you to do many excellent exercises which are impossible to do with exercise machines.	• Machines allow you to exercise to muscular failure without the need of a spotter.
• Free weights develop better concentration and more self-discipline, self-confidence and self-esteem. They will empower you better than exercise machines can. ✓	• Machines are sometimes safer than free weights for certain rehabilitation exercises.
• You hardly ever have to wait for free weights, even in a busy gym. ✓	

Disadvantages of Free Weights	Disadvantages of Exercise Machines
• Free weights can be difficult to balance and control. • Changing weights is time-consuming, and a general pain in the you-know-what. • Some exercises (especially for the legs) can be very inefficient, or even impossible to do, with free weights. • Beginning exercisers need a competent, alert spotter. • More experienced exercisers, when exercising to muscular failure with free weights, also require competent, alert spotters.	• Some exercise machines are badly designed, or just plain dangerous. • Most exercise machines are built for average sized people. Many are not adjustable enough, making them inefficient...or downright dangerous...for shorter and taller persons. • Many exercise machines lock you into one position. If this position happens to be incorrect for **your** body, or a particular joint, it could cause an injury. • Because the weights are controlled for you, exercise machines do not develop the secondary and small stabilizing muscles very well. • Exercise machines do not develop balance and coordination. • Exercise machines do not develop concentration, self-discipline, self-confidence, and self-esteem as well as do free weights. • Many exercise machines make exercise easier because they allow you to use the minimum amount of muscle during an exercise. This reduces the total amount of actual work being done. • If the gym is busy, you will probably have to wait longer for an exercise machine than you will for free weights.

Get That Feeling

Exercisers who use only exercise machines (or very light free weights) develop no "feel" for the exercises. Because machines control the balance and guide the movement of the weights for you, you can actually do the exercises without even thinking about what you are doing, much less concentrating on what you are doing. Therefore, it is much more difficult to develop a mind-to-body connection using only exercise machines.

Because of this lack of mind-to-body connection, some exercisers who only use exercise machines (or very light free weights) cannot even tell you which muscle(s) they are supposed to be exercising (feeling). In other words, they don't know what they are doing.

Once again, **how can you possibly expect to be successful at something** (exercise in this case) **if you don't know what you are doing?** It is like trying to be successful in school without comprehending what you read. It just won't work. My four years in the sixth grade are proof of that.

Who Chooses What

A very interesting, well-designed study was done several years ago to see which personality type used exercise machines, and which type would choose to use free weights. After exercising for one month with only machines, and then one month only with free weights, the exercisers were allowed to choose whichever type of exercise they preferred. As it turns out (surprise, surprise), the passive subjects chose to exercise with machines, while the more aggressive subjects chose free weights. Interestingly, the subjects with the highest IQs chose a **combination** of free weights and machines.

Of course, this is nothing more than exercise trivia. I only included it here because I have always used a combination of free weights and exercise machines. I hope you are now suitably impressed. However, using a combination of free weights and exercise machines cannot actually raise your IQ. I am, once again, living proof of that.

The Good and the Not Too Bad

Lat machine pull-downs can never take the place of pull-ups using your own body weight, but they do offer a greater range of motion, a greater variety of angles to work the back muscles, and the possibility of using much higher reps. Pull-downs are also great for developing the strength you need to eventually be able to do pull-ups.

But I can do pull-ups anywhere there is something strong enough for me to hang from. I can, therefore, effectively exercise my biceps and back in the park, on playgrounds, in a basement...practically anywhere. If you can't do pull-ups, then you have to find a pull-down machine somewhere.

The same goes for the squat versus the leg press. The squat is, very simply, one of the best all-around exercises you can do. Nearly every muscle in your body has to work hard in order to hold the weight steady on your shoulders, balance the weight during the squats, and keep your entire body stable during the exercise. When done properly, squats will make you work and breathe really hard...making it also one of the best fat-burning exercises you can do. You can do squats with someone sitting on your shoulders, or while holding any kind of weight, or even without any extra weight.

On the other hand, leg presses offer much more versatility, as far as foot positions and angles for working your various leg muscles goes, but first you have to find a leg press machine somewhere.

As you can see, I am not against all exercise machines. The good ones play a very important role in every well-designed exercise program and they are great for adding a little variety to your workout. In fact, every so often I will exercise exclusively with exercise machines for two or three weeks, just for a change of pace. It is mentally refreshing, and my body also reacts positively to the change.

I am against most exercise machines if you are attempting to lose body fat. Why? Very simply: because you can do more total work in the same amount of time when you primarily use free weights.

It's Off to Work We Go

If a person is going do bench presses on a machine, they first sit down comfortably. Then they select the weight they want by placing the pin in the desired place. On some machines they then push a foot lever to bring the bench press handles in front of them. When they finish bench pressing, they lower the weight with the foot lever again and sit comfortably until it is time for their next set (usually about five minutes later). Not much work is going on here, except for the couple of bench presses.

However, if you do dumbbell bench presses, you first have to walk over to the dumbbell rack, pick up the dumbbells, and carry them back to the bench. Now you sit down, raise (curl) the dumbbells up to your shoulders, and slowly lay back on the bench (a slow ½ abdominal crunch with weights). Now you do the dumbbell bench press for the required number of reps, having to balance them and keep them under control during the entire exercise. Now you have to sit up again (another slow ½ abdominal crunch with weights), lower the weights, stand up, and take the dumbbells back to the rack to exchange them for a lighter or heavier pair for your next set. Then you begin the whole process all over again. Lots of work going on here and, over an entire exercise session, you would be amazed how much more energy (calories) you burn with these seemingly unimportant movements. You are using your time more efficiently again.

Why Then?

So if free weights are so much better than exercise machines, why are the gyms full of machines? There are five main reasons for this:

1. They fill up the gym, making it look professional, impressive…and really pretty.
2. Most potential customers will not join a gym if it does not have lots of shiny exercise machines.
3. Exercise machines can make exercise easier, so less motivated customers will continue to exercise…and remain paying customers longer.
4. Exercise instruction is greatly simplified, so you can instruct more customers with fewer, less motivated and less qualified staff…which some gyms still do…unfortunately.
5. The need for concentrated supervision is greatly reduced.

The Best

For your further exercise education, the following are my choices for the best machine exercises for each major body part, mostly because these exercises are too complicated, or even impossible to do with free weights, or because they add an extra dimension to an exercise which is not possible using free weights.

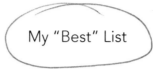

My "Best" List

Back
Cable lat machine pull-downs (various grips)
Seated cable rowing (various grips)
Horizontal back extensions (using your own bodyweight)
Smith machine bent-over-rows
Smith machine deadlifts

Chest
Pec Dek (used correctly, of course)

Shoulders
Cable upright rowing (done correctly, of course)
Lateral raises

Legs
Smith machine squats (various foot positions)
Leg press (various foot positions)
Leg extensions (various foot positions)
Leg curls (various foot positions)
Standing, seated, and leg-press calf raises (various foot positions)

Arms
Triceps cable pushdowns (various grips)
Biceps cable curls (various grips)

Not Recommended

I do not throw out any exercise, technique, equipment or method of training because they are "old fashioned" or "not in style." I disregard them only if:

- They do not work at all.

- They do not contribute significantly to reaching a specific goal.

- There is something better to take its place.

I personally do not recommend some exercises for the following reasons:

1. They may be ineffective, or even counterproductive, for a particular exercise goal.

2. They may require too much flexibility for most people to be able to do them safely and correctly.

3. They may require too much coordination for many people to be able to perform them safely and correctly.

4. They take up too much time for the results you will receive from them, i.e., they are not time efficient.

5. They make your workouts easier and longer, rather than shorter and more intense.

The Worst

The following are some of my choices for the worst exercises with both machines and free weights. By this I do not mean that any of these are inherently "bad" exercises. What I mean is that they are (many times) improperly taught, or incorrectly performed, or used by the wrong people at the wrong times, for the wrong reasons.

For instance, for a beginner/intermediate exerciser with little or no pectoral (chest) development, cable crossovers are a complete waste of time. For an advanced bodybuilder with well-developed pectorals, preparing for a competition, it can be an extremely useful exercise.

I fully realize that many of these exercises are considered standard, basic exercises in many gyms, but I have questioned this for many years and I am still convinced that some of these "basic" exercises are too difficult for many exercisers to perform safely and correctly. I say this with conviction, after having seen hundreds of people all over the world performing these exercises incorrectly, many times even under the tutelage of "certified" instructors. For some or all of the above reasons, you will not find these exercises included in this **CTTC** Exercise Program.

My "Worst" List

- All one-arm and one-legged exercises (except for one-legged calf raises)

- Deltoid front raises with a barbell or dumbbells

- Barbell presses behind the neck

- Lat machine pull-downs behind the neck

- Cable crossovers for the chest

- Adductor and abductor machines for the inner and outer thighs

- Any machine for the lower back which uses weights for extra resistance

- Any machine which uses weights to directly work your gluteus (butt) muscles

- Side-bends with or without weights

- Twisting exercises for the waist which use weights for extra resistance, or those which are done (even without extra weight) by **rapidly** twisting either your upper body or your lower body back and forth

- Leg (or knee) raises for the "lower" abdominals. First of all, a separate "lower abdominal" muscle does not exist. Second, to count all the exercisers I have ever seen who perform these exercises correctly (except for gymnasts), I would not even have to take off my shoes and socks. Hey...I graduated from the University of Iowa. Counting was a post-graduate course there.

- Any abdominal machine (or bench)...especially those that use weights for extra resistance

Hormones Again

Generally, your results will be better, and come more quickly, if you avoid machines that try to duplicate exercises which can be more effectively done with free weights, or by using your own bodyweight. Remember, hormones are the driving forces behind all reactions in your body, and compound free weight exercises will cause the greatest hormonal responses. These are large-muscle exercises such as bench presses, barbell rowing, and squats...not exercises like one arm dumbbell curls and bent over dumbbell flyes, which isolate single muscles or smaller muscle groups.

It's Not Rocket Science

The **CTTC** Exercise and Nutrition Programs correctly combine the four basic factors that are essential to **any** exercise program whose intended purpose is to build a strong, well-conditioned, shapely body, lose and/or control body fat, and increase health. These four factors are:

1. **Quality resistance exercise** using predominantly free weights to develop both functional and survival strength (explained in Chapter 15), as well as to develop shapely lean body mass (muscle), which is **essential** for keeping body fat levels under control…permanently.

2. **Quality Cardio-Aerobics** to develop functional and survival cardiovascular endurance (also explained in Chapter 15), and to **help** keep body fat levels under control…permanently.

3. **A sensible and practical eating plan** (explained in Chapter 12), which will support factors #1 and #2 above…and build health.

4. **A sensible and practical nutritional supplementation plan** (also explained in Chapter 12), which will support and enhance factors #1, #2, and #3 above.

CTTC at Work

Anyone, or any program, that claims you need none, or only some of these four essential factors to effectively, efficiently and permanently reach these health and fitness goals, is simply full of the stuff that this book is cutting through. You must have all four of them to be **optimally** successful at what you are attempting to accomplish.

RELY ON SCIENCE…NOT SCIENCE FICTION

Now let's finally get started on the **CTTC** Exercise and Nutrition Programs.

WAIT…I FORGOT THE EXERCISE PICTURES!

No, I didn't. Sorry, but there are no "begin – middle – end" exercise photographs in this book. What! You spent all that money on this crummy book and there are no exercise photos? What a rip-off. How the heck are you supposed to know how to perform the exercises without any photos to look at?

Back to School

Here's a novel idea. I'm actually going to ask you to read, study, visualize and learn how to do these exercises correctly. It has been my experience that when exercise books use photos (or drawings) to illustrate how the exercises should be done, most people give the photos a cursory glance, and then they actually believe that they know how to do the exercises correctly.

As you are about to find out, it is not quite that easy. You are also about to understand why I keep harping on "it's not **what** you do, but **how** you do it" throughout this book. **How you do it** is the difference between **successful, result-producing exercise** and just moving weights (or your body) around for a certain amount of time.

Four Factors to Success

How important is learning how to do the exercises correctly? I consider the four major factors in successful, result-producing exercise to be approximately as follows:

1. A Quality Exercise program: **40%**
2. Correct execution of the exercises: **20%**
3. Proper nutrition: **40%**
4. Nutritional supplementation: **10%**

Levels of Ambition

If you are doing none of these things correctly, you are missing out on at least 70% of your possible results. Now you know why so many people see little, or no results from all their hard work in the gym. Then there are the exercisers who are actually satisfied with 30% (or even less) results from their exercise programs. If only a 30% result is your level of ambition and you are happy with that…fine… but then you wouldn't be reading this book, would you?

If you only have a Quality Exercise program, you will be still be missing out on about 40% of your possible results. I give you 10% for execution here only because anything is better than nothing. The same goes for your nutrition. 10% for the average American diet is probably too much, but hey…I'm just a nice guy.

The same is true for proper nutrition. Without the other three factors also being in order, you can hear at least 40% of your possible results go down the drain with a big swoooosh!

With a Quality Exercise program, correct execution of the exercises (which you will learn in the following chapters), and proper nutrition (Chapter 12), you can realize 90% of your possible results. I seriously can't understand why anyone would be willing to settle for less, especially now that it is being handed to you on a silver platter…well, in this book (with no exercise pictures) anyway.

Add basic nutritional supplements to the formula (also Chapter 12), and the only way you can get better results is if you decide to become an elite athlete, which is OK too, if that is what you aspire to be.

Bad Math

OK, the intellectuals think they have caught me here, but I am fully aware that the numbers add up to 110%. That is because these four factors are synergistic, which means that each one of them increases the effectiveness of the other three. Having all four of them working together is like supercharging your body…or getting 110% out of your exercise and nutrition programs.

Cheating

I'm mind reading again. When you begin studying the **Explanation of the Exercises,** you are often going to think to yourself, "But I've never seen anyone do the exercises like this. I often see experienced exercisers with nice bodies using much looser exercise form." You are absolutely right. However, they are either naturals and would look like that no matter what they did (and don't you just hate people like that), or they have already gone through this stage of learning. I also do not use perfect exercise form all the time…most of the time, yes…but not all the time.

However, like anything worthwhile in life, you have to learn how to do something **correctly** before you can **effectively** do it incorrectly. In military school I learned that you first have to know exactly how the rules work before you can learn how to break them properly, that is, without getting into trouble…although my records will show that I was rather slow in learning this lesson too.

Patience

The same is true with exercise. With a half century of exercise experience, I have learned how to safely and effectively "bend" the rules of exercise to my advantage. However, if you attempt this without first learning the **correct** way of doing things, your results will suffer, and you will suffer…from lack of satisfactory results and inevitable injuries. Be patient. Like most good things, learning to exercise **correctly** takes time. Take it from this old dog (who can still run with the young ones): the superior (and lasting) results are more than worth it.

This is where the real work begins. Enjoy your successes!

Remember…

The decision to change something in your life does not take a week, a month, or a year.

It is made in an instant!

Chapter 8

CTTC Workout Number 1

Tempo

The tempo for most of the exercises in **CTTC Workout #1** is two seconds concentric (the active part of moving a weight, i.e., actively pulling or pushing it) and two seconds eccentric (the passive part of moving a weight, i.e., lowering the weight).

This tempo is a piston action, which means that the up and down movement of the weight should be continuous and smooth, without any stops at the top or bottom of the exercise.

In reality, you will occasionally have to pause during an exercise and take a few deep breaths before continuing. This is not only allowed, but is encouraged. If you need more oxygen during an exercise, it means that you are working hard, and that is good.

Intensity

When an exercise calls for only one set, you should use a weight that will make the last few repetitions (reps) of the exercise very difficult, but still allow the use of correct exercise form. These are usually warm-up sets for the following sets (or exercise), so the object is to increase the blood flow into that particular muscle or body-part, and to warm up the joints involved in the following sets or exercise.

When an exercise calls for more than one set, you should use a weight that will make the last repetition (rep) of each set absolutely the last rep that you can possibly do with relatively good exercise form. In other words, if the exercise calls for three sets of 15-12 reps (written: 3 x 15-12), you should use a weight on your first set that will allow you to do at least 12 or 13 reps with perfect exercise form. The next couple of reps should be very difficult to complete. Your exercise form can be a little bit looser for these couple of reps, including the last rep. The last rep (#15) should be the last rep that you can possibly do without someone helping you.

If you can do more than 15 reps, then the weight is too light, and if you cannot complete 14 reps, then the weight is too heavy. Ideally, on the first set the 15th rep should be the last one you could possibly do. On the 2nd set, it would be the 13th or 14th rep, and on the 3rd set the 12th or 13th rep should be the last one you could possibly do without someone helping you. You may have to add weight, reduce the weight, or use the same weight on each set of each exercise in order to accomplish this. Only careful experimentation on your part can tell you which of these you need to do, and when.

Of course, if you are not already an experienced exerciser, you will have to slowly build up to this level of intensity. This is partially built into the progression described in Chapter 11, **"Adapting the CTTC Workouts,"** but you will still need to apply these recommendations to your own personal situation.

Rest Periods:

The length of the rest periods between sets is **extremely** important. Have a watch with you (see Chapter 6, **"Don't Forget to Accessorize"**) and do not rest any longer than is given in the workout description. You should be breathing hard from the end of the warm-up until you are into your cool-down. Between sets, breathe as was described in Chapter 7. If you are not breathing hard enough between sets, increase the weight and/or shorten your rest periods.

The Exercises:

Do not change the order of the exercises. They are in this order for very specific reasons.

Do not substitute or alter the exercises unless it is absolutely unavoidable. They have been very carefully chosen for very specific reasons. If you do not have access to a particular piece of exercise equipment, then choose a substitute exercise that resembles the original exercise as closely as possible.

Do not add exercises, sets, or more repetitions than are called for in the **CTTC** Workouts. These have also been carefully calculated.

Do not do "forced reps." A forced rep is one where someone helps you to do another repetition when you can no longer complete the rep on your own. Forced reps are counterproductive to this exercise program.

Do not take longer rest periods than are given. In fact, when your cardiovascular fitness has improved enough for you to be able to shorten the rest periods without sacrificing strength or exercise form, please do so. However, this shortening of rest periods does not apply to the highest level of Cardio-Aerobics in **CTTC Workout #3**. Once you have reached this level, there is no advantage to be gained by shortening the "thirty seconds of medium effort" any more.

Note: Of course, once in a while it will happen that the piece of equipment that you need to use is occupied by someone else when you need it. If it is not possible to alternate with the person, then choose a substitute exercise that resembles the original exercise as closely as possible. This is preferable to having to wait too long between exercises. You have to keep your breathing and your heart rate elevated in order to enjoy the maximum benefits of the **CTTC** Exercise Program.

In order for you to get 100% out of the **CTTC** Exercise Program, you will have to follow these guidelines as closely as possible. The more you deviate from these guidelines, the less you will get out of this program. It is that simple.

CTTC Workout Number 1

Monday

CTTC **Workout #1** - 4 weeks long	**Exercise Tempo:** Piston Action, 2 seconds concentric, no pause, 2 seconds eccentric	
Monday: Back, Biceps, and Waist		
1. Warm-Up	Build up to 85% of MHR for the last minute.	10 minutes
2. Lat Machine Pull-downs to Chest - Wide Grip	45 seconds rest between sets.	3 x 15 -12
3. Bent Over Dumbbell Rowing – Elbows Out	45 seconds rest between sets.	3 x 15 -12
4. Seated Rowing - Close Parallel Grip – Elbows In	45 seconds rest between sets.	3 x 15 -12
5. Seated Incline Dumbbell Hammer Curls	30 seconds rest between sets.	3 x 15 -12
6. a- Lying Back Extensions – Bodyweight Only alternated with **b-** Crunches – Bodyweight Only	No rest between sets.	2 x 15 2 x 25
7. Cardio-Aerobics	10 intervals of 10 seconds all-out effort followed by 50 seconds of minimum effort.	10 minutes
8. Cool-Down	Moving and Stretching	10 minutes

NOTES

1st workout of the month	Time it took to complete the workout	Observations or comments about this workout
2nd workout of the month	Time it took to complete the workout	Observations or comments about this workout
3rd workout of the month	Time it took to complete the workout	Observations or comments about this workout
4th workout of the month	Time it took to complete the workout	Observations or comments about this workout

OTHER NOTES

Explanation of the Exercises

Monday

1. Warm-Up:

Do any type of movements which will increase your heart rate and increase your body temperature. Just make sure that the exercise does not use your arms (this would tire them too much for the workout which follows), and that you are able to keep control of your pulse rate. Power-walking, jogging, treadmills, elliptical walkers, steppers, bicycling and exercise bicycles (home-trainers) are all good examples. Follow the Warm-Up progression for your particular group (situation) as it is described in **CTTC Workout # 1** in Chapter 11, **"Adapting the CTTC Workouts."**

2. Lat Machine Pull-Downs to Chest – Wide Grip:

This exercise is for the large back muscles (latissimus dorsi, or lats for short), which extend from your armpits all the way down to your waist. When developed, they will make your shoulders and upper back appear wider and make your waistline appear smaller. Ah…the wonders of illusion! They will also conceal your ribs so that you don't look like a plate of uncooked spare ribs from behind.

Positioning: Grasp the bar with an overhand grip (palms of your hands facing away from you). Your hands should be wide enough so that when you have pulled the bar **halfway** down to your chest, your upper arms are parallel to the floor, forming a straight line through your shoulders, from one elbow to the other. Your forearms should then be parallel to each other and 90° to your upper arms. In other words, your arms should form a wide "u" like this: l_o_l. In case you are wondering, that is your head in the middle of the wide "u".

Hang completely stretched, also allowing your shoulders to completely extend upward (by your ears), and look forward and slightly upward. If you are doing pull-downs, sit so that your thighs are held down very securely by the pads on the machine. Your butt should not be able to rise up when you begin to pull the bar down. You should be sitting directly beneath, or slightly back from the overhead pulley. Your body should be completely relaxed at the beginning of the exercise, letting the weight stretch out your shoulders and spine.

Exercise Technique: Pull first your shoulders (by squeezing your shoulder blades down and together), and then your elbows down slowly (two seconds) until the bar touches the middle of your chest, a few inches below your collar bones.

As you begin to pull, you should continue to look forward and slightly upward. Your upper body should assume a slightly arched (curved) position as you bring your chest forward and up to meet the bar. You will automatically assume this position if you make sure to pull your shoulders and elbows back and down as you pull the bar down. As you continue to pull the bar down, you should lean back

slightly while keeping your back in the arched position. This **slight** lean-back should not be more than about 20°.

If you feel as if your shoulder blades are going to touch each other when the bar touches your chest, then you are doing the exercise correctly. If you cannot achieve this position, then you are using too much weight. Use less weight and perform the exercise correctly.

Note: Do not think of pulling with your hands. Concentrate on pulling first with your shoulders and then with your elbows. You should think of your hands as hooks whose only purpose is to hang onto the bar. Your elbows and shoulders should determine the direction and the distance of the pull.

Slowly return (two seconds) to the beginning position, following the same exercise form in reverse. Make sure that you completely straighten your arms and extend your shoulders upwards when you reach the beginning position again.

Note: If you are strong enough, substitute pull-ups for some, or all of the sets of pull-downs. The exercise technique is the same for both exercises.

Breathing: Breathe in slowly as you begin pulling your shoulders and elbows down. You should complete breathing in as the bar touches your chest. Breathe out slowly as you return to the starting position.

Do not: bring your head down, pull your elbows or your shoulders forward, round your back, let your chest sink in or bring your knees forward and up (if you are doing pull-ups). Do not forcefully lean back, or jerk your body in order to get the weights moving. If you have to do any of these things in order to get the bar to your chest, you are using too much weight. Use less weight and perform the exercise correctly. Also do not let the weight drop back to the beginning position. Keep control of the weight at all times. Remember, lowering the weight slowly is always at least half the exercise, therefore half the results.

3. Bent Over Dumbbell Rowing – Elbows Out:

This exercise is for the several smaller muscles that run from the back of one shoulder, across your upper back, to the back of the other shoulder. When developed, these muscles will fill in the valley between your shoulder blades so that they don't stick out like pygmy angels' wings. When these muscles are strong, they will pull your shoulders back and push your chest forward, thereby improving you posture and, once again, making your waistline appear smaller. We continue to build our illusion.

Positioning: Take two dumbbells of the same weight. Bend your knees slightly to take some stress off your lower back. Bend over at the waist until your upper body is parallel with the floor or **slightly** higher. Let the dumbbells hang straight down, with your knuckles facing forward. Allow your shoulders to hang down, completely relaxed, but keep your back (spine) straight. Keeping your head slightly up and looking forward (instead of down at the floor) will help to put your back in the correct position. Make sure that your lower back stays slightly arched and stable during the entire exercise.

Exercise Technique: Lift first your shoulders (by squeezing your shoulder blades together), and then your elbows, straight out to the side and up, slowly (two seconds). When you are almost at the end of the pull, and your upper arms are parallel to the floor, they should form a straight line through your shoulders, from one elbow to the other. Your forearms should then be parallel to each other and 90° to your upper arms. In other words, your arms should form a wide upside down "u". From this point, you should continue to lift (not swing) your elbows until they can go no higher.

Note: Do not think of pulling with your hands or arms. Concentrate on pulling first with your shoulders and then with your elbows. Let the dumbbells hang straight down from your elbows, and keep your knuckles facing forward. You should think of your hands as hooks whose only purpose is to hang onto the dumbbells. Your elbows and shoulders should determine the direction and the distance of the pull.

If you feel as if your shoulder blades are going to touch each other when your elbows reach their highest point, then you are doing the exercise correctly. If you cannot achieve this position, you are using too much weight. Use less weight and perform the exercise correctly.

Slowly return (two seconds) to the beginning position, following the same exercise form in reverse.

Breathing: Breathe in slowly as you begin pulling your shoulders and your elbows up. You should complete breathing in as your elbows reach their highest point. Breathe out slowly as you return to the starting position.

Do not: let your back (spine) round or let your lower back relax. Do not let your elbows drift back towards the sides of your body. Do not bounce up and down, or jerk your body in order to get the weights moving. If you have to do any of these things in order to get your elbows up high enough, you are using too much weight. Use less weight and perform the exercise correctly. Also do not let the dumbbells simply drop back to the beginning position. Keep control of the dumbbells at all times. Remember, lowering the weights slowly is always at least half the exercise, therefore half the results.

Note: To help protect your lower back, I recommend wearing your lifting belt for this exercise (see Chapter 6, **"Don't Forget to Accessorize"**).

If you still feel uncomfortable or insecure, fold up a towel and put it on the end of an adjustable exercise bench. The bench should be set at a height where, when your forehead is on the towel, your back is parallel with the floor or **slightly** higher. This will relieve most of the stress on your lower back, thereby protecting it even more.

4. Seated Rowing – Close Parallel Grip – Elbows In:

This exercise does all of the things that exercises #2 and #3 do, but in one exercise. This combination of three exercises enables you to completely work your upper back in a very short amount of time. This is why the proper combination of exercises is so important to a Quality Exercise program. Efficient use of your time! Randomly throwing a bunch of exercises together just won't get the job done.

Positioning: Sit on the Seated Rowing bench and put your feet on the foot supports. Keep your knees slightly bent to take stress off your lower back. Take the parallel grip handles and sit upright. Allow your shoulders to stretch forward, completely relaxed, but keep your back (spine) straight. Keep your head up and looking forward. Make sure that your lower back stays slightly arched and stable during the entire exercise.

Exercise Technique: Pull first your shoulders (by squeezing your shoulder blades together), and then your elbows, back slowly (two seconds) until the handles (or your hands) touch your mid-section, underneath your ribs. Keep your elbows down, close to your body, and push your chest forward and up.

As you begin to pull, you should continue to look forward. Your upper body should assume a slightly arched (curved) position as you bring your chest forward and up. You will automatically assume this position if you make sure to pull your shoulders back and down as you pull the handles towards you. As you continue pulling the handles to your mid-section, you should lean back **slightly** while keeping your back in the arched position. This **slight** lean-back should not be more than about 20°.

I personally prefer a parallel grip where the handles are wide enough apart that they touch the sides of my midsection instead of the very close ones which touch the stomach area. This way, I can move my shoulders and elbows just a little further back and it is easier to push my chest forward and up.

If you feel as if your shoulder blades are going to touch each other when your hands touch your mid-section (or sides), underneath your ribs, then you are doing the exercise correctly. If you cannot achieve this position, you are using too much weight. Use less weight and perform the exercise correctly.

Note: Do not think of pulling with your hands or arms. Concentrate on pulling first with your shoulders and then with your elbows. You should think of your hands as hooks whose only purpose is to hang onto the bar. Your elbows and shoulders should determine the direction and the distance of the pull.

Slowly return (two seconds) to the beginning position, following the same exercise form in reverse. Make sure that you completely straighten your arms and extend your shoulders forward when you reach the beginning position again.

Breathing: Breathe in slowly as you begin pulling your shoulders and your elbows back. You should complete inhaling as your shoulders and your elbows reach their furthest point behind you. Breathe out slowly as you return to the starting position.

Do not let your back (spine) round. Do not lean forward or let your lower back relax. Do not let your elbows drift up and away from the sides of your body when pulling. Do not forcefully lean back, or jerk your body in order to get the weights moving. If you have to do any of these things in order to get your shoulders and elbows back far enough, you are using too much weight. Use less weight and perform the exercise correctly. Also do not let the weights simply drop back to the beginning position. Keep control of the weights at all times. Remember, lowering the weight slowly is always at least half the exercise, therefore half the results.

Note: To help protect your lower back, I recommend wearing your lifting belt for this exercise (see Chapter 6, **"Don't Forget to Accessorize"**).

5.) Seated Incline Dumbbell Hammer Curls:

This particular exercise works not only both heads of the biceps (the muscle on the front of your upper arms), but also the smaller underlying muscles which stabilize your elbows, as well as the muscles on the top of your forearms. Are you beginning to understand why the proper selection of exercises is so important to a Quality Exercise program?

Your biceps have assisted on all three of the back exercises above, so they are already warmed up. This saves you the time you would normally have to spend on a warm-up set for your biceps. This is another example of why the correct order of exercises is also so important to a Quality Exercise program. It makes for efficient, time-saving exercise.

Positioning: Set an adjustable exercise bench to a fairly high incline (45°-60°, depending on how flexible your shoulders are). Take two dumbbells of the same weight and sit on the bench, leaning back on the 45°-60° incline. Place your feet flat on the floor, fairly wide apart. Let the dumbbells hang straight down at your sides with the thumb side of your hands facing forward (as if you were holding a hammer) and touching the front plates of the dumbbells. Keep your head in line with your body. Make sure to press your shoulders and lower back against the bench, and to push your chest forward and up.

Exercise Technique: Push your feet forcefully against the floor and tighten your midsection to stabilize your body. Curl (lift) the dumbbells straight forward and up slowly (two seconds), moving only your forearms, until your forearms cannot move any further because they have been stopped by your upper arms. The plates of the dumbbells (on your thumb side) should almost be touching the front of your shoulders at this point.

Slowly return (two seconds) to the beginning position following the same exercise form in reverse. Make sure that you begin and end this exercise with your elbows completely straight. Remember, lowering the weights slowly is always at least half the exercise, therefore half the results.

Breathing: Breathe in slowly as you begin curling the dumbbells up. You should complete inhaling as the dumbbells reach their highest point (by your shoulders). Breathe out slowly as you return to the starting position.

Do not move your upper arms or allow your forearms to rotate. Do not bounce or swing the dumbbells to get them up. Do not bring your head or shoulders forward or allow your chest to sink in. Do not allow your lower back to arch away from (lose contact with) the bench. If you need to do any of these things in order to curl the dumbbells, then you are using too much weight. Use less weight and perform the exercise correctly. Also do not let the dumbbells simply drop back to the beginning position. Keep control of the dumbbells at all times.

6.   a- Lying Back Extensions – Bodyweight Only:

This exercise develops all the muscles, large and small, on both sides of your spinal column from the back of your head all the way down to your butt. And it will keep your spine flexible too…when you perform the exercise as I describe it here. If you do this exercise correctly, you will develop a back (especially a lower back) which is stronger and healthier than 99% of the "average" people, including other exercisers who do not do this exercise correctly.

Speaking of butts, when this exercise is done correctly, it is one of the best ones around for firming up your butt, without making it bigger.

For this exercise you do need a special exercise bench. Unfortunately, many gyms are getting rid of these "old style" benches and replacing them with modern "lower back machines." I personally do not believe that the modern lower back machines are as effective as the "old" back extension benches. If your gym does not have a back extension bench then you can do this exercise on a high bench, or a sturdy table. However, then you will have to have someone hold your legs down and you will need something to cushion your feet, knees, and hips. The exercise form (technique) is the same, no matter where you do the exercise.

Positioning: Lie down on the back extension bench and hook your heels, or lower legs, under the pads. Place your pelvis on the padded part at the front of the bench. Your upper hip bones (pelvis) should be supported on the bench so that your body can only bend at the waist…not from your hips (the top of your thighs). If you bend from the hips, you will be doing a "hip extension," not a "back extension." Let your upper body hang down over the front of the bench. Put your chin on your chest with your elbows close together in front of you and your hands cupping your ears.

Exercise Technique: You have to concentrate and visualize in order to perform this exercise correctly. Don't just hang down from your waist. Curl your upper body underneath the back extension bench (or table) by contracting your stomach muscles and rounding your back as much as possible. You must visualize your spinal cord as a rope going through your vertebrae. Now visualize someone standing behind you and pulling on the rope. Concentrate on each individual vertebra, beginning with the lowest one, slowly being pulled straight…one by one. As each vertebra is pulled, your back will slowly begin to straighten out. As your lower back becomes straight, your upper back should still be rounded, with your head down and your chin still on your chest. Your upper back now begins to slowly straighten, vertebra by vertebra. The last movement is raising your head and lifting your elbows out to the side.

The finish position is with your entire back arched, your head pulled back, and your elbows behind your head (trying to touch your shoulder blades together), hands still by your ears. You should also be squeezing your buns (butt) together as hard as possible at this point.

Return to the beginning position following the same exercise form in reverse. In other words, begin by slowly lowering your elbows and head until they are in the beginning position (chin on your chest, your elbows close together in front of you, and your hands cupping your ears), and then begin slowly rounding your upper back, vertebra by vertebra, until you are in the beginning position again. That is one repetition. Only fourteen more to go! Unless you already have a very strong lower back, it will take some time to build up to fifteen repetitions. Be patient...the rewards are definitely worth it.

Note: I am sure many of you have been told not to raise your upper body past horizontal when doing this exercise. The reason given is that this will compress the discs between the vertebras in your back. This is **not** true. If you perform the exercise correctly, this is impossible. There is no weight pressing down on the spinal column, and the human body is too well designed to allow you to over-compress a spinal disc with muscle power alone. However, if you **swing** your upper body up past horizontal, you can very easily injure your back, so don't do that. Do the exercise correctly.

Exception to the Rule: Some gyms only have back extension benches which are fixed at a 45° angle, or so. This makes the exercise easier. But, on these back extension benches, you should not raise your upper body past a straight position because, at this angle, gravity (weight) is already starting to compress your discs. At this point, further contraction of your lower back muscles **will** compress the spinal discs too much. But gravity is the evildoer here, not muscle strength.

This same principle is also valid for your knees and elbows. If you straighten a leg or arm slowly and controlled, it is impossible to hyper-extend a knee or elbow. You can only do that if you straighten your leg or arm rapidly and with force (jerking), or if you bounce the weight, or if you let the weight drop uncontrolled back to the beginning position of an exercise...so don't do any of these things. Do the exercises correctly and avoid problems.

Note: As you can already see, a two seconds up, two seconds down tempo on this exercise would be too fast. Do not worry about a precise tempo here. Perform this exercise slowly and correctly.

This is the most difficult exercise in the **CTTC** Exercise Program to perform correctly, but it is also the most important exercise for a strong and healthy back. When you progress to a level where you can correctly perform 2-3 sets of fifteen reps on this exercise, you will have eliminated the vast majority of lower back problems that you might otherwise encounter in your lifetime. Why? Because then you will have built an extremely strong support system (muscles, again) on both sides, and along the entire length of your spinal column. Plus, your spine will become, and remain, much more flexible. When you stop to think that more than 80% of people have lower back problems at some time during their lives, then this is not a result to be laughed at. That is why it is so important to learn and do this exercise correctly.

Breathing: Breathe in slowly as you begin to rise up from the bottom (hanging) position. You should finish inhaling when you are at the highest position of the exercise. Breathe out slowly as you return to the starting position. You should have finished exhaling as you reach the beginning position of the exercise.

With any exercise, as the exercise progresses, you will need more and more oxygen. Whenever you feel the need for more air, pause at the beginning position of the exercise (usually where either you or the weights are hanging) and take a few deep breaths, breathing as described in Chapter 7, **"The CTTC Workouts: Scientific Fitness versus Science Fiction."** This will energize you for the next few reps.

Do not swing your arms or your head back or swing your shoulders up to create momentum. Do not pull on your head or neck with your hands or lift your head and shoulders first when performing this exercise. If you need to do any of these things in order to lift your upper body, then your lower back muscles are not yet strong enough. In that case, do only the number of repetitions that you can correctly perform on the back extension bench and then, without resting, continue with **Back Extensions on the floor** or **Reverse Leg Raises on a Table**, as described in Chapter 13, **"At Home and on the Road."**

If, in the beginning, you cannot do any repetitions correctly, then begin with **Back Extensions on the floor** or **Reverse Leg Raises on a Table**, as described in Chapter 13, and slowly progress to using the back extension bench (or table) as your back continues to become stronger.

Note: Unfortunately, this exercise is impossible to perform correctly if you have too much body-fat. If the amount of body-fat around your abdominal area is such that you cannot attain the correct beginning position for this exercise, or you have too much difficulty breathing in the beginning position of this exercise, then you should not try to include this exercise in your workout until you have lost sufficient body-fat using the rest of the **CTTC** Exercise and Nutrition Program. Until that time, substitute **Back Extensions on the floor**, as described in Chapter 13.

b- Crunches – Bodyweight Only:

Ah yes, abdominal exercises. There has never been a body-part which has caused more confusion, more frustration, been the source of more myths and fairy tales, inspired more worthless exercises and worthless exercise equipment, and wasted more time than the abdominal muscles. The abdominals have also made millions of dollars more than any other muscle by selling these myths and fairy tales to "dreamers" all over the world…decade after decade.

Just do a couple of "special" abdominal exercises for a couple of minutes, two or three times a week, and you will not only "magically" lose **all** your excess body-fat (not just the body-fat around your waist), but you will also build a tight, supple athletic body at the same time.

If you believe the before and after pictures, these "special" exercises also give you great posture, a deep tan, a new wardrobe, a better hairstyle, and (for the ladies) improve your makeup as well. I have a Dr. Phil question for you here: "How is that working for **you**?" Is the body-fat just melting off like they promised you in the commercials? How is your tan doing? Have they (whoever "they" are) sent your new clothes yet, and how do you like your new makeup and hairstyle? What? That hasn't happened yet either? Go figure!

Sorry, but if you get sucked into something this stupid, you should have "I are a idiot." tattooed on your forehead. It will save the other con artists lots of time…not that they can't already see you coming from a mile away.

Then there is the other end of the spectrum. Every time I walk into a gym, I see rows of people who need to lose 20-40 pounds or more, doing endless repetitions of "right foot behind your head, left arm crossed over your body, left foot under your right butt, right arm behind your back, reverse twisting, abdominal vibrations"…usually also with the help of some kind of exotic "apparatus" (which, I assume, will also help to provide you with that deep tan, those new clothes, the new hairstyle, etc.). Then they switch sides and do more endless repetitions.

They have obviously been taught that the more convoluted the position they can put their body in, and the more vibrations they can do, the better they can exercise their abdominals and the more excess body-fat they will lose, especially around their waists. Or maybe they are hoping for a better wardrobe or a deeper tan.

Wake up people! It is NOT that complicated. Your main abdominal muscle (rectus abdominis) only has one function, and one function only, and that is, to bring the top of your pelvis and the bottom of your ribs closer together. That's it…period. OK…I lied! It also assists in stabilizing your midsection, your "core."

And if you still believe that endless repetitions of abdominal exercises is the way to go, look up the holders of the world record for sit-ups (past and present) in *The Guinness Book of World Records*. The holder of the record up to 1985, for instance, was Allen Jones, who did more than 27,000 non-stop sit-ups. However, in spite of this fantastic feat of abdominal endurance, my abdominals are more visible than those of Mr. Jones, even though (as you will read in Chapter 11) I very rarely do **any** direct exercises for my abdominals at all.

In fact, in spite of doing tens of thousands of sit-ups a week for months on end in order to build up to the 27,000 non-stop sit-ups record, Mr. Jones could still have been described as "plump," "pudgy"… or even "overfat" for a fanatic exerciser.

After Mr. Jones, the record went up to more than 60,000 sit-ups in twenty-four hours, by Louis Scripta Jr., who would have also **not** won a Best Abdominals competition.

So if thousands of sit-ups a day are not enough to give you a "trim, fat-free waistline," then what good will 100 do…or 200…or 300? What amount will give you these results? The answer is: **No amount will.** You need a **combination** of Quality Exercise, proper nutrition, and effective aerobics.

Crunches won't elevate your metabolism (and burn body-fat); breathing squats and high-rep leg presses, heavy back and chest work, and Cardio-aerobics do that. Add a practical, logical, intelligent nutrition program and you **will** achieve a "trim, fat-free waistline."

If you perform your abdominal exercises correctly you will not need to do hundreds of repetitions of a dozen different abdominal exercises, much less thousands. In fact, only 2-3 sets of 15-25 repetitions of abdominal crunches, **done correctly**, 1-2 times per week, will provide your abdominal area with 80% of all the exercise it needs. Crunches, done as I explain them here, work both the upper and the lower abdominals.

The other 20% is covered by one other exercise, which I will explain later. Once again, it is the **quality** of the exercise that counts, **not** the quantity.

What I also see in nearly every gym is a bunch of people jerking their bodies up and down on the floor (using a movement of only a couple of inches) like they are having some sort of a mini-seizure. This is not a race. Do the exercise slowly and controlled. Concentrate on what you are doing, and feel your abdominal muscles working with each repetition. If you perform your crunches slowly and concentrated like this, I guarantee that you will not be able to do lots of repetitions. **More is not better…better is better!**

Crunches are probably the second most difficult exercise in the **CTTC** Exercise Program to perform properly, so let's learn how to do them correctly. Then we can get the **best results** with the least amount of work…and the least amount of wasted time.

Positioning: Lie on your back with your shoulders against the floor and with your legs raised so that your hips and your knees both form 90° angles. In other words, your thighs should be vertical (straight up and down) and your lower legs should be horizontal (parallel with the floor). Put your chin on your chest, squeeze a towel or other object between your knees to prevent unnecessary movement of your legs, and lay your hands on your belly (so you can feel your abdominals working). Now forcefully press the small of your back flat against the floor and raise your shoulders up until you feel your abdominal muscles begin to contract. This is the correct starting position for crunches.

Exercise Technique: Curl your upper body slowly (two seconds) towards your knees. Concentrate on lifting each vertebra, one by one, from the floor, starting with your upper back, and visualize touching your lower ribs to your pelvis. Concentrate on tilting your lower pelvis up to meet your lower ribs. Continue until your body cannot curl any further. This is the finish position of the exercise.

Slowly return (two seconds) to the beginning position, following the same exercise form in reverse.

Breathing: Breathe out forcefully as you curl your upper body up. At the finish position, you should have exhaled as much of the air in your lungs as possible. Slowly breathe in as you return to the beginning position.

Do not swing your arms, your head, your legs, or your shoulders to create momentum. Do not pull on your head or neck with your hands (they should be on your belly anyway). Do not allow your lower back to lose contact with the floor, or allow your shoulders to touch the floor when you return to the beginning position (thereby allowing your abdominal muscles to momentarily relax). Also do not allow your upper body to simply drop back to the beginning position. Keep your movements under control at all times. Remember, lowering slowly is always at least half the exercise, therefore half the results.

Note: In order to achieve satisfactory results from abdominal exercises, you first have to be able to do the exercises correctly. If you are too over-fat, it will be physically impossible for you to correctly perform abdominal exercises, so why waste a lot of time on them?

If you hold a large ball (representing your stomach) on the inside of your elbow (representing your waist) and then try to curl your arm, not much will happen. You will be able to do less than 30% of the curl because the ball will prevent your arm from bending any further. This is exactly how the body-fat inside and outside your abdominal area will prevent you from performing abdominal exercises correctly if you are too over-fat.

Not exhaling **forcefully** as you curl your upper body up will have exactly the same effect, even if you are not over-fat. The air in your lungs will act like the ball, preventing you from doing the crunches correctly.

So if you are too over-fat, don't waste your time trying to do lying crunches at this point. It will only discourage and depress you. Instead, do **Standing Crunches** (explained next). These are done standing (duh), and will provide you with a way to work your abdominals that will result in a feeling of success (instead of frustration) until you have progressed to the point where you can correctly perform lying crunches.

Note: One of the more trendy exercise fads, as I write this, is doing exercises (including crunches) on a large exercise ball. The proponents of exercise balls say that you get a better, more intense contraction when doing crunches like this…and they are absolutely right…**if** you do the crunches correctly. However, as you should be beginning to understand by now, exercising correctly is a little more complex than just mindlessly pushing a weight up, pulling it down, or indiscriminately moving your body around.

Most of the people that I have seen using these balls do the exercises incorrectly, making the exercises easier instead of more effective.

> You have to be able to do an exercise correctly before you can effectively get any "extra" benefits from adding something to the exercise.

If you want to learn how to safely and effectively use a chainsaw, you don't begin by putting on a pair of roller skates. Well, you can, but you are going to wind up missing a few body parts before you are finished and, when you are finished, you will still not be able to use a chainsaw properly.

If you can't do crunches correctly on the floor, why do you think doing them on an unstable ball is going to be a better solution? Learn the basic exercise correctly before you experiment with different variations.

Note to all exercisers: Some exercises for other body parts will also cause your abdominal muscles to contract in order to stabilize your midsection. Consciously contract your abdominals during these exercises. It will help to strengthen your abdominals every time you do, which means…less time you need to spend doing boring abdominal exercises.

c- Standing Crunches:

Positioning: Stand straight, with your knees slightly bent. Place your hands on a table, bench, or other stable object that is approximately waist high. Now you follow the same directions as for normal crunches.

Exercise Technique: You must concentrate on slowly (two seconds) tilting the bottom of your pelvis forward and up as you pull the bottom of your rib cage down. Both movements should be done by consciously contracting your abdominal muscles. Concentrate! Pressing down on the table with your hands, and compressing the body-fat inside your abdominal area will give your abdominal muscles all the resistance they need until you have lost enough excess body-fat to enable you to do lying crunches correctly.

Slowly return (two seconds) to the beginning position, following the same exercise form in reverse.

Breathing: Breathe out forcefully as you curl your upper body down and tilt the bottom of your pelvis forward and up. At the finish position, you should have exhaled as much of the air in your lungs as possible.

Slowly (two seconds) breathe in as you return to the beginning position.

Note: You can turn **Standing Crunches** into a more effective exercise by not only maximally contracting your abdominal muscles as you forcefully exhale but, at the same time, also maximally contracting **all** the muscles in your body.

7. Cardio-Aerobics:

You should still be breathing hard and your heart rate should still be elevated from doing the Back Extensions and Crunches. Therefore, you should begin your Cardio-aerobics immediately after completing these. Follow the Cardio-aerobics progression for your particular group (situation) as it is described in **CTTC Workout # 1** in Chapter 11, **"Adapting the CTTC Workouts."**

Your choice of exercises is limited by the fact that Cardio-aerobics requires that you be able to change resistance very quickly, from one that requires an all-out effort, to one than requires a minimum-to-medium effort on your part. Not all machines are able to do this quickly enough, so you will be limited to whichever machines are available to you that also meet this requirement. Exercise bicycles and treadmills are usually the best choices, depending on how quickly you can change the resistance on them. Sprints on an indoor or outdoor track are even better, providing you have access to either of these, of course. A level field, or a quiet street, is also a possibility.

When weather permits, outdoor Cardio-aerobics definitely gets my vote. Alternating sprinting with jogging/walking, or all-out bicycling with lower intensity bicycling is a great way to go. You are outside in the fresh air (hopefully) and sunshine (hopefully), which will make the time you spend exercising go by even more quickly…always a good thing, in my opinion.

Your choice of exercises may also be limited by old injuries, problems with your joints, or some other factor.

Do not jump into this intense form of aerobics if you are not physically prepared for it, nor should you abruptly terminate a Cardio-aerobics session without slowly tapering off.

8. Cool-Down:

Continue the exercise you used for your Cardio-aerobics for a couple of minutes longer at a lower intensity. This is the first part of your cool-down and allows your heart to slowly and safely return to a lower pulse rate. Then walk around easily, continuing to breathe deeply, as described in Chapter 7.

During this time, you should also use your elastic band (see Chapter 6, "Don't Forget to Accessorize") to continually stretch your chest, arms, and shoulders. Next, occasionally stop to stretch your legs and your spine.

After your heart rate has returned to a more normal level, you can lie down or sit on the floor to more effectively stretch your legs and lower back. After you have finished doing this, stand up and thoroughly stretch your shoulders and calves one more time.

I will not go into detail about stretching, because that would be another book. You will need to find a system of stretching which suits you personally. I will only say that the most flexible I ever became (and I am not naturally flexible) was when I was using **Hatha Yoga** techniques to develop maximal flexibility for gymnastics. Yoga is also extremely beneficial to your mental, emotional, and spiritual well-being, and is a great stress-buster to boot. Give it a try. I know you will like it. Do not shorten your cool-down or omit it altogether. Do not stand still, sit, or lie down immediately after completing a Cardio-aerobics session. Always taper off slowly.

CTTC Workout Number 1

Wednesday

CTTC **Workout #1** - 4 weeks long	**Exercise Tempo:** Piston Action, 2 seconds concentric, no pause, 2 seconds eccentric	
Wednesday: Legs		
1. Warm-Up	Build up to 85% of MHR for the last minute.	10 minutes
2. Leg Extensions	Warm-Up	1 x 25
3. Leg Curls – Seated or Lying	Warm-Up	1 x 20
4. Smith Machine Barbell Squats	1½ minutes rest between sets.	3 x 20
5. Leg Curls – Seated or Lying	30 seconds rest between sets.	2 x 15 -12
6. Leg Extensions	30 seconds rest between sets.	2 x 20 -15
7. Cardio-Aerobics	10 intervals of 10 seconds all-out effort followed by 50 seconds of minimum effort.	10 minutes
8. Standing Calf Raises – Bodyweight Only	30 seconds rest between sets.	1 set each of 30, 25, & 20 reps
9. Cool-Down	Moving and Stretching	10 minutes

NOTES

1st workout of the month	Time it took to complete the workout	Observations or comments about this workout
2nd workout of the month	Time it took to complete the workout	Observations or comments about this workout
3rd workout of the month	Time it took to complete the workout	Observations or comments about this workout
4th workout of the month	Time it took to complete the workout	Observations or comments about this workout

OTHER NOTES

Explanation of the Exercises

Wednesday

1. Warm-Up: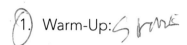

Do any type of movements which will increase your heart rate and increase your body temperature. Just make sure that the exercise does not use your arms (this would tire them too much for the workout which follows), and that you are able to keep control of your pulse rate. Power-walking, jogging, treadmills, elliptical walkers, steppers, bicycling, and exercise bicycles (home-trainers) are all good examples. Follow the Warm-Up progression for your particular group (situation) as it is described in **CTTC Workout # 1** in Chapter 11, **"Adapting the CTTC Workouts."**

2. Leg Extensions:

This exercise is one of the best for firming up the muscles on the front of your thighs (quadriceps, or quads). It is also one of the best exercises for keeping your knees strong and healthy.

Ladies: This is a great exercise for creating firm and beautifully shaped legs.

Positioning: Sit on the Leg Extension machine so that the backs of your knees are not being pinched by the front edge of the seat when your legs are in the beginning position for the exercise, i.e., lower legs hanging down. Your knees should be in a direct line with the pivot point of the Leg Extension machine, not in front of it or behind it. Now adjust the foot pad (if possible) so that the pad rests comfortably on the front of your ankles when your feet (toes) are pulled up towards your shins. Do not point your toes.

Note: If you have good knees, you can begin the exercise with slightly less than a 90° angle in your knees (where your knees are bent more than halfway). Even so, I do not recommend having less than a 90° angle in your knees if you ever use heavier weights for lower repetitions on this exercise.

If you have knee problems, I recommend performing this exercise with less than a 90° angle in your knees only if you are exercising with **very light** weights in order to maintain a good range of motion in your knee joints, or as a warm-up. Otherwise, you should only use less than a 90° angle in your knees under supervision of a qualified instructor or health professional.

Exercise Technique: Tighten your abdominals, press your butt down onto the seat, and slowly extend (two seconds) your lower legs until your knees are completely locked out straight. If you cannot achieve this position, you are using too much weight. Use less weight and perform the exercise correctly.

Slowly return (two seconds) to the beginning position, following the same exercise form in reverse. Remember, lowering the weight slowly is always at least half the exercise, therefore half the results.

Note: I personally prefer to change my leg positions (wide, medium, or legs together) with each set. However, never use a position that causes pain in your knees. The leg positions should always feel fairly natural, never forced.

Breathing: Breathe in slowly as you extend your legs. Breathe out slowly as you lower your legs.

Do not kick, jerk, bounce, or swing your legs to start them moving. If you need to do any of these things to extend your lower legs, you are using too much weight. Use less weight and perform the exercise correctly. Also do not allow your legs to simply drop back to the beginning position. Keep your movements under control at all times.

3. Leg Curls – Seated or Lying:

This exercise is one of the best for firming up the muscles on the back of your thighs (leg biceps, or hamstrings). It is also another one of the best exercises for keeping your knees strong and healthy.

Ladies: This is another great exercise for creating firm and beautifully shaped legs.

Positioning: Sit or lie down on the Leg Curl machine. Hook your heels under the foot pad after adjusting it so that the foot pad fits comfortably on the back of your lower legs, just above your heels. Your knees should be in a direct line with the pivot point of the Leg Curl machine, not in front of it or behind it. Pull your feet (toes) up towards your shins. In other words, do not point your toes.

Exercise Technique: From a position where your knees are completely straight, slowly curl (two seconds) your lower legs down if you are sitting, or up if you are lying down. Curl your legs until your knees cannot bend any further. If you cannot achieve this position, you are using too much weight. Use less weight and perform the exercise correctly.

Slowly return (two seconds) to the beginning position, following the same exercise form in reverse.

Note: Here I also personally prefer to change my leg positions (wide, medium, or legs together) with each set. However, never use a position that causes pain in your knees. The leg positions should always feel fairly natural, never forced.

Breathing: Breathe in slowly as you curl your legs. Breathe out slowly as you straighten your legs.

Do not kick, jerk, bounce, or swing your legs to start them moving. If you need to do any of these things to curl your legs, you are using too much weight. Use less weight and perform the exercise correctly. Also do not allow your legs to simply drop back to the beginning position. Keep your movements under control at all times. Remember, lowering the weight slowly is always at least half the exercise, therefore half the results.

Note to the ladies: Shapely, well-developed leg biceps (hamstrings) will make your butt appear smaller. Then you will be able to ask your boyfriend/husband, "Honey, do these hamstrings make my butt look big?" and he will finally be able to answer honestly, "No dear." Results: Gorgeous leg biceps and a smaller looking butt for you, and he can give an honest answer that won't land him in the doghouse. Another relationship is saved, thanks to exercise. It's enough to bring tears to your eyes, isn't it?

4. Smith Machine Barbell Squats:

A "Smith Machine" (see Chapter 14, **"At Home and on the Road"**) is an ominous looking piece of apparatus which used to be found only in hardcore bodybuilding gyms. Now they not only turn up in better-equipped fitness clubs, but even in home gyms. Why? Because they are so darned versatile, that's why. A Smith Machine makes certain "impossible" exercises possible. It also allows you to **safely** perform free weight exercises (breathing squats in this case) without having to have a training partner. It is a terrific piece of equipment…when used properly.

The **"breathing squat"** is, without a doubt, one of the very best all-around exercises you can do. It strengthens, firms, and shapes your quadriceps, your leg biceps, and your butt (gluteus maximus, or glutes). Done **properly**, it strengthens and keeps your knees healthy. It strengthens your back from the bottom of your neck all the way down to your butt, and it will help to strengthen your abdominals as well. It is the best exercise to safely build dense, healthy bone mass and prevent osteoporosis (loss of bone mass), especially of the spine. It is one of the best, most efficient exercises for elevating your metabolism and, therefore, one of the best exercises to increase the burning of body-fat. How many more reasons do you have to hear before you accept the fact that you definitely need to do this exercise?

Positioning: Place your hands on the barbell, a little wider than shoulder width apart. Step under the barbell and place it behind your head, high up on your shoulders. Keep your shoulders pulled back (by squeezing your shoulder blades together) and your elbows pointed down. Your back should be straight and remain so during the entire exercise. Look forward and **slightly** upward during the entire exercise. Place your feet approximately shoulder width apart, or **slightly** wider, and turned out at a natural angle (whatever that is for you). Your stance should feel natural and comfortable.

Thanks to the Smith Machine, you are able to place your feet **slightly** in front of the barbell. This will take much of the stress off of your lower back when doing squats because it eliminates the need to lean forward to balance the weight as you squat down. This also places more emphasis on your frontal thighs and less on your glutes…which is a good thing unless you are actually trying to build a bigger butt. This particular way of squatting will actually make your hips appear more slender. We are creating more illusion. This is good.

This "feet forward" position takes some stress off the knees and also does not require the ankle and hamstring flexibility that normal free-weight squats do. If you are doing free-weight squats, you may need to put your heels on a one-inch thick board or other stable object. This also makes balancing during the exercise much easier.

Exercise Technique: Grasp the bar tightly with your hands. Contract your abdominals and your back muscles, as well as all the other muscles in your body. Now begin slowly descending (two seconds) to a position where the tops of your upper legs (thighs) are parallel, or **slightly** under parallel, to the floor. Your knees should move slightly forward, but remain in a line directly over your feet. Do not allow them to move to the outside or to the inside during the exercise. Keep your hips and butt under your upper body during the exercise (don't stick them out behind you), especially when you are rising out of the squat.

Slowly return (two seconds) to the beginning position, following the same exercise form in reverse, but do not straighten your knees completely when you reach the beginning position again. Keep constant tension on your thighs throughout the entire set.

Concentrate on pushing evenly with your feet (not just with your heels or the balls of your feet), and keeping your hips and butt under your upper body. Feel the muscles on the front of your thighs working hard. Pushing on the barbell with your hands (as if you were trying to press it up) will take some pressure of the bar off your shoulders and will also help you to contract all the muscles in your back (thereby helping to keep it straight), especially as you ascend out of the parallel squat position.

Note: The intensity on this exercise is a little different than for the others. Due to the safety factor, we do not want to "make the last repetition (rep) of each set absolutely the last rep that you can possibly do." With breathing squats, the last repetition should be done with the same perfect exercise form as you used on the first few repetitions. The purpose of this exercise is to develop firm, strong, shapely legs…not massive, muscular legs. It is also designed to elevate your metabolism, improve your cardiovascular condition, and to increase your body's ability to use body-fat…and all that from one exercise. That is efficient exercising. The emphasis should be on working the leg muscles hard, and breathing hard…not on crushing yourself under a massive amount of weight.

Breathing: Breathe in slowly as you descend to the parallel squat position. Hold your breath as you begin to ascend out of the parallel position. After you begin moving upward (about halfway), begin breathing out forcefully.

One problem involved with holding your breath while exerting force is that it momentarily raises blood pressure. However, this is only a concern if you already have a serious problem with your blood pressure and, as I have repeatedly said, this book is written for exercisers who do not have special medical problems. However, if you do have high blood pressure, do not hold your breath.

Doing twenty reps per set on this exercise will necessitate your having to pause at the completion of some of the reps to take a couple of extra deep breaths. This is good. The last several repetitions of a set may even require that you take several deep breaths after every rep. Good. Take all the deep breaths you need to finish twenty reps. This is Quality Exercise, not a race.

For instance, you could do the first five reps by taking one deep breath between each repetition. From rep #5 to rep #10, take two deep breaths between each repetition. From rep #10 to rep #15, take three deep breaths, and from rep #15 to rep #20, you may have to take as many as four deep breaths between each repetition. I know this is hard work, which is why you don't see many people doing breathing squats, but believe me, the results are more than worth it.

Do not look down, round your upper or your lower back, bend forward, or let your shoulders move forward. Also do not allow your knees to move outward or inward as you squat. Keep them in a line directly over your feet. Do not move your butt and hips back as you push with you legs to come out of the parallel position. If you need to do any of these things to rise up, you are using too much weight. Use less weight and perform the exercise correctly. Absolutely do not drop quickly into the squat position. Keep your movements under control at all times.

Note: To help protect your lower back, I recommend wearing your lifting belt for this exercise (see Chapter 6, **"Don't Forget to Accessorize"**).

Note: You should be starting to realize by now why gyms have mirrors. It is not easy to remember all these things, visualize them, concentrate on them, and then actually do them. Your gym should have mirrors, so use them. If you train at home and don't have mirrors…get some!

5. Leg Curls **– seated or lying:** (same as in exercise #3 above)

6. Leg Extensions: (same as in exercise #2 above)

7. Cardio-Aerobics:

You should still be breathing hard and your heart rate should still be elevated from doing this leg workout. Therefore, you should begin your Cardio-aerobics immediately after completing your last set of Leg Extensions. Follow the Cardio-aerobics progression for your particular group (situation) as it is described in **CTTC Workout # 1** in Chapter 11, **"Adapting the CTTC Workouts"**.

Continue the exercise you used for your Cardio-aerobics for a couple of minutes longer at a lower intensity. This is the first part of your cool down and allows your heart to slowly and safely return to a lower pulse rate.

Do not jump into this intense form of aerobics if you are not physically prepared for it, nor should you abruptly terminate a Cardio-aerobics session without slowly tapering off.

8. Standing Calf Raises – Bodyweight Only:

This exercise will develop the muscles on the back of your lower legs (gastrocnemius, or calves). It is one of the best exercises for building, shaping, and delineating your calves.

Guys: This exercise makes the difference between looking great in shorts or having people go "cluck, cluck" and throw bird seed at you as you walk by.

Ladies: This exercise is the key to gorgeous, shapely, sexy calves…especially in high heels! It sure beats having your legs look like two toothpicks stuck in the floor.

Positioning: Stand with the balls of your feet on a step or other stable, raised surface. Your heels should be free, hanging over the step, and your knees should be locked out (straight). Your feet should be approximately shoulder width apart, with your toes pointing slightly out at a natural angle (whatever that is for you). Your stance should feel natural and comfortable.

Exercise Technique: Lower your heels slowly (two seconds) as far as possible, making sure that you get a maximum stretch in your calves at the bottom of the movement. Then slowly (two seconds) rise up on the balls of your feet, as high as possible. Keep your knees straight and keep your weight on the big toe side of the balls of your feet, so that your ankles stay in straight lines with your legs.

Note: If you are not wearing very supple shoes, then do this exercise wearing only your (clean) socks…and the rest of your exercise clothing, of course. Wearing only your socks would definitely distract the other people in the gym. If you are exercising at home…no problem…unless it scares your pets.

Seriously, if your shoes are too stiff, you will not be able to stretch or contract your calves maximally, thereby losing much of the effectiveness of this exercise.

Breathing: Breathe in slowly as you rise up on the balls of your feet, and breathe out slowly as you lower your heels.

Do not let your ankles turn out by letting your weight shift over to the little toe side of the balls of your feet. Do not bend your knees. Do not jerk, bounce, or allow your heels to simply drop into the stretch position. Keep your movements under control at all times.

Note: You should make a habit of stretching your calves at different times during the day, every day, for a minute or so each time. This will not only insure that your ankles and Achilles tendons become, and remain, flexible but will also assure you of beautifully shaped calves. This is especially important for women who spend a lot of time in high heels!

Flexible ankles and Achilles tendons will improve your posture (when you are not wearing high heels), thereby taking strain off your lower back. Taking strain off your lower back will save you an enormous amount of energy during the day, in addition to improving the health of your lower back. Anyone who spends a lot of time on their feet will appreciate what I am saying here.

Later, after you have gone through the **CTTC** Exercise Program at least once (without any adaptations), you may want, or need, to do this exercise on a **Standing Calf Raise Machine**, using extra weight. Please…be my guest. The Positioning and the Exercise Technique are exactly the same as for this calf exercise.

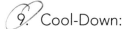 **9.** Cool-Down:

Walk around easily and continue to breathe deeply, as described in Chapter 7, **"The CTTC Workouts: Scientific Fitness versus Science Fiction."** Occasionally stop to stretch your legs, your spine, and your calves.

After your heart rate has returned to a more normal level, you can lie down or sit on the floor to more effectively stretch your legs and lower back. After you have finished doing this, stand up and thoroughly stretch your calves one more time.

Do not shorten your cool-down or omit it altogether. Do not stand still, sit, or lie down immediately after completing a Cardio-aerobics session. Always taper off slowly.

CTTC Workout Number 1

Friday

CTTC **Workout #1** - 4 weeks long	**Exercise Tempo:** Piston Action, 2 seconds concentric, no pause, 2 seconds eccentric	
Friday: Chest, Triceps, and Shoulders		
1. Warm-Up	Build up to 85% of MHR for the last minute.	10 minutes
2. 45°- 60° Incline Dumbbell Bench Press – Palms Facing – Elbows Out	45 seconds rest between sets.	3 x 15 -12
3. Flat Dumbbell Bench Press – Palms Facing – Elbows Out	45 seconds rest between sets.	3 x 15 -12
4. Cable Triceps Pushdowns - Parallel Grip – With Rope	30 seconds rest between sets	3 x 15 -12
5. Dumbbell Lateral Raises	30 seconds rest between sets.	3 x 15 -12
6. Seated Twisting Dumbbell Presses	30 seconds rest between sets.	2 x 15 -12
7. Cardio-Aerobics	10 intervals of 10 seconds all-out effort followed by 50 seconds of minimum effort.	10 minutes
8. Cool-Down	Moving and Stretching	10 minutes

NOTES

1st workout of the month	Time it took to complete the workout	Observations or comments about this workout
2nd workout of the month	Time it took to complete the workout	Observations or comments about this workout
3rd workout of the month	Time it took to complete the workout	Observations or comments about this workout
4th workout of the month	Time it took to complete the workout	Observations or comments about this workout

OTHER NOTES

Explanation of the Exercises

Friday

1. Warm-Up:

Do any type of movements which will increase your heart rate and increase your body temperature. Just make sure that the exercise does not use your arms (this would tire them too much for the workout which follows), and that you are able to keep control of your pulse rate. Power-walking, jogging, treadmills, elliptical walkers, steppers, bicycling, and exercise bicycles (home-trainers) are all good examples. Follow the Warm-Up progression for your particular group (situation) as it is described in **CTTC Workout # 1** in Chapter 11, **"Adapting the CTTC Workouts."**

2. 45°- 60° Incline Dumbbell Bench Press – Palms Facing – Elbows Out:

This exercise emphasizes the development of the upper portion of your chest muscles (pectoralis major, or pecs). It will fill in the area just underneath your collarbones, thereby giving your chest a higher, fuller look. This exercise will also make your shoulders appear wider and make your waist appear smaller.

Positioning: Set an adjustable exercise bench to approximately a 45°-60° incline. Take two dumbbells of the same weight and sit on the bench. Lift the dumbbells to your shoulders and lean back on the 45°-60° incline. Hold the dumbbells with the palms of your hands facing each other and your elbows pointing down and out, away from your body. Place your feet flat on the floor, fairly wide apart. Keep your head in line with your body. Make sure to press your lower back and shoulders against the bench, and to push your chest forward and up.

Note: I vary the incline every time I do incline chest exercises. Sometimes I even use a different incline for each set that I do in my chest workout.

Exercise Technique: Push your feet forcefully against the floor and tighten your midsection to stabilize your body. Press the dumbbells slowly up (two seconds) so that when they are at the **halfway point** your upper arms are parallel to the floor, forming a straight line through your shoulders, from one elbow to the other, with the palms of your hands still facing each other. Your forearms should then be parallel to each other and 90° to your upper arms. In other words, your arms should form a wide "u" like this: l_o_l.

Continue pressing them up until your arms are completely straight and your shoulders are extended up and off of the bench as far as they will go. At this point, the dumbbells should be touching each other above your chest, and your chest muscles should remain contracted (tensed).

Slowly return (two seconds) to the beginning position following the same exercise form in reverse.

Breathing: Hold your breath as you press the dumbbells up. Breathe out forcefully as the dumbbells begin to reach their highest position. Breathe in slowly as you lower the dumbbells. You should finish inhaling as your elbows reach their lowest position.

Note: Many instructors will tell you to exhale as you press the dumbbells up. I don't agree with this because the chest muscles attach to the rib cage, which moves when you breathe. If you exhale as you press up, your rib cage will no longer provide a stable base for your chest muscles to pull against. The less stable the base, the less force you will be able to exert.

For example, stand facing a wall and push against it. What happens? You can't exert any force because you do not have a stable base (your body) to push from. It moves while you are trying to push. Now have someone stand behind you and stabilize your back as you push against the wall. You can use much more force now, can't you?

One problem involved with holding your breath while exerting force is that it momentarily raises blood pressure. If you do have high blood pressure, do not hold your breath.

Do not bring your head forward. Do not allow your lower back to arch away from (lose contact with) the bench. Do not let your hands rotate or let your elbows move forward. Do not jerk or bounce the weights at the bottom of the exercise to start the pressing action. If you need to do any of these things in order to press the dumbbells up, you are using too much weight. Use less weight and perform the exercise correctly. Also do not let the dumbbells simply drop down to the bent arm position. Keep the dumbbells under control at all times.

3. Flat Dumbbell Bench Press – Palms Facing – Elbows Out:

This exercise develops the entire pectoralis major (chest muscle). It will make your entire chest and your shoulders appear fuller and wider, thereby helping to make your waist appear smaller.

Positioning: Take two dumbbells of the same weight and sit on a flat exercise bench. Lift the dumbbells to your shoulders and slowly lie back on the bench. Hold the dumbbells with the palms of your hands facing each other and your elbows pointing down and out, away from your body. Place your feet flat on the floor, fairly wide apart. Keep your head in line with your body. Make sure to press your lower back and shoulders against the bench, and to push your chest up.

Exercise Technique: Push your feet forcefully against the floor and tighten your midsection to stabilize your body. Press the dumbbells slowly up (two seconds) so that when they are at the **halfway point** your upper arms are parallel to the floor, forming a straight line through your shoulders, from one elbow to the other. Your forearms should then be parallel to each other and 90° to your upper arms. In other words, your arms should form a wide "u" like this: l_o_l.

Continue pressing them up until your arms are completely straight and your shoulders are extended up and off of the bench as far as they will go. At this point, the dumbbells should be touching each other above your chest, and your chest muscles should remain contracted (tensed).

Slowly return (two seconds) to the beginning position following the same exercise form in reverse.

Breathing: Hold your breath as you press the dumbbells up. Breathe out forcefully just as the dumbbells reach their highest position. Breathe in slowly as you lower the dumbbells. You should finish inhaling as your elbows reach their lowest position.

Do not lift your head or allow your lower back to arch away from (lose contact with) the bench. Do not let your hands rotate or your elbows move forward. Do not jerk or bounce the weights at the bottom of the exercise to start the pressing action. If you need to do any of these things in order to press the dumbbells up, you are using too much weight. Use less weight and perform the exercise correctly. Also do not let the dumbbells simply drop down to the bent arm position. Keep the dumbbells under control at all times.

4. Cable Triceps Pushdowns - Parallel Grip – With Rope:

This exercise works all three heads of the triceps (the muscle on the back of your upper arms).

Ladies: This is the best exercise to firm up that part of your arm which may wave more than your hand does.

Your triceps have assisted on both of the chest exercises above, so they are already warmed up. This saves you the time you would normally have to spend on a warm-up set for your triceps. Proper order of exercises...again.

Triceps Pushdowns are done on an overhead cable machine, like the one you used for Lat Machine Pull- Downs to Chest. However, this time you will use a rope attachment instead of a metal bar. The triceps pushdown rope attachment is simply a thick rope which hangs from its middle and has large knots...or something else...on the ends to keep your hands from slipping off as you push down.

Positioning: Stand about a foot back from where the overhead cable hangs straight down and take hold of the rope attachment with the thumb sides of your hands pointing up. Pull your upper arms down until your elbows are just in front, but still touching your body. Bend your knees slightly and bend **slightly** forward at the waist. Keep looking straight ahead. Now tighten your entire body to lock it in this position. Your elbows should now be completely bent, hands by your upper chest and almost touching each other. From this position, only your lower arms should move.

Exercise Technique: Squeeze the rope hard and slowly push down (two seconds) with your hands. Make sure that your upper arms do not move. As you continue to push down, your hands will naturally begin to drift away from each other. When your elbows are almost straight, begin to rotate your hands forcefully inward (palms down), and let your hands move further away from each other. When your elbows are completely locked, your hands should be **slightly** more than shoulder width apart, with palms turned down, as if you were holding a straight bar instead of a rope. Concentrate on forcefully contracting (flexing) your triceps (the muscles on the back of your upper arms) extra hard at this point.

Note: At the very end of the pushdown (as you rotate your hands inward) your upper arms will automatically begin to also rotate inward. This is a natural movement, so allow it to happen. This will result in a harder contraction of your triceps, so it is a good thing.

Slowly return (two seconds) to the beginning position following the same exercise form in reverse.

Breathing: Exhale slowly as you push the rope down. You should finish exhaling as your elbows straighten completely. Inhale slowly as you return to the beginning position.

You will notice that as you exhale, your abdominals will also begin to contract strongly. Therefore, consciously tighten your abdominals as much as possible during this exercise. It's like getting a free set of crunches as a bonus, which means…less time you need to spend doing boring abdominal exercises.

Do not let your upper arms, upper body, or head move during the exercise. Do not jerk or bounce the weight to start the pushing action. If you need to do any of these things in order to push the rope down, you are using too much weight. Use less weight and perform the exercise correctly. Also do not let the weight simply drop back to the beginning position. Keep the weight under control at all times. Remember, lowering the weight slowly is always at least half the exercise, therefore half the results.

Note: Instead of a rope, I personally use a towel looped through a handgrip (handle) for this exercise. Since the towel has no knots to prevent my hands from slipping, I have to grip the towel really hard. This way my forearms also get a good workout, thereby saving me the time I would otherwise have to spend specifically exercising them. As you know by now, I am all for saving time when exercising, especially when it also **increases** my results.

5. Dumbbell Lateral Raises:

This exercise will develop the side section of the deltoids (the muscle on the side of your shoulders). This will make your shoulders wider, which will make your waist appear smaller. Round, fully developed deltoids give your shoulders a beautiful shape. Lateral Raises also help to develop the muscles of your upper back to some degree.

Note: The deltoid muscle has three different sections: front, side, and back. The front section is worked enough with all types of pressing movements. The back section is worked enough with all types of exercises that you do for your back…**if** you do the back exercises correctly. This means that we only have to do specific exercises for the middle (side) section of the deltoids. Efficient exercise …that's what we want.

Ladies: Shapely, round deltoids are a must when you wear sleeveless tops or strapless dresses, not to mention a bathing suit.

Guys: Deltoids are one of the most important muscles for that wide-shoulder, narrow-waist look, whether you are wearing normal clothes or a bathing suit. This exercise will also prevent that embarrassing situation where people try to hang their hats and coats on your bony shoulders.

Positioning: Select two dumbbells of the same weight. Stand with your feet approximately shoulder width apart and knees slightly bent. Lean your upper body **slightly** forward and let the dumbbells hang in front of your thighs, with the palms of your hands facing each other and your elbows slightly bent. Push your butt back a little and arch your lower back. Contract your abdominal, leg, butt, and back muscles to stabilize your body in this position. Look straight ahead. Yes, I know …this position looks really stupid…but it works!

Exercise Technique: Lift both arms slowly sideways (two seconds) until your upper arms are parallel with the floor, forming a straight line through your shoulders, from one elbow to the other. Your elbows should remain **slightly** bent throughout the exercise. This will place the dumbbells out to the side and **slightly** in front of your shoulders when they are at the highest point of the exercise (shoulder height). Allow your shoulders to rotate forward **slightly** as you lift your arms so that the dumbbells remain parallel to the floor at all times. Thinking of pouring water out of the front of the dumbbells at their highest point will put them in the correct position, but make sure that the rotation comes from your shoulders, not from your wrists.

Slowly return (two seconds) to the beginning position, following the same exercise form in reverse.

Breathing: Breathe in slowly as you lift the dumbbells. You should finish inhaling when your upper arms are parallel with the floor. Slowly exhale as you return the dumbbells to the beginning position.

Do not allow your body or head to move from the beginning position. Do not bend your elbows more than slightly. Do not allow the dumbbells to rotate up as you raise them. Do not allow your upper arms to move forward or backward as you raise them. Do not raise the dumbbells more than shoulder height, or very **slightly** above shoulder height, at most. Do not bounce, jerk, or swing the dumbbells to start them moving. If you need to do any of these things in order to lift the dumbbells, you are using too much weight. Use less weight and perform the exercise correctly. Also do not let the dumbbells simply drop back to the beginning position. Keep the dumbbells under control at all times. Remember, lowering the weights slowly is always at least half the exercise, therefore, half the results.

Note: To help protect your lower back, I recommend wearing your lifting belt for this exercise (see Chapter 6, **"Don't Forget to Accessorize"**).

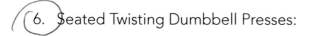

6. Seated Twisting Dumbbell Presses:

This exercise works all three sections of the deltoid muscle, plus the triceps and the muscles of the upper back. More work with less exercise. That is our goal.

Positioning: Take two dumbbells of the same weight and sit on an exercise bench. Place your feet flat on the floor, fairly wide apart. Lift the dumbbells up to your shoulders and hold them with the palms of your hands facing each other and your elbows pointing forward and down. Lean **slightly** forward with your upper body, keeping the natural curve in your lower back. Keep looking straight ahead.

Exercise Technique: Push your feet forcefully against the floor and tighten your midsection to stabilize your upper body. Press the dumbbells slowly up (two seconds) and simultaneously bring your elbows to the side so that when you are at the **halfway point** in the exercise your upper arms are parallel to the floor, forming a straight line through your shoulders, from one elbow to the other. In other words, your arms should form a wide "u" like this: l_o_l. The dumbbells should rotate out as your elbows move out to the side, away from your body.

Halfway through the exercise, the dumbbells should be in a line with each other, with the palms of your hands facing forward. Continue pressing the dumbbells up and rotating them until they will not rotate any further. At this point, the backs of your hands should be almost facing each other and your arms should be as straight as possible. Your shoulders should also be rotated out and pulled back as far as possible (by squeezing your shoulder blades together).

Note: Because of the rotation of the dumbbells and the position of your arms, it may not be possible to completely lock your elbows in the finish position. This is not a disaster. The contraction you should feel in your deltoids is much more important than completely straight arms, so concentrate on that. This exercise demonstrates how important flexibility is for correct exercise technique. At the finish position of this exercise your arms, hands, and shoulders will actually be behind your head, with your upper body still leaning **slightly** forward…if your shoulders are flexible enough. You really need a mirror to check your form on this exercise.

Slowly return (two seconds) to the beginning position, following the same exercise form in reverse.

Breathing: Breathe out slowly as you press the dumbbells up. You should finish exhaling as the dumbbells reach their highest point. Slowly inhale as you return to the beginning position.

Do not use a backrest to lean against. Do not lean back as you press the dumbbells up. Do not bring your shoulders forward when pressing the dumbbells up. Do not lose the natural curve in your lower back. Do not bounce or jerk the dumbbells to start them moving. If you need to do any of these things in order to press the dumbbells up, you are using too much weight. Use less weight and perform the exercise correctly. Also do not let the dumbbells simply drop back to the beginning position. Keep the dumbbells under control at all times.

Note: To help protect your lower back, I recommend wearing your lifting belt for this exercise (see Chapter 6, **"Don't Forget to Accessorize"**).

7. Cardio-Aerobics:

You should still be breathing hard and your heart rate should still be elevated from doing this chest, triceps, and shoulder workout. Therefore, you should begin your Cardio-aerobics immediately after completing your last set of Seated Twisting Dumbbell Presses. Follow the Cardio-aerobics progression for your particular group (situation) as it is described in **CTTC Workout #1** in Chapter 11, **"Adapting the CTTC Workouts."**

Do not jump into this intense form of aerobics if you are not physically prepared for it, nor should you abruptly terminate a Cardio-aerobics session without slowly tapering off.

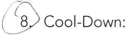 Cool-Down:

Continue the exercise you used for your Cardio-aerobics for a couple of minutes longer at a lower intensity. This is the first part of your cool-down and allows your heart to slowly and safely return to a lower pulse rate. Then walk around easily, continuing to breathe deeply, as described in Chapter 7.

During this time, you should also use your elastic band (see Chapter 6, **"Don't Forget to Accessorize"**) to continually stretch your chest, arms, and shoulders. Next, occasionally stop to stretch your legs and your spine.

After your heart rate has returned to a more normal level, you can lie down or sit on the floor to more effectively stretch your legs and lower back. After you have finished doing this, stand up and thoroughly stretch your shoulders and calves one more time.

Do not shorten your cool down or omit it altogether. Do not stand still, sit, or lie down immediately after completing a Cardio-aerobics session.

Chapter 9

CTTC Workout Number 2

Tempo:

2-1-3

The tempo for most of the exercises in **CTTC Workout #2** is two seconds concentric (the active part of moving a weight, i.e., actively pulling or pushing it), a one-second pause at the midpoint of the exercise where you should tense (contract) the working muscle(s) as hard as possible for one second, and three seconds eccentric (the passive part of moving a weight, i.e., lowering the weight).

You will occasionally have to pause during an exercise and take a few deep breaths before continuing. This is not only allowed, but is encouraged. If you need more oxygen during an exercise, it means that you are working hard, and that is good.

Intensity:

When an exercise calls for only one set, you should use a weight that will make the last few repetitions (reps) of the exercise very difficult, but still allow the use of correct exercise form. These are usually warm-up sets for the following sets (or exercise), so the object is to increase the blood flow into that particular muscle or body-part, and to warm up the joints involved in the following sets or exercise.

When an exercise calls for more than one set, you should use a weight that will make the last repetition (rep) of each set absolutely the last rep that you can possibly do with relatively good exercise form. In other words, if the exercise calls for three sets of 12 - 9 reps (written: 3 x 12 - 9), you should use a weight on your first set which will allow you to do at least nine or ten reps with perfect exercise form. The next couple of reps should be very difficult to complete. Your exercise form can be a little bit looser for these couple of reps, including the last rep. The last rep (#12) should be the last rep that you can possibly do without someone helping you.

If you can do more than twelve reps, then the weight is too light, and if you cannot complete eleven reps, then the weight is too heavy. Ideally, on the first set the 12th rep should be the last one you could possibly do. On the 2nd set, it would be the 10th or 11th rep, and on the 3rd set the 9th or 10th rep should be the last one you could possibly do without someone helping you. You may have to add weight, reduce the weight, or use the same weight on each set of each exercise in order to accomplish this. Only careful experimentation on your part can tell you which of these you need to do...and when.

Of course, if you are not already an experienced exerciser, you will have to slowly build up to this level of intensity. This is partially built into the progression described in Chapter 11, **"Adapting the CTTC Workouts,"** but you will still need to apply these recommendations to your own personal situation.

Rest Periods:

The length of the rest periods between sets is **extremely** important. Have a watch with you (see Chapter 6, **"Don't Forget to Accessorize"**) and do not rest any longer than is given in the workout description. You should be breathing hard from the end of the warm-up until you are into your cool down. Between sets, breathe as was described in Chapter 7. If you are not breathing hard enough between sets, then increase the weight and/or shorten your rest periods.

The Exercises:

Do not change the order of the exercises. They are in this order for very specific reasons.

Do not substitute or alter the exercises unless it is absolutely unavoidable. They have been very carefully chosen for very specific reasons. If you do not have access to a particular piece of exercise equipment, then choose a substitute exercise that resembles the original exercise as closely as possible.

Do not add exercises, sets, or more repetitions than are called for in the **CTTC** Workouts. These have also been carefully calculated.

Do not do "forced reps." A forced rep is one where someone helps you to do another repetition when you can no longer complete the rep on your own. Forced reps are counterproductive to this exercise program.

Do not take longer rest periods than are given. In fact, when your cardiovascular fitness has improved enough for you to be able to shorten to the rest periods without sacrificing strength or exercise form, please do so. However, this shortening of rest periods does not apply to the highest level of Cardio-aerobics in **CTTC Workout #3**. Once you have reached this level, there is no advantage to be gained by shortening the "30 seconds of medium effort" any more.

Note: Of course, once in a while it will happen that the piece of equipment that you need to use is occupied by someone else when you need it. If it is not possible to alternate with the person, then choose a substitute exercise which resembles the original exercise as closely as possible. This is preferable to having to wait too long between exercises. You have to keep your breathing and your heart rate elevated in order to enjoy the maximum benefits of the **CTTC** Exercise Program.

In order for you to get 100% out of the **CTTC** Exercise Program, you will have to follow these guidelines as closely as possible. The more you deviate from these guidelines, the less you will get out of this program. It is that simple.

CTTC Workout Number 2

Monday

CTTC **Workout #2** - 4 weeks long	**Exercise Tempo:** 2 seconds concentric, 1 second pause, 3 seconds eccentric	
Monday: Back, Biceps, and Waist		
1. Warm-Up	Build up to 85% of MHR for the last 3 minutes.	10 minutes
2. Lat Machine Pull-Downs to Chest - Close Parallel Grip – Elbows In	1 minute rest between sets.	1 x 15 3 x 12 -9
3. Bent Over Barbell Rowing – Shoulder-Width Grip – Elbows Neutral	1 minute rest between sets.	3 x 12 -9
4. Seated Incline Dumbbell Curls – Rotating	30 seconds rest between sets.	3 x 12 -9
5. a- Lying Back Extensions – Bodyweight Only alternated with **b-** Crunches – Bodyweight Only	No rest between sets.	2 x 12 2 x 20
6. Cardio-Aerobics	12 intervals of 10 seconds all-out effort followed by 40 seconds of minimum/ medium effort.	10 minutes
7. Cool-Down	Moving and Stretching	10 minutes

NOTES

1st workout of the month	Time it took to complete the workout	Observations or comments about this workout
2nd workout of the month	Time it took to complete the workout	Observations or comments about this workout
3rd workout of the month	Time it took to complete the workout	Observations or comments about this workout
4th workout of the month	Time it took to complete the workout	Observations or comments about this workout

OTHER NOTES

Explanation of the Exercises

Monday

1. Warm-Up:

Do any type of movements which will increase your heart rate and increase your body temperature. Just make sure that the exercise does not use your arms (this would tire them too much for the workout which follows), and that you are able to keep control of your pulse rate. Power-walking, jogging, treadmills, elliptical walkers, steppers, bicycling, and exercise bicycles (home-trainers) are all good examples. Follow the Warm-Up progression for your particular group (situation), as it is described in **CTTC Workout #2** in Chapter 11, **"Adapting the CTTC Workouts."**

2. Lat Machine Pull-Downs to Chest – Close Parallel Grip – Elbows In:

This exercise is also for the large back muscles (latissimus dorsi, or lats for short) which extend from your armpits all the way down to your waist.

Positioning: Grasp a close-parallel-grip bar (palms of your hands facing each other). Sit so that your thighs are held down very securely by the pads on the machine. Your butt should not be able to rise up when you begin to pull the bar down. You should be sitting directly beneath, or **slightly** back from the overhead pulley. Hang completely stretched, also allowing your shoulders to completely extend upward (by your ears), and look forward and slightly upward. Your body should be completely relaxed at the beginning of the exercise, letting the weight stretch out your shoulders and spine.

Exercise Technique: Pull first your shoulders (by squeezing your shoulder blades down and together), and then your elbows down slowly (two seconds) until the handles (or your hands) touch your lower chest on a line level with the bottom of your breast bone (sternum).

As you begin to pull, you should continue to look forward and slightly upward. Your upper body should assume a slightly arched (curved) position as you bring your chest forward and up to meet the handles. You will automatically assume this position if you make sure to pull your shoulders back and down as you pull the handles down. As you continue to pull the handles down, you should lean back **slightly** while keeping your back in the arched position. This **slight** lean-back should not be more than about 20°.

Note: Do not think of pulling with your hands. Concentrate on pulling first with your shoulders and then with your elbows. You should think of your hands as hooks whose only purpose is to hang onto the handles. Your elbows and shoulders should determine the direction and the distance of the pull.

On this exercise, your elbows move directly in front of you as you pull them down. When the handles touch your chest, your upper arms should be close to your sides, shoulders back and down, with your elbows as far behind your back as possible.

I personally prefer a parallel grip where the handles are somewhat wider apart, so they touch the **sides** of my chest, instead of the very close-grip handles which touch the center of my chest. This way, I can move my shoulders and elbows just a little further back and it is easier to push my chest forward and up.

If you feel as if your shoulder blades are going to touch each other when the handles touch your chest, then you are doing the exercise correctly. If you cannot achieve this position, then you are using too much weight. Use less weight and perform the exercise correctly.

Hold this position and **consciously** contract (tense) all your back muscles as hard as you can for 1 second.

Slowly return (three seconds) to the beginning position, following the same exercise form in reverse. Make sure that you completely straighten your arms and extend your shoulders upwards when you reach the beginning position again. Remember, lowering the weight slowly is always at least half the exercise, therefore half the results.

Breathing: Breathe in slowly as you begin pulling your shoulders and elbows down. You should complete breathing in as the handles touch your chest. Breathe out slowly as you return to the starting position.

Do not bring your head down, pull your shoulders forward, round your back, or let your chest sink in. Do not let your elbows move out to the side. Do not forcefully lean back, or jerk your body in order to get the weights moving. If you have to do any of these things in order to get the handles to your chest, you are using too much weight. Use less weight and perform the exercise correctly. Also do not let the weight drop back to the beginning position. Keep control of the weight at all times.

3. Bent Over Barbell Rowing – Shoulder-Width Grip – Elbows Neutral:

This exercise works your back from your neck all the way down to your butt. It will add thickness to your entire back, especially along your spinal column.

Positioning: Load a barbell with the appropriate amount of weight and take an overhand (palms facing down) grip, slightly wider than shoulder width. Bend your knees **slightly** to take some stress off your lower back. Bend over at the waist until your upper body is at a 30°-45° angle to the floor. Let the barbell hang straight down. Allow your shoulders to hang down, completely relaxed, but keep your back (spine) straight. Keeping your head slightly up and looking forward (instead of down at the floor) will help to put your back in the correct position. Make sure that your lower back stays slightly arched and stable during the entire exercise.

Exercise Technique: Lift first your shoulders (by squeezing your shoulder blades together) and then your elbows up and back. Slowly (two seconds) pull the bar up to your navel (bellybutton). Allow your elbows to follow a natural (neutral) path. They will angle out slightly away from your body as you pull, but that is OK, as long as they stay relatively close to the sides of your body.

Note: Do not think of pulling with your hands or arms. Concentrate on pulling first with your shoulders and then with your elbows.

If you feel as if your shoulder blades are going to touch each other when your elbows reach their highest point, then you are doing the exercise correctly. If you cannot achieve this position, you are using too much weight. Use less weight and perform the exercise correctly.

When the barbell reaches its highest point (touching your navel), hold this position and consciously contract (tense) all your back muscles as hard as you can for one second.

Slowly return (three seconds) to the beginning position, following the same exercise form in reverse.

Breathing: Breathe in slowly as you begin pulling your shoulders and your elbows up. You should complete breathing in as your elbows reach their highest point. Breathe out slowly as you return to the starting position.

Do not let your back (spine) round or let your lower back relax. Do not let your elbows drift out away from the sides of your body. Do not bounce up and down, or jerk your body in order to get the weights moving. If you have to do any of these things in order to get your elbows up high enough, you are using too much weight. Use less weight and perform the exercise correctly. Also do not let the barbell simply drop back to the beginning position. Keep the barbell under control at all times. Remember, lowering the weight slowly is always at least half the exercise, therefore half the results.

Note: To help protect your lower back, I recommend wearing your lifting belt for this exercise (see Chapter 6, **"Don't Forget to Accessorize"**).

If you feel uncomfortable or insecure using a barbell, you can do this exercise on a Smith Machine. I personally prefer this method because I can concentrate better on feeling my back muscles working, rather than worrying about my old lower back injuries.

If you still feel uncomfortable or insecure, fold up a towel and put it on the end of an adjustable exercise bench. The bench should be set at a height where, when your forehead is on the towel, your back is at a 30°-45° angle to the floor. This will relieve most of the stress on your lower back, thereby protecting it even more.

4. Seated Incline Dumbbell Curls – Rotating:

This exercise works not only both heads of the biceps (the muscle on the front of your upper arms), but also the smaller underlying muscles which stabilize your elbow.

Your biceps have assisted on both of the back exercises above, so they are already warmed up. This again saves you the time you would normally have to spend on a warm-up set for your biceps.

Positioning: Set an adjustable exercise bench to a fairly high incline (45°-60°), depending on how flexible your shoulders are). Take two dumbbells of the same weight and sit on the bench, leaning back on the 45°-60° incline. Place your feet flat on the floor, fairly wide apart. Let the dumbbells hang straight down at your sides with the palms of your hands facing each other (as if you were holding a hammer) and touching the front plates of the dumbbells. Keep your head in line with your body. Make sure to press your shoulders and lower back against the bench, and to push your chest forward and up.

Exercise Technique: Push your feet forcefully against the floor and tighten your midsection to stabilize your body. Curl (lift) the dumbbells forward and up slowly (two seconds) while simultaneously and continuously rotating your hands outward. Continue moving only your forearms until they cannot move any further because they have been stopped by your upper arms. The plates of the dumbbells (on your little finger side) should almost be touching your shoulders at this point, with your hands rotated out as far as possible.

When the dumbbells reach their highest point (almost touching your shoulders), hold this position and consciously contract (tense) your biceps as hard as you can for one second.

Slowly return (three seconds) to the beginning position, following the same exercise form in reverse. Make sure that you begin and end this exercise with your elbows completely straight.

Breathing: Breathe in slowly as you begin curling the dumbbells up. You should complete inhaling as the dumbbells reach their highest point (by your shoulders). Breathe out slowly as you return to the starting position.

Do not move your upper arms. Do not bounce or swing the dumbbells to get them up. Do not bring your head or shoulders forward, or allow your chest to sink in. Do not allow your lower back to arch away from (lose contact with) the bench. If you need to do any of these things in order to curl the dumbbells, then you are using too much weight. Use less weight and perform the exercise correctly. Also do not let the dumbbells simply drop back to the beginning position. Keep the dumbbells under control at all times.

5. a- Lying Back Extensions – Bodyweight Only:

These are done exactly as in **CTTC Workout #1**, except that when your upper body can not rise up any further, you hold this position and consciously contract (tense) your entire back as hard as you can for one second. Don't forget to also squeeze your buns together as hard as possible at this point.

Read the **Positioning** and **Exercise Technique** instructions for **Lying Back Extensions** in CTTC **Workout #1** again.

b- Crunches – Bodyweight Only:

These are done exactly as in **CTTC Workout #1**, except for a change in exercise tempo. In this workout, you do a two second concentric contraction (curling your upper body up). When your upper body can not curl up any further, hold this position and consciously contract (tense) your abdominals as hard as you can for one second.

Slowly return (three seconds) to the beginning position following the same exercise form in reverse.

Read the **Positioning** and **Exercise Technique** instructions for **Crunches** in **CTTC Workout #1** again.

6. Cardio-Aerobics:

You should still be breathing hard and your heart rate should still be elevated from doing the Back Extensions and Crunches. Therefore, you should begin your Cardio-aerobics immediately after completing these. Follow the Cardio-aerobics progression for your particular group (situation), as it is described in **CTTC Workout #2** in Chapter 11, **"Adapting the CTTC Workouts."**

7. Cool-Down:

Continue the exercise you used for your Cardio-aerobics for a couple of minutes longer at a lower intensity. This is the first part of your cool down and allows your heart to slowly and safely return to a lower pulse rate. Then walk around easily, continuing to breathe deeply, as described in Chapter 7.

During this time, you should also use your elastic band (see Chapter 6, **"Don't Forget to Accessorize"**) to continually stretch your chest, arms, and shoulders. Next, occasionally stop to stretch your legs and your spine.

After your heart rate has returned to a more normal level, you can lie down or sit on the floor to more effectively stretch your legs and lower back. After you have finished doing this, stand up and thoroughly stretch your shoulders and calves one more time.

Do not shorten your cool down or omit it altogether. Do not stand still, sit, or lie down immediately after completing a Cardio-aerobics session. Always taper off slowly.

CTTC Workout Number 2

Wednesday

CTTC **Workout #2** - 4 weeks long	**Exercise Tempo:** 2 seconds concentric, 1 second pause, 3 seconds eccentric	
Wednesday: Legs		
1. Warm-Up	Build up to 85% of MHR for the last 3 minutes.	10 minutes
2. Leg Extensions	Warm-Up	1 x 25
3. Leg Curls – Seated or Lying	Warm-Up	1 x 20
4. Leg Presses	1½ minutes rest between sets.	1 set each of 30, 25, & 20 reps.
5. Leg Curls – Seated or Lying	30 seconds rest between sets.	2 x 15 -12
6. Leg Extensions	30 seconds rest between sets.	2 x 20 -15
7. Cardio-Aerobics	12 intervals of 10 seconds all-out effort followed by 40 seconds of minimum/medium effort.	10 minutes
8. Standing Calf Raises – One Legged – Bodyweight Only – Alternating Legs	No rest between sets.	1 set each of 25, 20, & 15 reps.
9. Cool-Down	Moving and Stretching	10 minutes

NOTES

1st workout of the month	Time it took to complete the workout	Observations or comments about this workout
2nd workout of the month	Time it took to complete the workout	Observations or comments about this workout
3rd workout of the month	Time it took to complete the workout	Observations or comments about this workout
4th workout of the month	Time it took to complete the workout	Observations or comments about this workout

OTHER NOTES

Explanation of the Exercises

Wednesday

1. Warm-Up:

Do any type of movements that will increase your heart rate and increase your body temperature. Just make sure that you are able to keep control of your pulse rate. Power-walking, jogging, treadmills, elliptical walkers, steppers, bicycling, and exercise bicycles (home-trainers) are all good examples. Follow the Warm-Up progression for your particular group (situation) as it is described in **CTTC Workout #2** in Chapter 11, **"Adapting the CTTC Workouts."**

2. Leg Extensions:

These are done exactly as in **CTTC Workout #1**, except for a change in exercise tempo. In this workout, you do a two-second concentric contraction (extending your lower legs). When your knees are completely locked, hold the position and consciously contract (tense) your thigh muscles as hard as you can for one second.

Slowly return (three seconds) to the beginning position, following the same exercise form in reverse.

Read the **Positioning** and **Exercise Technique** instructions for **Leg Extensions** in **CTTC Workout #1** again.

3. Leg Curls – Seated or Lying:

These are done exactly as in **CTTC Workout #1**, except for a change in exercise tempo. In this workout, you do a 2 second concentric contraction (curling your lower legs). When your knees cannot bend any further, hold the position and consciously contract (tense) your hamstrings (and your butt) as hard as you can for 1 second.

Slowly return (three seconds) to the beginning position following the same exercise form in reverse.

Read the **Positioning** and **Exercise Technique** instructions for **Leg Curls** in **CTTC Workout #1** again.

4. Leg Presses:

This exercise provides all the benefits of Smith Machine Squats (see **CTTC Workout #1**) with several added advantages. Leg Presses are more comfortable, more versatile, and you can safely use more weight than you can with any kind of squats. With Leg Presses, you can safely "make the last repetition (rep) of each set absolutely the last rep that you can possibly do." In fact, if you get stuck on the last rep of a set of Leg Presses, you can place your hands on your thighs to help your legs push the weight up.

Positioning: Place yourself comfortably on whichever Leg Press machine is available to you. They vary from sitting straight up to lying down. Some are adjustable. Keep in mind that the more you sit up, the more you will use your butt muscles. Place your feet on the platform about shoulder width apart and turned out at a natural angle (whatever that is for you).

Your feet should be at a point on the platform where, when you lower the weight and your upper legs are as low as you want them to come, your knees are bent at 90°, or slightly more. Stop lowering the weight just before your pelvis begins to rotate upward, thereby rounding your lower back. Your knees should remain in a line directly over your feet. Your stance should feel natural and comfortable.

Exercise Technique: If your Leg Press machine has handles, grasp them tightly with your hands. Contract your abdominals and your back muscles, as well as all the other muscles in your body. Press your lower back against the backrest. Now begin slowly lowering the weight (three seconds) to a position where your knees are bent at a 90° angle, or slightly more.

Never lower the weight so far that your pelvis begins to rotate upward, thereby rounding your lower back.

Slowly return (two seconds) to the beginning position following the same exercise form in reverse, but do not straighten your knees completely when you reach the beginning position again. When you have reached this position, hold it for one second and consciously contract (tense) your legs (and your butt) as hard as you can for one second. Keep constant tension on your legs throughout the entire set.

Breathing: Breathe in slowly as you lower the weight. Hold your breath as you begin to push out of the bottom position. After you begin moving the weight upward (about halfway), begin breathing out forcefully.

One problem involved with holding your breath while exerting force is that it momentarily raises blood pressure. If you do have high blood pressure, **do not** hold your breath.

Doing twenty-five reps per set on this exercise will necessitate your having to pause at the completion of some of the reps to take a couple of extra deep breaths. This is good. The last several repetitions of a set may even require that you take several deep breaths after every rep. Good. Take all the deep breaths you need to finish twenty-five reps.

Do not lower the weight so far that your pelvis begins to rotate upward, thereby rounding your lower back. Do not round your upper or your lower back. Do not allow your knees to move outward or inward as you press the weight. Keep them in a line directly over your feet. If you need to do any of these things to complete the Leg Press, you are using too much weight. Use less weight and perform the exercise correctly. Absolutely do not drop quickly into the bent-knee position. Keep control of your movements at all times. Remember, lowering the weight slowly is always at least half the exercise, therefore half the results.

Note: There are many variations of foot placements possible with Leg Presses. You can place your feet low and narrow, high and wide, middle and middle, low and wide, high and narrow, and so on. Each of these foot placements will put the stress on a slightly different part of your legs, hips, and butt. After you have successfully completed the entire **CTTC** Exercise Program, you can begin to experiment with these different foot placements to find the one, or ones, which best suit your particular needs.

Basically, the higher your feet, the more your glutes (butt) are involved. The lower your feet, the more your quads (frontal thighs) are involved. The wider your feet, the more your inner thighs are involved; and the narrower your feet, the more your outer thighs are involved. Don't worry, if you do the exercise correctly, you will feel exactly where the stress is…especially the next day.

Note: To help protect your lower back, I recommend wearing your lifting belt for this exercise (see Chapter 6, **"Don't Forget to Accessorize"**).

5. Leg Curls – Seated or Lying: (same as in exercise #3 above)

6. Leg Extensions: (same as in exercise #2 above)

7. Cardio-Aerobics:

You should still be breathing hard and your heart rate should still be elevated from doing this leg workout. Therefore, you should begin your Cardio-aerobics immediately after completing your last set of Leg Extensions. Follow the Cardio-aerobics progression for your particular group (situation) as it is described in **CTTC** Workout #2 in Chapter 11, **"Adapting the CTTC Workouts."**

Continue the exercise you used for your Cardio-aerobics for a couple of minutes longer at a lower intensity. This is the first part of your cool-down and allows your heart to slowly and safely return to a lower pulse rate.

Do not jump into this intense form of aerobics if you are not physically prepared for it, nor should you abruptly terminate a Cardio-aerobics session without slowly tapering off.

8. Standing Calf Raises – One Legged – Bodyweight Only – Alternating Legs:

These are done exactly as in **CTTC** Workout #1, except for a change in exercise tempo, and a slight change in **Positioning**.

In this workout, your toes should point straight ahead (not out at an angle) and you are exercising one leg at a time. You do a two-second concentric contraction (rising up on the balls of your feet). When you cannot raise up any higher, hold the position and consciously contract (tense) your calf as hard as you can for one second.

Slowly return (three seconds) to the beginning position following the same exercise form in reverse. When your heel reaches the lowest position possible, allow a maximum stretch for one second.

Alternate back and forth between legs (after each set) without resting until you have completed all six sets (three sets for each leg).

Read the **Positioning** and **Exercise Technique** instructions for **Standing Calf Raises** in CTTC **Workout #1** again.

9. Cool-Down:

Walk around easily, continuing to breathe deeply, as described in Chapter 7, **"The CTTC Workouts: Scientific Fitness versus Science Fiction."** Occasionally stop to stretch your legs, your spine, and your calves.

After your heart rate has returned to a more normal level, you can lie down or sit on the floor to more effectively stretch your legs and lower back. After you have finished doing this, stand up and thoroughly stretch your calves one more time.

Do not shorten your cool down or omit it altogether. Do not stand still, sit, or lie down immediately after completing a Cardio-aerobics session. Always taper off slowly.

CTTC Workout Number 2

Friday

CTTC **Workout #2** - 4 weeks long	**Exercise Tempo:** 2 seconds concentric, 1 second pause, 3 seconds eccentric.	
Friday: Chest, Triceps, and Shoulders		
1. Warm-Up	Build up to 85% of MHR for the last 3 minutes.	10 minutes
2. 30°- 45° Incline Barbell Bench Press – Wide Grip – Elbows Out	1 minute rest between sets	1 x 15 2 x 12 - 9
3. Flat Barbell Bench Press – Shoulder-Width Grip – Elbows Neutral	1 minute rest between sets.	3 x 12 - 9
4. Cable Triceps Pushdowns – Shoulder-Width Grip - Curved Bar	30 seconds rest between sets.	3 x 12 - 9
5. Dumbbell Upright Rowing	30 seconds rest between sets.	1 x 15 2 x 12 - 9
6. Seated Barbell Press – Elbows Out	30 seconds rest between sets.	2 x 12 - 9
7. Cardio-Aerobics	12 intervals of 10 seconds all-out effort followed by 40 seconds of minimum/medium effort.	10 minutes
8. Cool-Down	Moving and Stretching	10 minutes

NOTES

1st workout of the month	Time it took to complete the workout	Observations or comments about this workout
2nd workout of the month	Time it took to complete the workout	Observations or comments about this workout
3rd workout of the month	Time it took to complete the workout	Observations or comments about this workout
4th workout of the month	Time it took to complete the workout	Observations or comments about this workout

OTHER NOTES

Explanation of the Exercises

Friday

1. Warm-Up:

Do any type of movements which will increase your heart rate and increase your body temperature. Just make sure that the exercise does not use your arms (this would tire them too much for the workout which follows), and that you are able to keep control of your pulse rate. Power-walking, jogging, treadmills, elliptical walkers, steppers, bicycling, and exercise bicycles (home-trainers) are all good examples. Follow the Warm-up progression for your particular group (situation) as it is described in **CTTC Workout #2** in Chapter 11, **"Adapting the CTTC Workouts."**

2. 30°- 45° Incline Barbell Bench Press – Wide Grip – Elbows Out:

This exercise emphasizes the development of the upper portion of your chest muscles.

Positioning: Set an adjustable incline bench press bench (if available) to approximately a 30°-45° incline. Sit on the bench, leaning back on the 30°-45° incline. Place your feet flat on the floor, fairly wide apart. Keep your head in line with your body. Make sure to press your lower back and shoulders against the bench, and to push your chest forward and up.

Note: I vary the incline every time I do incline chest exercises. Sometimes I even use a different incline for each set that I do in my chest workout.

Grasp the barbell with an overhand grip (palms facing away from you). Your hands should be far enough apart so that, when you are at the **halfway point** in the exercise, your upper arms are parallel to the floor, forming a straight line through your shoulders, from one elbow to the other. Your forearms should then be parallel to each other and 90° to your upper arms. In other words, your arms should form a wide "u" like this: l_o_l.

Exercise Technique: Push your feet forcefully against the floor and tighten your midsection to stabilize your body. Take the barbell off the supports and lower it slowly (three seconds) until the bar touches your upper chest (just below your collar bones).

Immediately press the barbell up slowly (two seconds) until your arms are completely straight and your shoulders are extended up and off of the bench as far as they will go.

When the barbell reaches its highest point, hold this position and consciously contract (tense) your chest muscles as hard as you can for 1 second.

Breathing: Breathe in slowly as you lower the barbell. You should finish inhaling as the barbell touches your upper chest. Now hold your breath as you press the barbell up. Breathe out forcefully just as the barbell reaches its highest position.

One problem involved with holding your breath while exerting force is that it momentarily raises blood pressure. If you do have high blood pressure, **do not** hold your breath.

Do not bring your head forward. Do not allow your lower back to arch away from (lose contact with) the bench. Do not let your elbows move forward. Do not jerk or bounce the weights off of your chest to start the pressing action. If you need to do any of these things in order to press the barbell up, you are using too much weight. Use less weight and perform the exercise correctly. Also do not let the barbell simply drop down to your chest. Keep the barbell under control at all times. Remember, lowering the weight slowly is always at least half the exercise, therefore, half the results.

Note: If you feel uncomfortable or insecure using a free-weight barbell, you can do this exercise on a Smith Machine. However, your results will suffer in the long run if you use the Smith Machine exclusively.

3. Flat Barbell Bench Press – Shoulder-Width Grip – Elbows Neutral:

This exercise develops the entire pectoralis major (chest muscle), as well as your triceps.

Positioning: Lie down on a bench press bench. Grasp the barbell with an overhand grip (palms facing away from you), and with your hands approximately shoulder width apart. Place your feet flat on the floor, fairly wide apart. Keep your head in line with your body. Make sure to press your lower back and shoulders against the bench, and to push your chest up.

Exercise Technique: Push your feet forcefully against the floor and tighten your midsection to stabilize your body. Take the barbell off the supports and lower it slowly (three seconds) until the bar touches the middle of your chest at about the nipple line.

Immediately press the barbell up slowly (two seconds) until your arms are completely straight and your shoulders are extended up and off of the bench as far as they will go.

When the barbell reaches its highest point, hold this position and consciously contract (tense) your chest muscles as hard as you can for one second.

Allow your elbows to follow a natural (neutral) path. They will angle slightly out away from your body as you do the exercise, but that is OK, as long as they do not drift out too wide.

Breathing: Breathe in slowly as you lower the barbell. You should finish inhaling as the barbell touches the middle of your chest. Now hold your breath as you press the barbell up. Breathe out forcefully just as the barbell reaches its highest position.

One problem involved with holding your breath while exerting force is that it momentarily raises blood pressure. If you do have high blood pressure, **do not** hold your breath.

Do not lift your head or allow your lower back to arch away from (lose contact with) the bench. Do not let your elbows move out too wide. Do not jerk or bounce the weights off of your chest to start the pressing action. If you need to do any of these things in order to press the barbell up, you are using too much weight. Use less weight and perform the exercise correctly. Also do not let the barbell simply drop down to your chest. Keep the barbell under control at all times. Remember, lowering the weight slowly is always at least half the exercise, therefore half the results.

Note: If you feel uncomfortable or insecure using a barbell, you can do this exercise on a Smith Machine. However, your results will suffer in the long run if you use the Smith Machine exclusively.

4. Cable Triceps Pushdowns – Shoulder-Width Grip – Curved Bar:

This exercise works all three heads of the triceps (the muscle on the back of your upper arms).

Your triceps have assisted on both of the chest exercises above, so they are already warmed up.

These Cable Triceps Pushdowns are very similar to the ones you did in **CTTC Workout #1**, except that instead of a rope attachment, you will now use a short, slightly curved triceps bar. The slight curve will take some strain off of your wrists while providing a little different feel to the contraction of your triceps.

Positioning: Stand about a foot back from where the overhead cable hangs straight down and take hold of the triceps bar with a shoulder width grip, or slightly narrower, palms facing down. Pull your upper arms down until your elbows are just in front, but still touching your body. Bend your knees slightly and bend **slightly** forward at the waist. Keep looking straight ahead. Now tighten your entire body to lock it in this position. Your elbows should now be completely bent, hands by your upper chest. From this position, only your lower arms should move.

Exercise Technique: Push the triceps bar down slowly (two seconds). Make sure that your upper arms do not move. Continue to push the triceps bar down until your elbows are completely locked. Hold this position and consciously contract (tense) your triceps as hard as you can for one second.

Slowly return (three seconds) to the beginning position following the same exercise form in reverse.

Breathing: Exhale slowly as you push the rope down. You should finish exhaling as your elbows straighten completely. Inhale slowly as you return to the beginning position.

You will notice that as you exhale, your abdominals will also begin to contract strongly, therefore, consciously tighten your abdominals as much as possible during this exercise. It's like getting a free set of crunches as a bonus, which means less time you need to spend doing boring abdominal exercises.

Do not let your upper arms, upper body, or head move during the exercise. Do not jerk or bounce the weight to start the pushing action. If you need to do any of these things in order to push the bar down, you are using too much weight. Use less weight and perform the exercise correctly. Also do not let the weight simply drop back to the beginning position. Keep the weight under control at all times. Remember, lowering the weight slowly is always at least half the exercise, therefore half the results.

5. Dumbbell Upright Rowing:

This exercise will develop the middle section of the deltoids (the muscle on the side of your shoulders) as well as the muscles in your upper back.

Positioning: Select two dumbbells of the same weight. Stand with your feet approximately shoulder width apart and knees slightly bent. Lean your upper body **slightly** forward and let the dumbbells hang in front of your thighs, with the backs of your hands facing forward. Push your butt back a little and arch your lower back. Contract your abdominal, leg, butt, and back muscles to stabilize your body in this position. Look forward and slightly upwards.

Exercise Technique: Lift both upper arms slowly sideways (two seconds) until your upper arms are parallel with the floor, forming a straight line through your shoulders, from one elbow to the other. This will place the dumbbells slightly in front of your shoulders when they are at the highest point of the exercise (shoulder height).

When your upper arms reach the highest point of the exercise (shoulder height or **slightly** higher), hold this position and consciously contract (tense) your upper back (by squeezing your shoulder blades together) and deltoid (shoulder) muscles as hard as you can for 1 second. This may pull your elbows (upper arms) slightly behind your shoulders, but that is OK. Allowing your elbows to move in front of your shoulders is **not** OK.

Slowly return (three seconds) to the beginning position, following the same exercise form in reverse.

Breathing: Breathe in slowly as you lift the dumbbells. You should finish inhaling when your upper arms are parallel with the floor. Slowly exhale as you return the dumbbells to the beginning position.

Do not allow your body or head to move from the beginning position. Do not allow the dumbbells to rotate up or down as you raise them. Do not allow your upper arms (elbows) to move forward or backward as you raise them. Do not raise your upper arms more than shoulder height, or **slightly** above shoulder height, at most. Do not bounce, jerk, or swing the dumbbells to start them moving. If you need to do any of these things in order to lift the dumbbells, you are using too much weight. Use less weight and perform the exercise correctly. Also do not let the dumbbells simply drop back to the beginning position. Keep the dumbbells under control at all times. Remember, lowering the weights slowly is always at least half the exercise, therefore half the results.

Note: To help protect your lower back, I recommend wearing your lifting belt for this exercise (see Chapter 6, **"Don't Forget to Accessorize"**).

6. Seated Barbell Press – Elbows Out:

This exercise works all three sections of the deltoid muscle, plus the triceps, and the muscles of the upper back.

Positioning: Grasp the barbell with an overhand grip (palms facing away from you). Lift the barbell up to your shoulders and hold it with your elbows pointing out to the sides and down. Carefully sit down on an exercise bench. Place your feet flat on the floor, fairly wide apart. Sit straight and push your chest forward and up. Keep the natural curve in your lower back and keep looking straight ahead.

Grasp the barbell with your hands far enough apart so that, when you are at the **halfway point** in the exercise, your upper arms are parallel to the floor, forming a straight line through your shoulders, from one elbow to the other. Your forearms should then be parallel to each other and 90° to your upper arms. In other words, your arms should form a wide "u" like this: l_o_l.

Exercise Technique: Push your feet forcefully against the floor and tighten your midsection to stabilize your body. As you press the barbell up slowly (two seconds), lean **slightly forward with your** upper body, but keep the natural curve in your lower back. Pull your elbows back as you press the barbell up. Continue pressing the barbell up until your arms are completely straight and your shoulders are pushed up as far as they will go. At this point, your shoulders should also be rotated out and pulled back as far as possible (by squeezing your shoulder blades together).

At the finish position of this exercise your arms, hands, and shoulders will actually be behind your head, with your upper body still leaning slightly forward…if your shoulders are flexible enough.

When the barbell reaches its highest point, hold this position and consciously contract (tense) your shoulder and upper back muscles as hard as you can for one second.

Now lower the barbell slowly (three seconds), following the same exercise form in reverse, until the bar touches your upper chest (just below your collar bones).

Breathing: Breathe out slowly as you press the barbell up. You should finish exhaling as the barbell reaches its highest point. Slowly inhale as you return to the beginning position.

Do not use a backrest to lean against. Do not lean back as you press the barbell up. Do not bring your shoulders forward when pressing the barbell up. Do not lose the natural curve in your lower back. Do not bounce or jerk the barbell to start it moving. If you need to do any of these things in order to press the barbell up, you are using too much weight. Use less weight and perform the exercise correctly. Also do not let the barbell simply drop back to the beginning position. Keep the barbell under control at all times. Remember, lowering the weights slowly is always at least half the exercise, therefore, half the results.

Note: To help protect your lower back, I recommend wearing your lifting belt for this exercise (see Chapter 6, **"Don't Forget to Accessorize"**).

7.) Cardio-Aerobics:

You should still be breathing hard and your heart rate should still be elevated from doing this chest, triceps, and shoulder workout. Therefore, you should begin your Cardio-aerobics immediately after completing your last set of Seated Barbell Presses. Follow the Cardio-aerobics progression for your particular group (situation) as it is described in **CTTC Workout #2** in Chapter 11, **"Adapting the CTTC Workouts."**

Do not jump into this intense form of aerobics if you are not physically prepared for it, nor should you abruptly terminate a Cardio-aerobics session without slowly tapering off.

8.) Cool-Down:

Continue the exercise you used for your Cardio-aerobics for a couple of minutes longer at a lower intensity. This is the first part of your cool-down and allows your heart to slowly and safely return to a lower pulse rate. Then walk around easily, continuing to breathe deeply as described in Chapter 7.

During this time, you should also use your elastic band (see Chapter 6, **"Don't Forget to Accessorize"**) to continually stretch your chest, arms, and shoulders. Next, occasionally stop to stretch your legs and your spine.

After your heart rate has returned to a more normal level, you can lie down or sit on the floor to more effectively stretch your legs and lower back. After you have finished doing this, stand up and thoroughly stretch your shoulders and calves one more time.

Do not shorten your cool-down or omit it altogether. Do not stand still, sit, or lie down immediately after completing a Cardio-aerobics session.

Chapter 10

CTTC Workout Number 3

Tempo:

The tempo for most of the exercises in **CTTC Workout #3** is an explosive concentric movement (the active part of moving a weight, i.e., actively pulling or pushing it), no pause, and a four-second eccentric movement (the passive part of moving a weight, i.e., lowering the weight).

Explosive movement does **not** mean **jerking** the weight. It means applying maximum force in a controlled manner right from the beginning of each repetition. First you tense (contract) the muscle(s) you are exercising by applying some force (pushing or pulling) against the weight you will be moving. When your muscles are tensed, then try to **accelerate** the weight through the full range of motion by applying as much force as you can.

The first few concentric repetitions will be quite rapid (one second, or even less), but should still be controlled, and done with correct exercise form. You want to **purposely** move the weight, not just throw it around. As the set continues, the concentric repetitions will automatically slow down, but you should continue to attempt to accelerate the weight as quickly as possible.

The eccentric part of the exercises should continue to take four seconds, no matter what the speed of the concentric movements are.

You will occasionally have to pause during an exercise and take a few deep breaths before continuing. This is not only allowed, but is encouraged. If you need more oxygen during an exercise, it means that you are working hard, and that is good.

Intensity:

When an exercise calls for only one set, you should use a weight that will make the last few repetitions (reps) of the exercise very difficult, but still allow the use of correct exercise form. These are usually warm-up sets for the following sets (or exercise), so the object is to increase the blood flow into that particular muscle or body-part, and to warm up the joints involved in the following sets or exercise.

When an exercise calls for more than one set, you should use a weight that will make the last repetition (rep) of each set absolutely the last rep that you can possibly do with relatively good exercise form. In other words, if the exercise calls for three sets of 8-6 reps (written: 3 x 8-6), you should use a weight on your first set that will allow you to do at least five or six reps with perfect exercise form. The next couple of reps should be very difficult to complete. Your exercise form can be a little bit looser for these couple of reps, including the last rep. The last rep (#8) should be the last rep that you can possibly do without someone helping you.

If you can do more than eight reps, then the weight is too light, and if you cannot complete six reps, then the weight is too heavy. Ideally, on the first set the 8th rep should be the last one you could possibly do. On the 2nd set, it would be the 7th rep, and on the 3rd set the 6th rep should be the last one you could possibly do without someone helping you. You may have to add weight, reduce the weight, or use the same weight on each set of each exercise in order to accomplish this. Only careful experimentation on your part can tell you which of these you need to do…and when.

Of course, if you are not already an experienced exerciser, you will have to slowly build up to this level of intensity. This is partially built into the progression described in Chapter 11, **"Adapting the CTTC Workouts,"** but you will still need to apply these recommendations to your own personal situation.

Rest Periods:

The length of the rest periods between sets is **extremely** important. Have a watch with you (see Chapter 6, **"Don't Forget to Accessorize"**) and do not rest any longer than is given in the workout description. You should be breathing hard from the end of the warm-up until you are into your cool-down. Between sets, breathe as was described in Chapter 7. If you are not breathing hard enough between sets, then increase the weight and/or shorten your rest periods.

The Exercises:

Do not change the order of the exercises. They are in this order for very specific reasons.

Do not substitute or alter the exercises unless it is absolutely unavoidable. They have been very carefully chosen for very specific reasons. If you do not have access to a particular piece of exercise equipment, then choose a substitute exercise that resembles the original exercise as closely as possible.

Do not add exercises, sets, or more repetitions than are called for in **CTTC** Workouts. These have also been carefully calculated.

Do not do "forced reps." A forced rep is one where someone helps you to do another repetition when you can no longer complete the rep on your own. Forced reps are counterproductive to this exercise program.

Do not take longer rest periods than are given. In fact, when your cardiovascular fitness has improved enough for you to be able to shorten the rest periods without sacrificing strength or exercise form, please do so. However, this shortening of rest periods does not apply to the highest level of Cardio-aerobics in **CTTC Workout #3**. Once you have reached this level, there is no advantage to be gained by shortening the "thirty seconds of medium effort" any more.

Note: Of course, once in a while it will happen that the piece of equipment that you need to use is occupied by someone else when you need it. If it is not possible to alternate with the person, then choose a substitute exercise that resembles the original exercise as closely as possible. This is preferable to having to wait too long between exercises. You have to keep your breathing and your heart rate elevated in order to enjoy the maximum benefits of the **CTTC** Exercise Program.

In order for you to get 100% out of the **CTTC** Exercise Program, you will have to follow these guidelines as closely as possible. The more you deviate from these guidelines, the less you will get out of this program. It is that simple.

CTTC Workout Number 3

Monday

CTTC **Workout #3** - 4 weeks long After these 4 weeks, take one week free from **all** exercise before beginning with CTTC **Workout #1** again.	**Exercise Tempo:** Explosive concentric, no pause, 4 seconds eccentric	
Monday: Back and Biceps		
1. Warm-Up	Build up to 85% of MHR for the last 5 minutes.	10 minutes
2. Lat Machine Pull-Downs to Chest – Wide Grip	1 minute rest between sets.	1 x 15 2 x 8 - 6
3. Lat Machine Pull-Downs to Chest – Shoulder Width Curl Grip – Elbows In	1 minute rest between sets.	2 x 8 - 6
4. Bent Over Barbell Rowing – Wide Grip – Elbows Out	1 minute rest between sets.	2 x 8 - 6
5. Bent Over Rowing - Shoulder Width Curl Grip – Elbows In	1 minute rest between sets.	2 x 8 - 6
6. Barbell Curls – Shoulder Width Grip	1 minute rest between sets.	2 x 8 - 6
7. Cardio-Aerobics	15 intervals of 10 seconds all-out effort followed by 30 seconds of medium effort.	10 minutes
8. Cool-Down	Moving and Stretching	10 minutes

NOTES

1st workout of the month	Time it took to complete the workout	Observations or comments about this workout
2nd workout of the month	Time it took to complete the workout	Observations or comments about this workout
3rd workout of the month	Time it took to complete the workout	Observations or comments about this workout
4th workout of the month	Time it took to complete the workout	Observations or comments about this workout

OTHER NOTES

Explanation of the Exercises

Monday

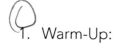

1. Warm-Up:

Do any type of movements that will increase your heart rate and increase your body temperature. Just make sure that the exercise does not use your arms (this would tire them too much for the workout which follows), and that you are able to keep control of your pulse rate. Power-walking, jogging, treadmills, elliptical walkers, steppers, bicycling, and exercise bicycles (home-trainers) are all good examples. Follow the Warm-Up progression for your particular group (situation) as it is described in **CTTC Workout #3** in Chapter 11, **"Adapting the CTTC Workouts."**

2. Lat Machine Pull-Downs to Chest – Wide Grip:

These are done exactly as explained in **CTTC Workout #1**, with the exception of the exercise tempo and the rest periods between the sets.

Here in **CTTC Workout #3**, the exercise tempo is an explosive concentric movement, no pause, followed by a four-second eccentric movement.

You should take one-minute rest periods between sets. When your cardiovascular fitness has improved enough for you to be able to shorten the rest periods without sacrificing strength or exercise form, please do so.

Read the **Positioning** and **Exercise Technique** instructions for Lat Machine Pull-Downs to Chest – Wide Grip in **CTTC Workout #1** again.

3. Lat Machine Pull-Downs to Chest – Shoulder-Width Curl Grip – Elbows In:

This exercise is also for the large back muscles (latissimus dorsi, or lats for short), which extend from your armpits all the way down to your waist. It also works the biceps very hard.

These are done exactly like Pull-Downs to Chest – Close Parallel Grip, as explained in **CTTC Workout #2**, with the exception of the grip, exercise tempo, and the rest periods between the sets.

Here you take a shoulder-width curl grip (the palms of your hands are facing you) and in **CTTC Workout #3**, the exercise tempo is an explosive concentric movement, no pause, followed by a four-second eccentric movement.

You should take one-minute rest periods between sets. When your cardiovascular fitness has improved enough for you to be able to shorten the rest periods without sacrificing strength or exercise form, please do so.

Read the **Positioning** and **Exercise Technique** instructions for Pull-Downs to Chest – Close Parallel Grip in **CTTC Workout #2** again.

4. Bent Over Barbell Rowing – Wide Grip – Elbows Out:

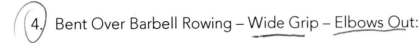

This exercise is for the several smaller muscles that run from the back of one shoulder, across your upper back, to the back of the other shoulder.

This exercise is done exactly like Bent Over Dumbbell Rowing – elbows out in **CTTC Workout #1**, with three exceptions: the equipment (a barbell), the exercise tempo, and the rest periods between sets.

Positioning: Grasp the barbell with an overhand grip (palms of your hands facing down). Your hands should be wide enough so that when you have pulled the bar **halfway** up to your chest, your upper arms will be parallel to the floor, forming a straight line through your shoulders, from one elbow to the other. Your forearms should then be parallel to each other and 90° to your upper arms. In other words, your arms should form a wide upside down "u". Continue pulling until the barbell touches the middle of your chest.

The exercise tempo in **CTTC Workout #3** is an explosive concentric movement, no pause, followed by a four-second eccentric movement.

You should take one-minute rest periods between sets. When your cardiovascular fitness has improved enough for you to be able to shorten the rest periods without sacrificing strength or exercise form, please do so.

Read the **Positioning** and **Exercise Technique** instructions for Bent Over Dumbbell Rowing – elbows out in **CTTC Workout #1** again.

Note: To help protect your lower back, I recommend wearing your lifting belt for this exercise (see Chapter 6, **"Don't Forget to Accessorize"**).

5. Bent Over Barbell Rowing – Shoulder Width Curl Grip – Elbows In:

This exercise works your back from your neck all the way down to your butt. It will add thickness to your entire back, especially along your spinal column.

This exercise is done exactly like Bent Over Barbell Rowing – Shoulder-Width Grip – elbows neutral in **CTTC Workout #2**, except for the grip, the exercise tempo, and the rest periods between sets.

Here you use a shoulder-width curl grip (palms of your hands facing up), and your elbows should stay as close to the sides of your body as possible as you pull them up and back.

The exercise tempo in **CTTC Workout #3** is an explosive concentric movement, no pause, followed by a four-second eccentric movement.

You should take one-minute rest periods between sets. When your cardiovascular fitness has improved enough for you to be able to shorten the rest periods without sacrificing strength or exercise form, please do so.

Read the **Positioning** and **Exercise Technique** instructions for Bent Over Barbell Rowing – Shoulder-Width Grip – elbows neutral in **CTTC Workout #2** again.

Note: To help protect your lower back, I recommend wearing your lifting belt for this exercise (see Chapter 6, **"Don't Forget to Accessorize"**).

6.) Barbell Curls – Shoulder Width Grip:

This exercise works both heads of the biceps (the muscle on the front of your upper arms).

Your biceps have assisted on all of the back exercises above, so they are already warmed up. This again saves you the time you would normally have to spend on a warm-up set for your biceps.

Positioning: Actually, the width of your hands on this exercise should be **slightly** less than shoulder width and, yes, it does make a difference. If it didn't, I wouldn't waste my time mentioning it.

So pick up a straight barbell (yes…that also makes a difference) with your hands **slightly** less than shoulder-width apart. Stand straight, with your feet shoulder-width apart and your knees slightly bent. Your elbows should be just in front, but still touching the sides of your body. Keep looking straight ahead. Now tighten your entire body to lock it in this position. Your elbows should be completely straight.

Exercise Technique: Curl (lift) the barbell up, moving only your forearms, until your forearms cannot move any further because they have been stopped by your upper arms. Your upper body should not move.

The exercise tempo in **CTTC Workout #3** is an explosive concentric movement, no pause, followed by a four-second eccentric movement.

Make sure that you begin and end this exercise with your elbows completely straight.

Breathing: Breathe in as you begin curling the barbell up. You should complete inhaling as the barbell reaches its highest point (by your shoulders). Breathe out slowly as you return to the starting position.

Do not move your upper arms or your body. Do not bounce or swing the barbell to get it up. Do not swing your shoulders or your body back to get the barbell started, or to finish the curl. If you need to do any of these things in order to curl the barbell, then you are using too much weight. Use less weight and perform the exercise correctly. Also do not let the barbell simply drop back to the beginning position. Keep the barbell under control at all times. Remember, lowering the weights slowly is always at least half the exercise, therefore, half the results.

Tip: If you want to work your forearms at the same time (and why wouldn't you?), begin this exercise by letting the barbell roll down your hands until you are holding it with only the tips of your fingers. Now slowly roll the barbell back up, with your fingers, until you are gripping it hard with your whole hand again. The next step is to curl your wrists up while still gripping the barbell as hard as you can. You begin to curl the barbell with your upper arms when your wrists can curl no further. Until that point, your lower arms should not move. Keep your wrists in this position for the remainder of the repetition, and then repeat the exercise for the rest of the 6-8 reps.

You should take one-minute rest periods between sets. When your cardiovascular fitness has improved enough for you to be able to shorten the rest periods without sacrificing strength or exercise form, please do so.

Note: To help protect your lower back, I recommend wearing your lifting belt for this exercise (see Chapter 6, **"Don't Forget to Accessorize"**).

7. Cardio-Aerobics:

You should still be breathing hard and your heart rate should still be elevated from doing this back and biceps workout. Therefore, you should begin your Cardio-aerobics immediately after completing these. Follow the Cardio-aerobics progression for your particular group (situation), as it is described in **CTTC Workout #3** in Chapter 11, **"Adapting the CTTC Workouts."**

8. Cool-Down:

Continue the exercise you used for your Cardio-aerobics for a couple of minutes longer at a lower intensity. This is the first part of your cool-down and allows your heart to slowly and safely return to a lower pulse rate. Then walk around easily, continuing to breathe deeply, as described in Chapter 7.

During this time, you should also use your elastic band (see Chapter 6, **"Don't Forget to Accessorize"**) to continually stretch your chest, arms, and shoulders. Next, occasionally stop to stretch your legs and your spine.

After your heart rate has returned to a more normal level, you can lie down or sit on the floor to more effectively stretch your legs and lower back. After you have finished doing this, stand up and thoroughly stretch your shoulders and calves one more time.

Do not shorten your cool-down or omit it altogether. Do not stand still, sit, or lie down immediately after completing a Cardio-aerobics session. Always taper off slowly.

CTTC Workout Number 3

Wednesday

CTTC **Workout #3** - 4 weeks long After these 4 weeks, take one week free from **all** exercise before beginning with CTTC **Workout #1** again.	**Exercise Tempo:** Explosive concentric, no pause, 4 seconds eccentric ✓	
Wednesday: Legs		
1. Warm-Up	Build up to 85% of MHR for the last 5 minutes.	10 minutes
2. Leg Extensions	Warm-Up	1 x 25
3. Leg Curls – Seated or Lying	Warm-Up	1 x 20
4. Smith Machine Barbell Squats	1½ minutes rest between sets.	1 set each of 20, 15, & 10 reps.
5. Leg Presses	1½ minutes rest between sets.	1 set each of 12, 10, & 8 reps.
6. Cardio-Aerobics	15 intervals of 10 seconds all-out effort followed by 30 seconds of medium effort.	10 minutes
7. Leg Press Calf Raises	1 minute rest between sets.	1 set each of 25, 20, 15, & 10 reps.
8. Cool-Down	Moving and Stretching	10 minutes

NOTES

1st workout of the month	Time it took to complete the workout	Observations or comments about this workout
2nd workout of the month	Time it took to complete the workout	Observations or comments about this workout
3rd workout of the month	Time it took to complete the workout	Observations or comments about this workout
4th workout of the month	Time it took to complete the workout	Observations or comments about this workout

OTHER NOTES

Explanation of the Exercises

Wednesday

1. Warm-Up:

Do any type of movements that will increase your heart rate and increase your body temperature. Just make sure that you are able to keep control of your pulse rate. Power-walking, jogging, treadmills, elliptical walkers, steppers, bicycling, and exercise bicycles (home-trainers) are all good examples. Follow the Warm-Up progression for your particular group (situation) as it is described in **CTTC Workout #3** in Chapter 11, **"Adapting the CTTC Workouts."**

2. Leg Extensions:

This is a warm-up set, so do the Leg Extensions exactly as in **CTTC Workout #1**.

VERY IMPORTANT: Do **not** use an explosive concentric movement (raising the weight) on this exercise.

Read the **Positioning** and **Exercise Technique** instructions for Leg Extensions in **CTTC Workout #1** again.

3. Leg Curls – Seated or Lying:

This is a warm-up set, so do the Leg Curls exactly as in **CTTC Workout #1**.

VERY IMPORTANT: Do **not** use an explosive concentric movement (raising the weight) on this exercise.

Read the **Positioning** and **Exercise Technique** instructions for Leg Curls in **CTTC Workout #1** again.

4. Smith Machine Barbell Squats:

These are done exactly as explained in **CTTC Workout #1**, with the exception of the exercise tempo and the rest periods between the sets.

Here in **CTTC Workout #3**, the exercise tempo is a four-second eccentric movement (lowering the weight), no pause, followed by an explosive concentric movement (pushing the weight up).

You should take 1½ minute rest periods between sets. When your cardiovascular fitness has improved enough for you to be able to shorten the rest periods without sacrificing strength or exercise form, please do so.

Read the **Positioning** and **Exercise Technique** instructions for Smith Machine Barbell Squats in **CTTC Workout #1** again.

Note: To help protect your lower back, I recommend wearing your lifting belt for this exercise (see Chapter 6, **"Don't Forget to Accessorize"**).

5. Leg Presses:

These are done exactly as explained in **CTTC Workout #2**, with the exception of the exercise tempo and the rest periods between the sets.

Here in **CTTC Workout #3**, the exercise tempo is a four-second eccentric movement (lowering the weight), no pause, followed by an explosive concentric movement (pushing the weight up).

You should take 1½ minute rest periods between sets. When your cardiovascular fitness has improved enough for you to be able to shorten the rest periods without sacrificing strength or exercise form, please do so.

Read the **Positioning** and **Exercise Technique** instructions for Leg Presses in **CTTC Workout #2** again.

Note: To help protect your lower back, I recommend wearing your lifting belt for this exercise (see Chapter 6, **"Don't Forget to Accessorize"**).

6. Cardio-Aerobics:

You should still be breathing hard and your heart rate should still be elevated from doing this leg workout. Therefore, you should begin your Cardio-aerobics immediately after completing your last set of Leg Presses. Follow the Cardio-aerobics progression for your particular group (situation) as it is described in **CTTC Workout #3** in Chapter 11, **"Adapting the CTTC Workouts."**

Continue the exercise you used for your Cardio-aerobics for a couple of minutes longer at a lower intensity. This is the first part of your cool down and allows your heart to slowly and safely return to a lower pulse rate.

Do not jump into this intense form of aerobics if you are not physically prepared for it, or abruptly terminate a Cardio-aerobics session without slowly tapering off.

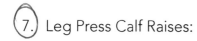 **7.** Leg Press Calf Raises:

Because you can use heavier weights, this exercise will add some size, as well as shape, to your calves.

Positioning: Place yourself on a Leg Press Machine with the balls of your feet on the lowest part of the foot platform. Your heels should be hanging over, and your knees should be locked out (straight). Your feet should be approximately shoulder width apart, with your toes pointing either straight ahead or slightly out at a natural angle (whatever that is for you). For a little variety, you can change your foot position with each set. In any case, your stance should feel natural and comfortable.

Exercise Technique: These are done exactly like Standing Calf Raises, as explained in **CTTC Workout #1**, with the exception of the exercise tempo and the rest periods between the sets.

Here in **CTTC Workout #3**, the exercise tempo is a four-second eccentric movement (lowering the weight), no pause, followed by an explosive concentric movement (pushing the weight up).

You should take one-minute rest periods between sets. When your cardiovascular fitness has improved enough for you to be able to shorten the rest periods without sacrificing strength or exercise form, please do so.

Read the **Exercise Technique** instructions for Standing Calf Raises in **CTTC Workout #1** again.

8. Cool-Down:

Walk around easily, continuing to breathe deeply as described in Chapter 7, **"The CTTC Workouts: Scientific Fitness versus Science Fiction."** Occasionally stop to stretch your legs, your spine, and your calves.

After your heart rate has returned to a more normal level, you can lie down or sit on the floor to more effectively stretch your legs and lower back. After you have finished doing this, stand up and thoroughly stretch your calves one more time.

Do not shorten your cool-down or omit it altogether. Do not stand still, sit, or lie down immediately after completing a Cardio-aerobics session. Always taper off slowly.

CTTC Workout Number 3

Friday

CTTC Workout #3 - 4 weeks long After these 4 weeks, take one week free from **all** exercise before beginning with **CTTC Workout #1** again.	**Exercise Tempo:** Explosive concentric, no pause, 4 seconds eccentric.	
Friday: Chest, Triceps, Shoulders, and Waist		
1. Warm-Up	Build up to 85% of MHR for the last 5 minutes.	10 minutes
2. 45° Incline Barbell Bench Press – Shoulder-Width Grip – Elbows Neutral	1 minute rest between sets.	1 set each of 15, 10, & 8 reps.
3. Flat Barbell Bench Press – Wide Grip – Elbows Out	1 minute rest between sets.	3 x 8 - 6
4. Barbell Upright Rowing – Shoulder-Width Grip	1 minute rest between sets.	3 x 8 - 6
5. Standing Barbell Press – Elbows Out	1 minute rest between sets.	2 x 8 - 6
6. The following exercises should be done consecutively. • Repeat this sequence 2 times. a. Lying Back Extensions – done very slowly – 4 seconds up, 1 second pause, 4 seconds down	No rest.	10
b. Seated Trunk Twists – hold for 2 seconds on each side, on each rep.	No rest.	10 x each side
c. Crunches – done slowly – with a 1 second pause	No rest	15
7. Cardio-Aerobics	15 intervals of 10 seconds all-out effort followed by 30 seconds of medium effort.	10 minutes
8. Cool-Down	Moving and Stretching	10 minutes

NOTES

1st workout of the month	Time it took to complete the workout	Observations or comments about this workout
2nd workout of the month	Time it took to complete the workout	Observations or comments about this workout
3rd workout of the month	Time it took to complete the workout	Observations or comments about this workout
4th workout of the month	Time it took to complete the workout	Observations or comments about this workout

OTHER NOTES

Explanation of the Exercises

Friday

1. Warm-Up:

Do any type of movements that will increase your heart rate and increase your body temperature. Just make sure that the exercise does not use your arms (this would tire them too much for the workout which follows), and that you are able to keep control of your pulse rate. Power-walking, jogging, treadmills, elliptical walkers, steppers, bicycling, and exercise bicycles (home-trainers) are all good examples. Follow the Warm-Up progression for your particular group (situation) as it is described in **CTTC Workout #3** in Chapter 11, **"Adapting the CTTC Workouts."**

2. 45° Incline Barbell Bench Press – Shoulder-Width Grip – Elbows Neutral:

This exercise emphasizes the development of the upper portion of your chest muscles, as well as your triceps.

This exercise is done exactly like Flat Bench Barbell Bench Press – Shoulder-Width Grip – elbows neutral in **CTTC Workout #2**, except for the incline and the exercise tempo.

Here we use an incline bench set at 45° instead of a flat exercise bench. The exercise tempo in **CTTC Workout #3** is a four-second eccentric movement (lowering the weight until the bar touches the middle of your chest at about the nipple line), no pause, followed by an explosive concentric movement (pushing the weight up).

You should take one-minute rest periods between sets. When your cardiovascular fitness has improved enough for you to be able to shorten the rest periods without sacrificing strength or exercise form, please do so.

Read the **Positioning** and **Exercise Technique** instructions for Flat Bench Barbell Bench Press – Shoulder-Width Grip – elbows neutral in **CTTC Workout #2** again.

3. Flat Barbell Bench Press – Wide Grip – Elbows Out:

This exercise develops the entire pectoralis major (chest muscle).

This exercise is done exactly like 30°-45° Incline Barbell Bench Press – Wide Grip – Elbows Out in **CTTC Workout #2**, except for the incline and the exercise tempo.

Here we use a flat exercise bench instead of an incline. The exercise tempo in **CTTC Workout #3** is a four-second eccentric movement (lowering the weight to the middle of your chest, between the nipple line and your collar bones), no pause, followed by an explosive concentric movement (pushing the weight up).

You should take one-minute rest periods between sets. When your cardiovascular fitness has improved enough for you to be able to shorten the rest periods without sacrificing strength or exercise form, please do so.

Read the **Positioning** and **Exercise Technique** instructions for 30°-45° Incline Barbell Bench Press – Wide Grip – elbows out in **CTTC Workout #2** again.

4. Barbell Upright Rowing – Shoulder-Width Grip:

This exercise will develop the middle section of the deltoids (the muscle on the side of your shoulders) as well as the muscles in your upper back.

This exercise is done exactly like Dumbbell Upright Rowing in **CTTC Workout #2**, except for the equipment, the exercise tempo, and the rest periods between the sets.

Here we use a straight barbell instead of dumbbells. The exercise tempo in **CTTC Workout #3** is an explosive concentric movement (lifting the weight), no pause, followed by a four-second eccentric movement (lowering the weight).

You should take one-minute rest periods between sets. When your cardiovascular fitness has improved enough for you to be able to shorten the rest periods without sacrificing strength or exercise form, please do so.

Read the **Positioning** and **Exercise Technique** instructions for Dumbbell Upright Rowing in **CTTC Workout #2** again. Make sure that your grip on the barbell is wide enough that, when your upper arms are parallel with the floor (the highest point of the exercise), they form a straight line through your shoulders, from one elbow to the other. Having your elbows (upper arms) slightly behind your shoulders at this point is OK. Allowing your elbows to move in front of your shoulders is **not** OK.

Note: To help protect your lower back, I recommend wearing your lifting belt for this exercise (see Chapter 6, **"Don't Forget to Accessorize"**).

5. Standing Barbell Press – Elbows Out:

This exercise works all three sections of the deltoid muscle, plus the triceps and the muscles of the upper back.

This exercise is done exactly like the Seated Barbell Press in **CTTC Workout #2**, except for the exercise tempo, the rest periods between the sets, and the fact that that you are standing instead of sitting.

The exercise tempo in **CTTC Workout #3** is an explosive concentric movement (pushing the weight up), no pause, followed by a four-second eccentric movement (lowering the weight).

You should take one-minute rest periods between sets. When your cardiovascular fitness has improved enough for you to be able to shorten the rest periods without sacrificing strength or exercise form, please do so.

Read the **Positioning** and **Exercise Technique** instructions for the Seated Barbell Press in **CTTC Workout #2** again. The only difference is that, instead of sitting, you will now be standing with your feet **slightly** more than shoulder width apart. Don't forget to tighten your midsection to stabilize your body.

Note: To help protect your lower back, I recommend wearing your lifting belt for this exercise (see Chapter 6, **"Don't Forget to Accessorize"**).

6.   a- Lying Back Extensions – Bodyweight Only:

These are done exactly as in **CTTC Workout #1**, except that when your upper body can not rise up any further, hold this position and consciously contract (tense) your entire back as hard as you can for one second. Don't forget to also squeeze your butt together as hard as possible at this point.

VERY IMPORTANT: Do **not** use an explosive concentric movement (raising your back) on this exercise.

Read the **Positioning** and **Exercise Technique** instructions for Lying Back Extensions in **CTTC Workout #1** again.

b- Seated Trunk Twists – Bodyweight Only:

This exercise takes the place of all those "crooked" crunches, "sideways" sit-ups, "lateral" leg raises, and other exotic abdominal exercises that you can see people **trying** to do in gyms all over the world. Unless you are a fanatic bodybuilder or an elite athlete who uses these particular muscles in your sport, these exercises are mostly a waste of time.

All these exercises work the external and internal oblique muscles, which are located on each side of your waist. But these muscles are also used somewhat during crunches, to assist your abdominals in bringing your pelvis closer to your ribs. So now you do **more** crunches, but add a twist to them, thereby **half** working your abdominals and **half** working your obliques. That's really **not** using your exercise time efficiently…especially when the every-day purpose of the obliques is to twist your body from the waist when you are standing or sitting up straight.

Let's see now, how many times during your day do you sit up from a lying position and simultaneously twist your upper body…unless you are lying on the couch and have to reach for a beer on the coffee

Now, how many times during your day do you have to **powerfully** twist your upper body to reach for something while you are standing or sitting? Maybe…never?

And then we have the infamous side bends while holding a dumbbell, or using some other form of resistance. Most people seem to think that this exercise is done by quickly dropping their body down on the side where they are holding the dumbbell, and then partially straightening up again. They don't seem to realize that they are actually attempting to exercise the muscles on **the other side** of their bodies and, therefore, they need to straighten up and continue to bend completely over to that side in order to effectively work those muscles. Let's see now, how many times during your day (or ever) do you bend straight over sideways to pick up something heavy? Also maybe…never?

Last, but certainly not least, why would you ever want to develop a muscle which could actually make your waist appear wider and/or make you look like you have a "spare tire" around your waist? You are then busy destroying the illusion instead of creating the illusion. You don't want to build these muscles, you want to strengthen them so that they become tight (toned) and strong, but flexible…and stay that way. Leave these exercises to the athletes who do need them for their particular sports.

In **CTTC Workout #1** I said that crunches (when done correctly) "will provide your abdominal area with 80% of all the exercise it needs". The remaining 20% is covered by **Seated Trunk Twists**.

When done correctly, **Seated Trunk Twists** will strengthen, tighten, and "tone" all the muscles of your midsection (or your "core" as the latest fad exercise programs like to call it), thereby actually making your waist smaller. It will do much more to help to flatten your stomach…especially that hard-to-affect lower abdominal area (pot belly)…than all those knee raises, leg raises, reverse crunches, and other "lower abdominal" exercises that I see hundreds of exercisers doing… mostly incorrectly!

Seated Trunk Twists will also increase and maintain the twisting flexibility of your entire spinal column and will strengthen the smaller muscles which help to support and rotate your spine. This will help to keep your spine young and healthy.

That's a lot of really great results from an easy exercise that few people use in their exercise programs. Of those who do, very few do this exercise correctly. What a waste of a truly terrific exercise.

Positioning: Take a broomstick, a barbell without any weights on the ends, or some other "stick-like" object, and sit down straddling an exercise bench. The "stick" must not be heavy. Your knees should be on each side of the bench so that they cannot move sideways. Sit perfectly straight, look straight ahead, and squeeze the bench with your knees. Place the stick behind your head, resting on your shoulders. Grasp the ends of the stick with your hands, or hang your wrists over the top of the stick at the ends. The stick should be long enough so that your arms will be almost straight when you are in this beginning position. Keep your head in a straight line with your body.

Exercise Technique: Beginning with your lower back, slowly twist your upper body to the left (or right) as far as possible. When your lower back will twist no further, continue twisting with your shoulders. When your shoulders will twist no further, continue twisting with your head. When your head will twist no further, hold this position for two seconds and consciously contract all the muscles you are using to twist your upper body.

Slowly return to the beginning position, following the same exercise form in reverse. Twist your upper body to the other side, following the same exercise form.

Breathing: Breathe out slowly as you begin twisting to the side. You should complete exhaling as you complete the twisting. Breathe in slowly as you return to the starting position. Follow the same breathing pattern as you twist to the other side.

Do not jerk or swing your upper body. Do not allow your legs or hips to move. Do not allow your head or upper body to bend forward. Do not push or pull the "stick" with your hands when you are twisting your shoulders. This is another exercise which has to be done slowly in order to be maximally effective.

c- Crunches – Bodyweight Only:

These are done exactly as in **CTTC Workout #1**, except for a change in exercise tempo. In this workout, you do a three-second concentric contraction (curling your upper body up). When your upper body can not curl up any further, hold this position for one second and then consciously contract (tense) your abdominals, as hard as you can, once more before you lower your upper body back to the beginning position. Breathe out forcefully again during this second contraction. Your upper body will only move very slightly, but you will definitely feel a maximal contraction.

Slowly return (four seconds) to the beginning position following the same exercise form in reverse.

Read the **Positioning** and **Exercise Technique** instructions for Crunches in **CTTC Workout #1** again.

7. Cardio-Aerobics:

You should still be breathing hard and your heart rate should still be elevated from doing the Back Extensions, Trunk Twists, and Crunches. Therefore, you should begin your Cardio-aerobics immediately after completing these. Follow the Cardio-aerobics progression for your particular group (situation), as it is described in **CTTC Workout #3** in Chapter 11, **"Adapting the CTTC Workouts."**

Do not jump into this intense form of aerobics if you are not physically prepared for it, nor should you abruptly terminate a Cardio-aerobics session without slowly tapering off.

8. Cool-Down:

Continue the exercise you used for your Cardio-aerobics for a couple of minutes longer at a lower intensity. This is the first part of your cool-down and allows your heart to slowly and safely return to a lower pulse rate. Then walk around easily, continuing to breathe deeply as described in Chapter 7.

During this time, you should also use your elastic band (see Chapter 6, **"Don't Forget to Accessorize"**) to continually stretch your chest, arms, and shoulders. Next, occasionally stop to stretch your legs and your spine.

After your heart rate has returned to a more normal level, you can lie down or sit on the floor to more effectively stretch your legs and lower back. After you have finished doing this, stand up and thoroughly stretch your shoulders and calves one more time.

Do not shorten your cool-down or omit it altogether. Do not stand still, sit, or lie down immediately after completing a Cardio-aerobics session. Always taper off slowly.

CONGRATULATIONS!

If you have paid your dues by faithfully and conscientiously, following **The CTTC Exercise and Nutrition Programs** this far, you will have made spectacular gains in your levels of health and fitness. You will have also radically changed the shape and composition of your body and be in much better control of your body-fat. Well done! Now be sure to keep up the good work. Your results will continue to amaze you and your satisfaction with yourself will continue to grow.

After completing **CTTC Workout #3,** take **one complete week of rest** from all exercise. Enjoyable low-to-medium intensity exercise activities are allowed during this week. Adjust your food intake accordingly, i.e., eat a little less during this week…not differently…just a little less.

After this week of rest and recuperation, begin **CTTC Workout #1** again, but begin adapting the **CTTC** Workouts to better suit your personal goals and circumstances.

Chapter 11

ADAPTING THE CTTC WORKOUTS

This **CTTC** Exercise and Nutrition Program is designed to achieve superior health and fitness goals as well as to sculpt a more attractive body. If you follow this **CTTC** program faithfully and conscientiously, you will develop a very high level of cardiovascular fitness, strong and supple muscles, and a healthier, shapelier body. Depending on your present condition, available time, and degree of motivation, you may have to repeat this program one or more times. However, after your general goals have been reached, the workouts will need to become better adapted to your specific needs and specific goals.

I obviously have no way of knowing who will read this book. I don't know if you are skinny or over-fat, average or otherwise, healthy or unhealthy…or somewhere in between. I also can't know what your strong and weak points are. You will have to honestly determine these for yourself. Only then will you be able to effectively adapt the **CTTC** Workouts to better suit your personal needs.

Find Your Strengths

For example, I very rarely do any direct exercises for my abdominals (stomach muscles). Yes, you read that right. I very rarely do any direct exercises for my abdominals, and yes, I do have a six-pack (washboard stomach)…at sixty years young.

The reason I can do this is that I developed very strong stomach muscles when I was a diver and gymnast. Since then, my work as an acrobat, exercising with weights, and regularly taking part in various exercise activities have been enough to keep my stomach muscles healthy and strong. Because I use exercise machines very sparingly, my abdominals have to constantly contract to stabilize my torso while I am exercising other body parts.

Beer Gut Abs

When it is time to get into "beach shape" again, I will **occasionally** do a couple of sets of quality crunches, just to put the finishing touches on my abdominals again, but otherwise, why on earth would I want to build big, thick stomach muscles that hang over my belt like a beer gut when they are not tensed? I try to sculpt my body so that I like the way it looks when I stand relaxed. I am lazy, remember. Walking around flexed all day is much too much work for me. And if you are not trying to build big, thick stomach muscles, then why are you spending all that time doing abdominal exercises? Some exercisers even do abdominal exercises using extra weight. Why? To make their waists smaller? I don't think so.

Enough Is Enough

You should have realized by now that I really hate to waste time when I am exercising. I want to get it over with as quickly as possible so I can get back to doing things I really enjoy. Once you have developed strong and healthy abdominal muscles, you need only do the **minimum** amount of direct abdominal exercise needed to **maintain** them. If you are over-fat and one of your goals is to have visible abdominal muscles, the solution is **not** to do **more** abdominal exercises…it is to lose more excess body-fat. One-inch thick abs cannot be seen under a two-inch layer of flab.

Ten minutes of Cardio-aerobics will do ten times more to make your six-pack visible (or your waist smaller) than will another ten minutes of abdominal exercises. But also never forget that how, when, and what you eat will ultimately determine whether you will become the proud owner of a visible six-pack or not.

Please note: I am not saying here that everyone should develop visible abdominals. I am sure that some people even find them ugly. That is OK. I happen to like them…for myself. You don't have to like them, although I am quite sure that you would like to have a smaller, tighter waist. What I am saying here is that when you are at a point where you are satisfied with **any** body part, cut your exercise for that particular body part down to a **maintenance** level so you are not wasting time and energy exercising something that doesn't need it anymore. Spend that time on your weaker body parts. Exercise efficiently! Exercise intelligently!

More Examples

I also never do any direct exercises for my forearms. Once again, while I was a gymnast I developed very strong forearms by hanging onto the apparatus with a death grip…out of pure fear. Now, I never use anything to help me grip the equipment when I am exercising. I don't use hooks or straps when I do pulling exercises, and when I am using dumbbells or a barbell, I always forcefully squeeze the bar. This not only keeps my forearms strong, without extra exercise, but also helps my concentration and control of the exercise. However, you will not enjoy as much of this benefit if you use predominantly exercise machines.

My lower chest (pecs) responds easily to exercise, and I am satisfied with its present size and shape. My upper chest, however, is one of my least responsive body parts. For this reason, I do **only** chest exercises for my upper chest. The lower chest muscles are used secondarily and as stabilizing muscles in many exercises, and that is enough stimulation to **maintain** mine to my satisfaction. Prioritizing like this brings my upper and lower chest into better balance while, once again, saving me a lot of time in my exercise program.

Fortunately for me, the majority of the exercises I do for my upper chest (and some that I do for my shoulders) also directly involve my triceps (muscles in the back of the arms). Since my triceps also respond quite easily to exercise, and I am satisfied with their present size and shape, I very rarely need to do any direct exercises for them either.

Get Smart

These are all good examples of working **smarter** for **better** results, rather than working **longer** or **harder** for **possible** results.

While I am on this subject…I often see relatively thin exercisers (especially ladies with less than 25% body-fat) spending hours and hours, day after day, on treadmills, exercise bikes, etc. Well I have some great advice for you: **Get off!** This is a massive waste of time. You can keep your body-fat under control…**better**…with much **less** aerobics than this.

Sweat Where It Counts

I hope you are beginning to get the point here. I continually see people spending the same amount of time exercising their good body parts as they do their less satisfactory body parts. Some people even spend **more** time exercising their better body parts than they do their inadequate ones, because they are avoiding the confrontation. These exercisers are in denial. I guess they think that if they make their good body parts even better, no one will notice the inferior ones. Sorry…the contrast just makes the inferior ones look even more out of balance.

Minimum Effort

Once you are satisfied with a particular body part, you should do only the **minimum** amount of exercise needed to maintain that body part. Spend your time improving things that **need** improving. Doing this will have three major consequences.

1. Your body will become shapelier and better balanced.
2. This will happen more quickly.
3. You will be spending **less time** exercising…with **better results** to show for it.

Intelligent Exercise

This is the difference between exercising intelligently, or just doing a certain number of exercises…or just exercising for a certain amount of time. After you have completed the entire twelve-week **CTTC** Exercise Program for the first time **without any adaptations**, you can begin to alter the workouts to better suit your personal situation. Simply do fewer sets for the body parts with which you are already satisfied. Do not add sets for your less satisfactory body parts yet. Just concentrate and visualize better to make these sets more effective.

This is when you **really** begin to **exercise less**…with **better results** to show for it. More for less…I just love it when that happens!

Now let's examine who should be doing what and…just as importantly…who should **not** be doing what.

BEGINNING EXERCISERS

Beginners are persons who have **never** exercised. (or who have exercised with weights and/or aerobics for **less than** six months.

Welcome to the world of better fitness, better health, and a better quality of life. You have a very difficult task in front of you. After you begin the **CTTC** Exercise and Nutrition Programs and start enjoying all the benefits you have been missing up to now, you are going to have to temper your enthusiasm for exercising, or you will burn out. If you follow the guidelines, that will not happen.

INTERMEDIATE EXERCISERS

Intermediates are persons who have seriously exercised with weights and/or aerobics for **at least** six months.

ADVANCED EXERCISERS

Advanced exercisers are persons who have seriously exercised with weights **and** aerobics for **more than** one year.

If you have seriously followed a Quality Exercise program, which includes both cardiovascular building aerobics and exercising with reasonably heavy weights…for **more than** one year…you may be able to begin with **CTTC Workout #1** and continue through **CTTC** Workouts **#2** and **#3** without any adaptations.

Nevertheless, for safety's sake, I still recommend that you ease into each of the three **CTTC** Workouts the first time around. Always listen to your body and make adjustments according to your personal circumstances.

SENIOR EXERCISERS

If you are a fellow Senior Citizen, you will have to decide for yourself where to begin the **CTTC** Exercise Program. This is because the levels of health and fitness vary enormously within this group of people. I know some "young," healthy eighty-year-olds, as well as many "old," unhealthy fifty-year-olds. Heck, I have seen a fair share of "old," unhealthy thirty-year-olds, for that matter.

As a matter of fact, a good friend of ours is the oldest performing acrobat in the world. He is ninety-six years young and can still do several chin-ups with his legs in an "L" position, while using only two fingers. He can do other amazing feats of strength as well. He finds this to be completely "normal." I agree with him.

If you are healthy, active, and have consistently done some type of vigorous exercise for the past several years, you may be able to start with **CTTC** Workout #1, **Category Number 1**. The categories are explained at the beginning of each **CTTC** Workout in this chapter.

If you have not been consistently active for the past several years, or if you are over-fat, or if your health is not at a high level, I would strongly suggest that you begin with **CTTC** Workout #1, **Category Number 2**. The categories are explained at the beginning of each **CTTC** Workout in this chapter.

The debate goes on as to whether exercise can actually add years to your life…or not…but one thing is sure:

The CTTC Exercise and Nutrition Programs will add LIFE to your years!

SPECIAL MEDICAL PROBLEMS

Whether you are a Senior Citizen…or obese…or not…if you have special medical problems you should undertake **any** exercise program only under the supervision of a competent medical doctor/ therapist, or with a competent personal trainer working together with your doctor/therapist. **Do not** attempt this **CTTC** Exercise Program (or any other exercise program) without this supervision.

WHERE DO I BEGIN

First you need to decide which level of exerciser you are: Beginner, Intermediate, or Advanced.

Next, decide which one of the two categories of exercise you belong in: **Category #1**, or **Category #2**, depending on your personal situation.

The 2 categories are:

1. If you are **less than twenty** pounds over-fat (smaller, shorter persons), or **less than** forty pounds over-fat (larger, taller persons), but are otherwise in reasonably good health.

2. If you are a **non-exercising** Senior Citizen, or if you are **obese** but have no other life-threatening medical problems, or other physical problems (such as problems with your joints, tendons, etc) which could be exacerbated by these exercises.

For instance, if you are a Beginning or Intermediate exerciser belonging in **Category #1,** simply go to **The Adapted CTTC Workout #1 For Beginners/Intermediates** and follow the (adapted) **CTTC** Exercise Program for **Category #1** from there.

If you are a Beginning or Intermediate exerciser belonging in **Category #2,** simply go to **The Adapted CTTC Workout #1 For Beginners/Intermediates** and follow the (adapted) CTTC Exercise Program for **Category #2** from there.

If you are an **Advanced** exerciser, simply begin the CTTC Exercise Program, **without any adaptations**.

STILL NOT SURE?

If you have **any** doubts whatsoever, start with **The Adapted CTTC Workout #1 for Beginners/Intermediates, Category #2.**

RECOMMENDED

I do strongly recommend that you photocopy (or scan) each **CTTC** Workout that you are using, as well as the **Explanation of the Exercises** which correspond to that workout. Take these with you when you go to exercise.

This will not only prevent confusion during your workout, but you can also jot down notes and reminders to yourself for future reference. You should use these copies to keep track of the amount of weight you are using for each exercise and how much time it takes you to complete the workouts.

This is a great way to keep track of your progress. I always do this so I can look back and see which exercise program I was doing one month ago (or thirty years ago), how successful (or unsuccessful) it was, what I learned from it, how much weight I was using for the different exercises, how much I weighed at the time, and what my measurements were then. This treasure trove of information is one of the reasons I am able to write this book now.

THE ADAPTED CTTC WORKOUT #1

FOR BEGINNERS/INTERMEDIATES

CATEGORY #1

Beginners are persons who have **never** exercised, or who have exercised with weights and/or aerobics for **less than** six months.

Intermediates are persons who have seriously exercised with weights and/or aerobics for **at least** six months.

Category #1: If you are **less than** twenty pounds over-fat (smaller, shorter persons), or **less than** forty pounds over-fat (larger, taller persons), but are otherwise in **reasonably good health**, you should start **The Adapted CTTC Workout #1** as follows:

IMPORTANT NOTE: Use the first two weeks to experiment and find the correct weight to use on each of the exercises. Slowly add weight to the exercises, but without sacrificing correct exercise form.

First Week
- Warm-up – build up to only **70%** of your **MHR** for the **last minute**.
- Do only **one set** of each exercise. Experiment to find the correct weight to use on each exercise.
- Do only **three** intervals of **CTTC Workout #1** Cardio-aerobics.

Second Week
- Warm-up – build up to only **75%** of your **MHR** for the **last minute**.
- Do only **two sets** of each exercise (unless the exercise calls for only one set). Concentrate on exercise form.
- Do only **four** intervals of **CTTC Workout #1** Cardio-aerobics.

Third Week
- Warm-up – build up to **80%** of your **MHR** for the **last minute**.
- Do **all sets** of each exercise, but don't use too much weight. Your body is still learning the proper technique for each of the exercises.
- Do only **five** intervals of **CTTC Workout #1** Cardio-aerobics.

Fourth Week
- Warm-up – build up to **85%** of your **MHR** for the **last minute**.
- Do **all sets** of each exercise, still concentrating on correct exercise form.
- Do only **six** intervals of **CTTC Workout #1** Cardio-aerobics.

Start **The Adapted CTTC Workout #1** again. Do the complete program for **four** more weeks. Do **all** the sets of each exercise. Slowly begin adding weight to the exercises when possible, but always use perfect exercise technique (form). The intensity of your warm-ups and the Cardio-aerobics at the end of the workout should be as follows:

First Week
- Warm-up – build up to **85%** of your **MHR** for the **last minute**.
- Do only **seven** intervals of **CTTC Workout #1** Cardio-aerobics.

Second Week
- Warm-up – build up to **85%** of your **MHR** for the **last minute**.
- Do only **eight** intervals of **CTTC Workout #1** Cardio-aerobics.

Third Week
- Warm-up – build up to **85%** of your **MHR** for the **last minute**.
- Do only **nine** intervals of **CTTC Workout #1** Cardio-aerobics.

Fourth Week
- Warm-up – build up to **85%** of your **MHR** for the **last minute**.
- Do all **ten** intervals of **CTTC Workout #1** Cardio-aerobics.

```
┌─────────────────────────────────────────────────────┐
│                                                       │
│         THE ADAPTED CTTC WORKOUT #2                    │
│                                                       │
│         FOR BEGINNERS/INTERMEDIATES                    │
│                                                       │
│                CATEGORY #1                            │
│                                                       │
└─────────────────────────────────────────────────────┘
```

IMPORTANT NOTE: When starting **The Adapted CTTC Workout #2**, all exercisers should follow the same procedure as you did with **The Adapted CTTC Workout #1**. Use the first two weeks to experiment and find the correct weight to use on each of the exercises. Slowly add weight to the exercises, but without sacrificing correct exercise form.

- You should have repeated **The Adapted CTTC Workout #1** and, therefore, now be prepared for **The Adapted CTTC Workout #2**, with the following adaptations:

First Week
- Warm-up – build up to **85%** of your **MHR** for the last **two** minutes.
- Do only **one set** of each exercise. Experiment to find the correct weight to use on each exercise.
- Do only **five** intervals of **CTTC Workout #2** Cardio-aerobics.

Second Week
- Warm-up – build up to **85%** of your **MHR** for the last **two** minutes.
- Do only **two sets** of each exercise (unless the exercise calls for only one set). Concentrate on exercise form.
- Do only **six** intervals of **CTTC Workout #2** Cardio-aerobics.

Third Week
- Warm-up – build up to **85%** of your **MHR** for the last **two** minutes.
- Do **all sets** of each exercise, but don't use too much weight. Your body is still learning the proper technique for each of the exercises.
- Do only **seven** intervals of **CTTC Workout #2** Cardio-aerobics.

Fourth Week
- Warm-up – build up to **85%** of your **MHR** for the last **two** minutes.
- Do **all sets** of each exercise, still concentrating on correct exercise form.
- Do only **eight** intervals of **CTTC Workout #2** Cardio-aerobics.

Start **The Adapted CTTC Workout #2** again. Do the complete program for **four** more weeks. Do **all** the sets of each exercise. Slowly begin adding weight to the exercises when possible, but always use perfect exercise technique (form). The intensity of your warm-ups and the Cardio-aerobics at the end of the workout should be as follows:

First Week
- Warm-up – build up to **85%** of your **MHR** for the last **three** minutes.
- Do only **nine** intervals of **CTTC Workout #2** Cardio-aerobics.

Second Week
- Warm-up – build up to **85%** of your **MHR** for the last **three** minutes.
- Do only **ten** intervals of **CTTC Workout #2** Cardio-aerobics.

Third Week
- Warm-up – build up to **85%** of your **MHR** for the last **three** minutes.
- Do only **eleven** intervals of **CTTC Workout #2** Cardio-aerobics.

Fourth Week
- Warm-up – build up to **85%** of your **MHR** for the last **three** minutes.
- Do all **twelve** intervals of **CTTC Workout #2** Cardio-aerobics.

> THE ADAPTED CTTC WORKOUT #3
>
> FOR BEGINNERS/INTERMEDIATES
>
> CATEGORY #1

IMPORTANT NOTE: When starting **The Adapted CTTC Workout #3**, all exercisers should follow the same procedure as you did with **The Adapted CTTC Workouts #1 and #2.** Use the first two weeks to experiment and find the correct weight to use on each of the exercises. Slowly add weight to the exercises, but without sacrificing correct exercise form.

- You should have repeated **The Adapted CTTC Workout #2** and, therefore, now be prepared for **The Adapted CTTC Workout #3**, with the following adaptations:

First Week
- Warm-up – build up to **85%** of your **MHR** for the last **four** minutes.
- Do only **eight** intervals of **CTTC Workout #3** Cardio-aerobics.

Second Week
- Warm-up – build up to **85%** of your **MHR** for the last **four** minutes.
- Do only **nine** intervals of **CTTC Workout #3** Cardio-Aerobics.

Third Week
- Warm-up – build up to **85%** of your **MHR** for the last **four** minutes.
- Do only **ten** intervals of **CTTC Workout #3** Cardio-Aerobics.

Fourth Week
- Warm-up – build up to **85%** of your **MHR** for the last **four** minutes.
- Do only **eleven** intervals of **CTTC Workout #3** Cardio-Aerobics.

Start **The Adapted CTTC Workout #3** again. Do the complete program for **four** more weeks. Do **all** the sets of each exercise. Slowly begin adding weight to the exercises when possible, but always use perfect exercise technique (form). The intensity of your warm-ups and the Cardio-aerobics at the end of the workout should be as follows:

First Week
- Warm-up – build up to **85%** of your **MHR** for the last **five** minutes.
- Do only **twelve** intervals of **CTTC Workout #3** Cardio-aerobics.

Second Week
- Warm-up – build up to **85%** of your **MHR** for the last **five** minutes.
- Do only **thirteen** intervals of **CTTC Workout #3** Cardio-aerobics.

Third Week
- Warm-up – build up to **85%** of your **MHR** for the last **five** minutes.
- Do only **fourteen** intervals of **CTTC Workout #3** Cardio-aerobics.

Fourth Week
- Warm-up – build up to **85%** of your **MHR** for the last **five** minutes.
- Do all **fifteen** intervals of **CTTC Workout #3** Cardio-aerobics.

CONGRATULATIONS!

If you have paid your dues by faithfully and conscientiously following **The Adapted CTTC Exercise and Nutrition Programs** this far, you will have made spectacular gains in your levels of health and fitness. You will have also radically changed the shape and composition of your body, and be in much better control of your body-fat. Well done! Now be sure to keep up the good work. Believe it or not, the hardest part is now over. From this point on, the exercise will become more enjoyable (or tolerable), your satisfaction with yourself will continue to grow, and your results will continue to amaze you.

After completing **The Adapted CTTC Workout #3** this time, take **one complete week of rest** from all exercise. Enjoyable low-to-medium intensity exercise activities are allowed during this week. Adjust your food intake accordingly, i.e., eat a little less during this week…not differently…just a little less.

After this week of rest and recuperation, begin the (actual) **CTTC Workout #1** again and complete all three **CTTC** Workouts in twelve weeks, **without any adaptations**. After these twelve weeks, you should be ready to begin adapting the **CTTC** Workouts to better suit your personal goals and circumstances.

```
┌─────────────────────────────────────────────────┐
│                                                   │
│         THE ADAPTED CTTC WORKOUT #1               │
│                                                   │
│      FOR BEGINNERS/INTERMEDIATES                  │
│                                                   │
│              CATEGORY #2                          │
│                                                   │
└─────────────────────────────────────────────────┘
```

Category #2: If you are a **non-exercising Senior Citizen**, or if you are **obese** but have **no other life-threatening medical problems, or other physical problems** (such as problems with your joints, tendons, etc) which could be exacerbated by these exercises, you should begin **The Adapted CTTC Workout #1** as follows:

IMPORTANT NOTE: Use the first two weeks to experiment and find the correct weight to use on each of the exercises. Slowly add weight to the exercises, but without sacrificing correct exercise form.

First Week
- Warm-up – build up to only **45%** of your **MHR** for the **last minute**.
- Do only **one set** of each exercise. Experiment to find the correct weight to use on each exercise.
- Do **ten minutes** of aerobics at **45%** of your **MHR** in place of the Cardio-aerobics.

Second Week
- Warm-up – build up to only **50%** of your **MHR** for the **last minute**.
- Do only **two sets** of each exercise (unless the exercise calls for only one set). Concentrate on exercise form.
- Do **ten minutes** of aerobics at **50%** of your **MHR** in place of the Cardio-aerobics.

Third Week
- Warm-up – build up to only **55%** of your **MHR** for the **last minute**.
- Do **all sets** of each exercise, but don't use too much weight. Your body is still learning the proper technique for each of the exercises.
- Do **ten minutes** of aerobics at **55%** of your **MHR** in place of the Cardio-aerobics.

Fourth Week
- Warm-up – build up to only **60%** of your **MHR** for the **last minute**.
- Do **all sets** of each exercise, still concentrating on correct exercise form.
- Do **ten minutes** of aerobics at **60%** of your **MHR** in place of the Cardio-aerobics.

Start **The Adapted CTTC Workout #1** again. Do the complete program for **four** more weeks. Do **all** the sets of each exercise. Slowly begin adding weight to the exercises when possible, but always use perfect exercise technique (form). The intensity of your warm-ups and the Cardio-aerobics at the end of the workout should be as follows:

First Week
- Warm-up - build up to only **65%** of your **MHR** for the **last minute**.
- Do **ten minutes** of aerobics at **65%** of your **MHR** in place of the Cardio-aerobics.

Second Week
- Warm-up - build up to only **70%** of your **MHR** for the **last minute**.
- Do **ten minutes** of aerobics at **70%** of your **MHR** in place of the Cardio-aerobics.

Third Week
- Warm-up - build up to only **75%** of your **MHR** for the **last minute**.
- Do **ten minutes** of aerobics at **75%** of your **MHR** in place of the Cardio-aerobics.

Fourth Week
- Warm-up - build up to only **80%** of your **MHR** for the **last minute**.
- Do **ten minutes** of aerobics at **80%** of your **MHR** in place of the Cardio-aerobics.

THE ADAPTED CTTC WORKOUT #2

FOR BEGINNERS/INTERMEDIATES

CATEGORY #2

IMPORTANT NOTE: When starting **The Adapted CTTC Workout #2**, all exercisers should follow the same procedure as you did with **The Adapted CTTC Workout #1.** Use the first 2 weeks to experiment and find the correct weight to use on each of the exercises. Slowly add weight to the exercises, but without sacrificing correct exercise form.

- You should have repeated **The Adapted CTTC Workout #1** and, therefore, now be prepared for **The Adapted CTTC Workout #2**, with the following adaptations:

First Week
- Warm-up – build up to **85%** of your **MHR** for the **last minute**.
- Do only **one set** of each exercise. Experiment to find the correct weight to use on each exercise.
- Do only **three** intervals of the **CTTC Workout #1** Cardio-aerobics.

Second Week
- Warm-up – build up to **85%** of your **MHR** for the **last minute**.
- Do only **two sets** of each exercise (unless the exercise calls for only one set). Concentrate on exercise form.
- Do only **four** intervals of **CTTC Workout #1** Cardio-aerobics.

Third Week
- Warm-up – build up to **85%** of your **MHR** for the **last minute**.
- Do **all sets** of each exercise, but don't use too much weight. Your body is still learning the proper technique for each of the exercises.
- Do only **five** intervals of **CTTC Workout #1** Cardio-aerobics.

Fourth Week
- Warm-up – build up to **85%** of your **MHR** for the **last minute**.
- Do **all sets** of each exercise, still concentrating on correct exercise form.
- Do only **six** intervals of **CTTC Workout #1** Cardio-aerobics.

Start **The Adapted CTTC Workout #2** again. Do the complete program for **four** more weeks. Do **all** the sets of each exercise. Slowly begin adding weight to the exercises when possible, but always use perfect exercise technique (form). The intensity of your warm-ups and the Cardio-aerobics at the end of the workout should be as follows:

First Week
- Warm-up – build up to **85%** of your **MHR** for the last **two** minutes.
- Do only **seven** intervals of **CTTC Workout #1** Cardio-aerobics.

Second Week
- Warm-up – build up to **85%** of your **MHR** for the last **two** minutes.
- Do only **eight** intervals of **CTTC Workout #1** Cardio-aerobics.

Third Week
- Warm-up – build up to **85%** of your **MHR** for the last **two** minutes.
- Do only **nine** intervals of **CTTC Workout #1** Cardio-aerobics.

Fourth Week
- Warm-up – build up to **85%** of your **MHR** for the last **two** minutes.
- Do all **ten** intervals of **CTTC Workout #1** Cardio-aerobics.

THE ADAPTED CTTC WORKOUT #3

FOR BEGINNERS/INTERMEDIATES

CATEGORY #2

IMPORTANT NOTE: When starting **The Adapted CTTC Workout #3**, all exercisers should follow the same procedure as you did with **The Adapted CTTC Workouts #1 and #2.** Use the first two weeks to experiment and find the correct weight to use on each of the exercises. Slowly add weight to the exercises, but without sacrificing correct exercise form.

- You should have repeated **The Adapted CTTC Workout #2** and, therefore, now be prepared for **The Adapted CTTC Workout #3**, with the following adaptations:

First Week
- Warm-up – build up to **85%** of your **MHR** for the last **three** minutes.
- Do only **one set** of each exercise. Experiment to find the correct weight to use on each exercise.
- Do only **five** intervals of **CTTC Workout #2** Cardio-aerobics.

Second Week
- Warm-up – build up to **85%** of your **MHR** for the last **three** minutes.
- Do only **two sets** of each exercise (unless the exercise calls for only one set).
- Do only **six** intervals of **CTTC Workout #2** Cardio-aerobics.

Third Week
- Warm-up – build up to **85%** of your **MHR** for the last **three** minutes.
- Do **all sets** of each exercise, but don't use too much weight. Your body is still learning the proper technique for each of the exercises.
- Do only **seven** intervals of **CTTC Workout #2** Cardio-aerobics.

Fourth Week
- Warm-up – build up to **85%** of your **MHR** for the last **three** minutes.
- Do **all sets** of each exercise, still concentrating on correct exercise form.
- Do only **eight** intervals of **CTTC Workout #2** Cardio-aerobics.

After completing **The Adapted CTTC Workout #3**, start **The Adapted CTTC Workout #1** again. Do **all** the sets of each exercise. Slowly begin adding weight to the exercises when possible, but always use perfect exercise technique (form). The intensity of your warm-ups and the Cardio-aerobics at the end of the workout should be as follows:

First Week
- Warm-up – build up to **85%** of your **MHR** for the last **four** minutes.
- Do only **nine** intervals of **CTTC Workout #2** Cardio-aerobics.

Second Week
- Warm-up – build up to **85%** of your **MHR** for the last **four** minutes.
- Do only **ten** intervals of **CTTC Workout #2** Cardio-aerobics.

Third Week
- Warm-up – build up to **85%** of your **MHR** for the last **four** minutes.
- Do only **eleven** intervals of **CTTC Workout #2** Cardio-aerobics.

Fourth Week
- Warm-up – build up to **85%** of your **MHR** for the last **four** minutes.
- Do all **twelve** intervals of **CTTC Workout #2** Cardio-aerobics.

After completing **The Adapted CTTC Workout #1**, start **The Adapted CTTC Workout #2** again. Do **all** the sets of each exercise. Slowly begin adding weight to the exercises when possible, but always use perfect exercise technique (form). The intensity of your warm-ups and the Cardio-aerobics at the end of the workout should be as follows:

First Week
- Warm-up – build up to **85%** of your **MHR** for the last **five** minutes.
- Do only **eight** intervals of **CTTC Workout #3** Cardio-aerobics.

Second Week
- Warm-up – build up to **85%** of your **MHR** for the last **5** minutes.
- Do only **9** intervals of **CTTC Workout #3** Cardio-aerobics.

Third Week
- Warm-up – build up to **85%** of your **MHR** for the last **five** minutes.
- Do only **ten** intervals of **CTTC Workout #3** Cardio-aerobics.

Fourth Week
- Warm-up – build up to **85%** of your **MHR** for the last **five** minutes.
- Do only **eleven** intervals of **CTTC Workout #3** Cardio-aerobics.

After completing **The Adapted CTTC Workout #2**, start **The Adapted CTTC Workout #3** again. Do **all** the sets of each exercise. Slowly begin adding weight to the exercises when possible, but always use perfect exercise technique (form). The intensity of your warm-ups and the Cardio-aerobics at the end of the workout should be as follows:

First Week
- Warm-up – build up to **85%** of your **MHR** for the last **five** minutes.
- Do only **twelve** intervals of **CTTC Workout #3** Cardio-aerobics.

Second Week
- Warm-up – build up to **85%** of your **MHR** for the last **five** minutes.
- Do only **thirteen** intervals of **CTTC Workout #3** Cardio-aerobics.

Third Week
- Warm-up – build up to **85%** of your **MHR** for the last **five** minutes.
- Do only **fourteen** intervals of **CTTC Workout #3** Cardio-aerobics.

Fourth Week
- Warm-up – build up to **85%** of your **MHR** for the last **five** minutes.
- Do all **fifteen** intervals of **CTTC Workout #3** Cardio-aerobics.

CONGRATULATIONS!

If you have paid your dues by faithfully and conscientiously following **The Adapted CTTC Exercise and Nutrition Programs** this far, you will have made spectacular gains in your levels of health and fitness. You will also have radically changed the shape and composition of your body and be in much better control of your body-fat. Well done! Now be sure to keep up the good work. Believe it or not, the hardest part is now over. From this point on, the exercise will become more enjoyable (or tolerable), your satisfaction with yourself will continue to grow, and your results will continue to amaze you.

After completing **The Adapted CTTC Workout #3** this time, take **one complete week of rest** from all exercise. Enjoyable low-to-medium intensity exercise activities are allowed during this week. Adjust your food intake accordingly, i.e., eat a little less during this week…not differently…just a little less. After this week of rest and recuperation, begin the (actual) **CTTC Workout #1** again and complete all three **CTTC** Workouts in twelve weeks, **without any adaptations**. After these twelve weeks, you should be ready to begin adapting the **CTTC** Workouts to better suit your personal goals and circumstances.

NOTE TO ALL CATEGORIES OF EXERCISERS

- Once you have achieved the level of Cardio-aerobics in **CTTC Workout #3** (all fifteen intervals), continue to use this intensity of Cardio-aerobics **for all three** of the **CTTC** Workouts, in order to maintain a superior level of cardiovascular fitness.

- If you are a real cardio fanatic, you may increase this Cardio-aerobic time to fifteen minutes… but **more than fifteen minutes will negatively affect your recovery** and will result in less than optimal results from the **CTTC** Workouts.

- I do not recommend this intensity of cardiovascular exercise outside of the three **CTTC** Workouts. More than three times per week is just not necessary unless you are an elite or professional athlete.

- **Use common sense!** If you are overly tired, or recovering from an illness, etc., adapt your Cardio-aerobics accordingly. Substitute a less intense Cardio-aerobics program from **CTTC Workouts #1** or **#2**, or shorten the time of the Cardio-aerobics, or even stop doing the Cardio-aerobics until you have fully recovered (feel better). Always listen to your body and make adjustments according to your personal circumstances.

NOTE TO ALL EXERCISERS WHO ARE TRYING TO LOSE BODY-FAT

After having slowly progressed to doing the complete twelve-week **CTTC** Exercise Program **without any adaptations**, you will have already radically changed the shape and composition of your body. If you still have excess body-fat, then read the chapter on aerobics again (Chapter 3), and begin adding extra T-aerobics to your program as described at the end of that chapter.

CONSISTENT, EFFECTIVE, INTELLIGENT EXERCISE IS THE KEY

The **CTTC** Exercise and Nutrition Programs will work for anyone…if you are honest about your goals, possibilities, and expectations. Only then can you effectively adapt the **CTTC** Exercise and Nutrition Programs (or any exercise program for that matter) to successfully fulfill your exercise goals.

It requires some hard work for a short time, but then you will have to do **much less** in order to maintain your newfound shape and healthy body. Once you have reached this **maintenance level**, you should concentrate your exercise on further improvement of more specific aspects of your new body. You can then also adapt the **CTTC** Workouts for more variety.

For instance, you could substitute exercise machines for all free weights for a four-week period. You will then return to free weights inspired, motivated, and with renewed fervor.

You could also do your abdominal exercises at home on Tuesday and/or Thursday. In addition to shortening some of your **CTTC** Workouts even more, this will allow you to work your abdominals two times per week instead of only once. That should help to soothe those of you who are still terrified that only one abdominal exercise session per week is not enough. You can do the same with your (bodyweight only) calf exercises.

The important things are that you **continue** to exercise…that you **continue** to have satisfactory results…that you **continue** to achieve your goals…and that you **continue** to have goals.

Good luck!

I wish you colossal success with The CTTC Exercise and Nutrition Programs!

GAINING MUSCULAR WEIGHT

I am sure that the majority of people who read this book will be mostly interested in losing excess body-fat and creating a shapelier body…or adopting a more efficient program to maintain their present fitness level. However, there are those individuals (both men and women) who want to create a more athletic physique…without looking like a bodybuilder. Their problem is usually that they have difficulty adding shapely muscle to their frames.

This can be every bit as frustrating as trying to lose excess body-fat. Believe it or not, this can be even **more difficult** than losing excess body-fat. I know. I've been there too. These people don't get much sympathy from over-fat and former over-fat people, but this is a legitimate problem for them. Fortunately, they can use the **CTTC** Exercise and Nutrition Programs too…with the following adaptations.

- Drop **all** aerobics…except the warm-up from **CTTC Workout #1.**

- Cut the **CTTC Workout #1** warm-up down to **five** minutes.

- Use this warm-up for **all three** of the **CTTC** Workouts.

- **Double** the rest periods in all of the **CTTC** Workouts.

- Drop **all** exercise activities…if possible.

- Eat 1½ **grams of high-quality, lean protein per pound of LBW** (lean body weight), per day.

- **Eat BIG:** lots of nutrient dense calories…but from high-quality, health-building foods.

- **Eat six times per day**…every 2½ - 3 hours…using high-quality protein shakes or high-quality meal replacement shakes for two or three of the six meals….including your **After CTTC Workout Recovery Shake** (Chapter 12). And yes…I do know how difficult this can be. When I was really fanatic about gaining more muscle, I used to set my alarm clock so that I would wake up in the middle of the night. Why? So I could eat (or drink) another meal and then go back to sleep. Maybe a little zealous…but it sure worked.

- Sleep **at least** eight hours per night.

- **Take 10-20 minute naps during the day**…if at all possible.

- A 20-30 minute "muscle-building" nap **after each CTTC Workout** is especially beneficial.

- Stay physically, mentally, and emotionally **calm.**

- **Be as lazy as you can be**…except during your **CTTC** Workouts.

Think!

Once again, I often see exercisers in the gym…especially the younger guys who are skinny and are trying to gain muscular weight…and what are they doing? They are in the gym for two hours a day, five or six days a week, doing three or four exercises for each body-part, for four or five sets each! Believe it or not, some of them even add aerobics to this, burning even more energy that they can't afford to waste. Well here's a little advice for you. This is insane, so…**STOP!**

Think about this logically. Before you started exercising with weights, you were already expending too much energy to allow you to gain any kind of weight at all. **That's why you are skinny.** Now your plan to **gain** muscular weight is to expend **thousands of calories more** by exercising with weights for ten or twelve hours a week.

Do you seriously believe that this is going to work? In fact, even this modified **CTTC** Exercise Program may be too much for you…especially if you do not **rigorously** follow **The CTTC Nutrition Guidelines**. But don't panic. It will still form a great foundation for future gains and in the near future I will be offering another **CTTC** program, specifically designed to solve the problem of gaining muscular weight. So until then, remember:

Back to Logic…Again

Quality Exercise is a logical process. All exercise uses muscles…so you must:

1. **Stimulate the muscles** – exercise

2. **Feed the muscles** – health-building nutrition and proper supplementation

3. **Allow the muscles to fully recover between exercise sessions** – rest

Don't just attempt to get BIG … build fat-free muscle!

Chapter 12

FEEDING A HARDBODY

I want this to be primarily an exercise book, not a detailed nutrition guide. The reason is that a practical and effective exercise program should be your **FIRST** step to a stronger, healthier, and shapelier body, not a complex nutrition makeover. Not being aware of this is the main reason that fat-loss diets fail, even the good ones.

Without a Quality Exercise program, you will have disappointing results from any nutrition program, no matter how good it is, and when you see minimal results, you will eventually give up. Therefore, this chapter will cover only the basic, most important things you need to know in order to recover optimally from the CTTC Workouts, and to begin developing a practical, health and immunity building nutrition program. I will cover nutrition in much more detail in future CTTC publications.

If you follow the simple **CTTC Nutrition Program Guidelines** in this chapter, you will be well on your way to adopting a health-building, energizing, body fat-burning, way of eating. The vast majority of you will not have to do anything more than this in order to realize your health, fat-loss and exercise goals. Once again, most of this is not rocket science – it is common sense – so here we go.

Back to Fat

Since having your body fat under control is one of the major factors in being really healthy, let's start with the question, How do we get over-fat? The easy answer…and aren't we all looking for the easy answer to every problem in our lives…is that we eat too many calories. Sorry! Easy, "magic bullet" answers like this never work!

Ingested food doesn't just randomly go somewhere in your body after it has been digested and absorbed. The proteins, fats, and sugars are shunted to different places for different purposes… depending on several factors, some of which have already been discussed in Chapter 4.

- The total **number of calories** you eat will greatly determine whether you gain or lose weight.

- **What** you eat and **when** you eat it will greatly determine whether the weight you gain or lose will come from muscle, or from body fat.

Why We Get Over-fat

There are ten reasons we get fat. **All of them** have to be addressed if you are serious about building and keeping a strong, healthy, shapely, and fat-free body.

1. We don't exercise.
2. When we do exercise, we don't exercise correctly (Quality Exercise).
3. We eat too little of the good foods.
4. We eat too much of the bad foods.
5. We drink too little of the good beverages (especially pure, clean water).
6. We drink too much of the bad beverages.
7. We eat at the wrong times (especially the bad foods).
8. We drink at the wrong times (especially the bad beverages).
9. We don't eat (smaller, healthier, complete meals) often enough.
10. Our portions are too large.

Very important: Always remember that exercise is not a panacea for bad nutrition. President Clinton ran 20-25 miles a week, but still needed to have a quadruple bypass because he clocked many of those miles by running to fast-food restaurants. Bad nutrition is also the reason you see so many dedicated exercisers who never change. They always look the same, in spite of hundreds of hours in the gym or jogging thousands of miles. So let's talk about food…logically!

Food

Food should be your friend, not your enemy. Good food is necessary to build and keep your health.

The best nutritional plan for losing excess body fat, keeping it off, creating shapely muscle, and building health and a strong immune system, is to eat and drink as follows:

What to Eat

1. Higher amounts of first class, low-fat proteins.

2. Medium total fats (approximately 20% of total calories), with higher amounts of essential fatty acids (EFAs)…especially the Omega 3s.

3. Medium amounts of complex carbohydrates, with higher amounts of bulky, filling, fibrous carbohydrates, and lower amounts of starchy carbohydrates.

4. 25-35 grams of fiber, every day, which you will automatically get if you are eating the amounts of fibrous carbohydrates recommended above.

5. Lots of pure, clean water, all day long, every day.

How and When to Eat

As I often say in this book, **how** you do something is often just as important, if not more important, as **what** you do. You should endeavor to consume the above foods and drinks as follows:

1. **Always** eat a nutritious breakfast.

2. Eat small, nutritious meals every 3-4 hours. Eating large, infrequent meals will increase your fat-storing hormones and enzymes.

3. Eat 5-6 small meals per day (this includes shakes). Eating fewer than 4-5 properly-spaced, small meals a day will cause your body to absorb fats and carbohydrates faster, causing a more rapid production of excess body fat.

4. Eat some high-quality, low-fat protein at every meal.

5. Eat most of your starchy carbohydrates early in the day, tapering off at the end of your day.

6. If you do eat carbohydrates later in the evening, strive to make them high-fiber, difficult to digest, complex carbohydrates.

7. If you are attempting to lose body fat, eat **no** carbohydrates for 3-4 hours before going to bed.

8. Drink lots of pure, clean water. Divide your (estimated) lean-body weight (in pounds) by two. This is the amount of water (in fluid ounces) that you should drink every day…or 8-10 large glasses…or 3 quarts (women)…or 4 quarts (men). This is **in addition** to fluids that you get from other beverages…and food.

Very Simplified

Very simply, after you eat a **nutritious** meal, one of three things will happen, depending on how you ate:

1. If you are still a little bit hungry, you will lose body fat.

2. If you are just satisfied, you will maintain your present weight and body fat.

3. If you stuff yourself, you will gain body fat.

If you wake up in the morning and you are **not** hungry, you did one of three things:

1. You ate much too much at your last meal last night.

2. You ate your last meal much too late last night.

3. You ate much too much…much too late last night.

Think of a little feeling of hunger in your stomach as a good thing. It is your body saying, "Hey, I am burning some of my excess body fat. Great! Keep it up!" Don't misinterpret this. I am not talking about "going hungry" here. I am talking about a subtle feeling that your stomach is just a few bites away from being completely satisfied. There is a BIG difference…which will also show in your results.

To Lose…or Gain

Following these simple nutrition guidelines, in combination with the **CTTC** Exercise Program, will solve the vast majority of your health and body fat problems.

To either lose excess body fat, or to gain lean body mass (muscle), you should eat the same basic nutritious foods and use the same basic nutritional supplements.

If it is difficult for you to gain solid muscular weight, you should eat more often (minimum six times per day), and eat slightly larger portions than you would if you were attempting to lose excess body fat.

So how do you go about doing this? First, you have to know which nutritious foods we are talking about before you can incorporate them into your eating plan.

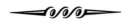

Proteins

- First class quality, low-fat proteins: Very simply, these are low-fat (except for some of the fish...but they contain the healthy EPA and DPA Omega 3 fats), high protein, unprocessed foods, such as the following:

Poultry	Fish	Dairy Products
White meat turkey (without skin)	Cod	Non-fat dairy products (yogurts, cheeses). Use skim milk in moderation because of the simple sugar (lactose) in milk.
White meat chicken (without skin)	Flounder & Sole	
Ostrich (without skin)	Halibut	
	Orange Roughy	
	Red Snapper	
Egg whites and egg yokes (1 egg yoke for every 3-4 egg whites)	Sea Bass	Low-fat cheeses and other low-fat dairy products...in moderation
	Tilapia	
	Trout (fish farm)	
Meats	Albacore Tuna (water packed, white-meat)	Always check the sugar content of non-fat and low-fat products. Some manufacturers simply replace the fat calories with calories from simple sugars.
Eye round steak	Atlantic Salmon	
Top round steak	Herring	
Top sirloin steak	Mackerel	
Round tip steak	Sardines	
Top loin steak		Superior-quality whey protein supplements
Flank steak	**Seafood**	
5% fat ground sirloin		You can flavor dairy products by liberally using all types of fresh or frozen berries.
Rib steak	Crabs	
Tenderloin steak	Lobster	
Buffalo steak	Scallops	
Venison	Mussels, oysters and clams	
	Shrimp	
	Octopus and squid (delicious)	

Fats

- Medium total fats (approximately 20% of total **calories**…not total **grams** of fat), with higher amounts of essential fatty acids (EFAs)…especially the Omega 3s:

The fats I recommend using are cold-pressed, unprocessed oils. Extra virgin olive oil is unprocessed and can be bought in the supermarket. It is an excellent oil. So is unprocessed canola oil. Safflower and sunflower oils can also be used sparingly, but only if they are unprocessed. You can probably only find these in specialty stores.

You have always heard that you have to have some fats in your diet. This is true, but they never tell you how much of which fats you actually need to have.

Your body can make almost all of the different kinds of fats that it needs. The exceptions are three groups of fats that your body absolutely has to get from the food you eat. That is why they are called **essential** fatty acids (EFAs). You get enough of two of these groups from your normal food, so we only really need to be concerned with getting enough of the third group, the Omega 3 fats. We can do this by simply taking 1-3 teaspoons of unprocessed, cold-pressed flaxseed oil per day, depending on whether you are a small, medium or large person.

Even the highly praised fish oils, the EPAs and DPAs, can be formed in the body from these Omega 3 fatty acids…but the reverse is not possible. Take your Omega 3s (flaxseed oil) daily. End of discussion.

Of course you can **also** take EPAs and DPAs if you wish, but they are much more expensive than flaxseed oil.

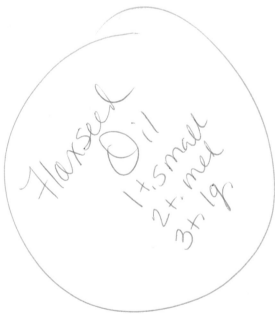

Carbohydrates

- Medium amounts of complex carbohydrates…with higher amounts of bulky, filling, fibrous carbohydrates and lower amounts of starchy carbohydrates.

Fibrous Carbohydrates, such as:	Starchy Carbohydrates, such as:
all salad greens	all legumes (beans, peas, lentils, etc.)
all salad vegetables	**whole grain** breads with **more than** three grams of fiber per slice
asparagus	**whole grain** pastas
broccoli	**whole grain** pitas and tortillas
cabbage	brown rice
carrots	unrefined cereals with **more than** three grams of fiber per serving
cauliflower	corn
celery	oat bran
green beans	steel-cut oatmeal
melons	rolled oats
onions (all colors)	potatoes
papaya	squash
peppers (all kinds and all colors)	sweet potatoes (the most nutritious of all "potato" sorts)
spinach	wheat bran
all sprouts	yams

Question: How much of each of the above foods do I need…and how much can I consume?

Answer: I don't know. Everyone is different. Only you can answer this question. However, there are certain foods of which you can eat unlimited quantities, such as the following:

- Lettuce and all other leafy salad greens and vegetables
- Broccoli
- Cauliflower
- Cucumbers
- Mushrooms
- Onions
- Peppers
- Sprouts
- Tomatoes

Make a salad with all these ingredients, throw some strips of chicken and a few hard-boiled egg whites in for your protein and add a low-calorie dressing. Now you have a terrific, health-building, low-calorie, filling meal, which you can divide over the whole day or combine with other meals.

Instead of fattening sauces, use lots of spices to liven up your food: basil, bay leaves, chili powders, cinnamon, cumin powder, curry powders (there are dozens of different ones), garlic, ginger, lemon juice, imitation butter, different mustards, mint leaves, nutmeg, oregano, pepper, low-sodium soy sauce, Tabasco, tomato paste, thyme, vanilla extract, vinegars, and so on.

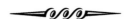

LBW (Lean Bodyweight)

Before you are able to answer the above question of "How much?" you first have to know what you are feeding. You want to be feeding everything in your body except your body fat. So now we have to find out how much of your bodyweight is non-fat. This is called your lean bodyweight or your LBW.

You have already read that the "average" man has about 25% body fat, and that the "average" woman has about 35% body fat. That's a starting point. There are all sorts of electrical impedance fat meters. They are even built into bathroom scales nowadays. There is ultrasound. There are anthropometric measurements, and many different mathematical formulas. Try as many different methods as you can. They will all give different readings, so take the average. Your gym should also be able to measure you by one or more methods. If you were in good shape at sometime during your adult life, also use that weight to approximate your present body fat level.

Let's assume that you have used three different methods and came up with 26%, 30%, and 34% body fat. We average them and come up with 30% body fat. If your total bodyweight is 150 pounds, then your lean bodyweight (LBW) is approximately 105 pounds (150 lbs. − 30% fat = 105 lbs). Since these are estimations, we will round it off to 100 lbs. to make our calculations easier. Now we know that we need to feed 100 lbs. of LBW. The forty-five pounds of body fat doesn't need any nutrition, and we don't want to feed our body fat anyway.

Protein

To feed your theoretic 100 lbs. of LBW, you need to eat approximately one gram of high-quality protein per pound, every day, spread out over your five or six meals. Proteins cannot be stored like fats and carbohydrates can. This will take care of the general repair and upkeep of your body and recovery from exercise activities. On **CTTC** Workout days you will need 1½ grams to ensure complete recovery from these workouts. I also make an attempt to stay closer to the 1½ gram level if I am seriously engaged in striving to lose excess body fat and/or gain muscle. If I am on a maintenance program, one gram per pound is usually sufficient.

Carbs

Your energy requirements, however, depend greatly on what type of metabolism your body has. Therefore, you can use the following guidelines to **estimate** your body's carbohydrate needs…**then adjust as individually needed**.

1. If you have a slow metabolism…i.e., you gain body fat easily…you should try consuming 2-2½ grams of complex carbohydrates per pound of LBW. This includes all carbohydrates from food **and** drinks.

2. If you have a regular metabolism…i.e., your bodyweight tends to remain the same most of the time (assuming that you are not too over-fat)…you should begin by consuming between 2½ and 3 grams of complex carbohydrates per pound of LBW. This includes all carbohydrates from food **and** drinks.

3. If you have been blessed with a fast metabolism you will have a low amount of body fat and have difficulty gaining weight…and the rest of us hate you for it. You can start with 3-3½ grams of complex carbohydrates per pound of LBW. This includes all carbohydrates from food **and** drinks.

Remember, a no-carb (or very low-carb) diet will cause you to lose muscle…and even more so if you are also exercising intensely and/ or doing a lot of aerobics and/or exercise activities.

I am talking about **complex** carbohydrates here. There is only one time when your body needs, and can effectively use, **simple** carbohydrates, but I will discuss that later.

To Fat or Not to Fat

As far as fats go, I always advise people to eat as few saturated fats and trans-fats as possible. I realize that this goes against some of the popular high-fat diets. Nevertheless, I still believe that there is a **big** health difference between the different types of fats and if you make an attempt to eat as few saturated and trans-fats as possible, you will still take in more than is good for you.

Less Fat…More Food

There are two other good reasons for doing this. The less of these unhealthy fats you eat, the more of the health-building fats (extra virgin olive oil, canola oil, and Omega 3 fats) you can consume in place of them. Best of all, the less fat you eat, the greater the volume of other foods you will **need** to eat in order to get enough calories. 400-500 calories of high-fat foods is not much food, while 400-500 calories of high-quality, low-fat protein and fibrous carbohydrates is a lot of food, especially if you are eating 4-5 meals a day. The average American diet is comprised of more than 40% fats, most of which are of the unhealthy varieties. And people wonder why Americans are becoming more over-fat and unhealthier every day. Go figure!

Counting Carbs

As you can see, the amounts of protein and fats that you eat should remain relatively constant. Therefore, with the CTTC Nutrition Program, you only need to adjust your complex carbohydrate intake in order to lose body fat, to gain muscle, or to be in harmony with your body's energy needs.

Beverages

The best health-building beverages to drink are:

1. Pure, clean water: Not drinking enough pure, clean water will actually help to make you over-fat. You need lots of water for your body to be able to effectively and efficiently burn excess body fat.
2. Green tea
3. Herbal teas
4. 100% pure, low-carbohydrate vegetable juices
5. Skim (non-fat) milk…unless you are lactose intolerant
6. Red wine with dinner: maximum two glasses for men and one glass for women

Recovery, Repair, Energy

These are the three results we should be looking for from the food and drinks we stuff in our mouths and pour down our throats…as well as good taste, of course!

There are three questions you should always ask yourself before you stuff any food or drink in your mouth.

1. What will my body do with this food until the next time it gets fed? If it is recovering from a CTTC Workout, it needs extra, high-quality protein for recovery and repair. If it is recovering from intense aerobic exercise, it needs extra complex carbohydrates to recover and replenish energy stores. If your body will not be recovering, repairing, or energizing, it needs a smaller portion of a complete meal to support normal bodily functions.

2. Is the food I am about to put in my body a quality, health-building food which will help me to reach my goals (especially my short-term goals), or will it sabotage what I am attempting to accomplish? It is your choice!

3. If I eat (or drink) this unhealthy food (fast-food, junk-food, sugared drink, etc.), how many hours of exercise is it going to take me to correct the mistake? Is it really going to be worth it?

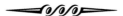

Not Suitable for Human Consumption

Just as important as what you should eat and drink is what you should NOT eat and drink. You should absolutely strive to stop eating and drinking the following:

- All beverages containing simple sugars. ~ SODA

- All foods and snacks containing lots of simple sugars.

- All high-fat foods. This also includes salad dressings, mayonnaise, sauces, etc. Substitute low-fat or non-fat products for these.

- All fried foods…period…no discussion.

- All white flour products. Dying white flour brown does not make it whole grain flour.

- All foods canned in oil, excessive sugar or excessive salt.

- All junk-foods. More than 30% of all calories in the diet of American adults come from junk-foods…not fast-foods…even though fast-foods get most of the blame for the obesity problem in America.

- Too much coffee (more than 2-3 cups per day). Substitute healthy teas the rest of the time.

- Alcoholic beverages. Even small amounts of alcohol will reduce your body's ability to use fats by up to 40% for several hours. A binge will also disrupt your sleep pattern for three or four nights.

Impotent

If you would just clean the above foods and beverages out of your house, you would never have to worry about becoming (or being) over-fat again. And don't try to con me…or yourself. You know darn good and well what foods and drinks I am talking about here: soft drinks sweetened with sugar, pies, cakes, cookies, candy, all kinds of chips and other junk-foods, fat cuts of meat, most lunch meats, bacon, sausages, hot dogs, cream "anything"…I will not insult your intelligence by continuing with this list of "nutritionally impotent foods." These "foods" will literally suck the healthy nutrients out of your body, thereby creating shortages, obesity, and disease.

> No fast-food or junk-food tastes as good as being healthy feels.

You Poor Thing

Before you start feeling too sorry for yourself…you don't know how lucky you are. My wife and I spend a lot of time in Europe where they have just begun to introduce low-fat and non-fat products to the market. It is very difficult to find some products, and impossible to find others. It is still difficult to even find skim milk in some countries in Europe. You have food choices in America that make it so much easier to control your body fat, improve your health, and still eat really well…so stop complaining. Just do it.

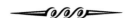

If at First You Don't Succeed…

Of course it is not practical, or even possible, to eliminate all bad things from your nutrition, but you should still **strive to eat and drink:**

- **As few simple carbohydrates as is humanly possible.** The average American consumes more than 150 pounds of sucrose (table sugar) every year. That is about 25% of all the calories in the average American diet – equivalent to nearly **eighty pounds of body fat** right there. When eaten together with fat, **simple sugars increase the amount of fat your body absorbs from the food you eat.** Double bacon cheeseburger, jumbo fries, and a sugar sweetened cola, anyone?

  Sugar sweetened soft drinks contain about one teaspoon of sugar per ounce of liquid. Half of the **excess calories** that people consume **come from what they drink**.

- I also do not recommend drinking fruit juices because of the high simple sugar (fructose) content. **Eat fruit…don't drink it.** It takes about five pounds of oranges to make just one quart of orange juice. You can drink a quart of orange juice in one sitting. Try eating five pounds of oranges in one sitting.

  If you want to have juices, drink low carbohydrate vegetable juices…not fruit juices. Too many simple carbohydrates, even from fruit juices, can disrupt your fat metabolism and raise your cholesterol and triglyceride levels, all of which are very bad. Bacon and orange juice for breakfast, anyone?

  Sorry, but here's another exception to a rule. **Do not drink carrot juice.** Carrot juice will raise your blood sugar as quickly as pure sugar will.

- **As little salt as possible.** Americans eat about five times more salt than is needed for optimal health…much of it hidden in foods. If they would put that much of a vitamin in a food, the FDA would ban the food.

  Too much salt will pull water out of your muscles (which are about 70% water) and re-deposit it just under your skin. One gram of sodium (salt) will hold 180 grams of water in your body. Does this bring the words "puffy" and "bloated" to mind?

- **As few processed food products as is humanly possible.** This includes margarines. Margarines are a synthetic food, so your body doesn't know what to do with it. Use **a little** butter instead.

- **As little fast-food as is possible**…and still have a life. When you do eat fast-food, be sure to pick the higher-protein, lower-fat, lower-carbohydrate choices. They are there. Find them and make good use of them when it is necessary.

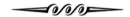

Nutritional Supplementation

Just as with comedy, when it comes to nutritional supplements, quality and timing is everything. A bad joke will always bomb…and so will a good joke delivered with bad timing. Bad quality supplements will always fail and high-quality supplements, taken at the wrong time or in the wrong amounts, can also slow down or even stop your progress.

The single best nutritional supplement you can take is a daily diet of nutritionally wholesome, health-building foods.

Now you are probably thinking that food is not a supplement. Unfortunately, for many people nutritionally wholesome, health-building food has become a supplement. Supplement means "in addition to." Many people's diets are now so unhealthy that wholesome, nutritious food would be **an addition** to what they normally eat.

Attempting to fix bad nutrition with dietary supplements is like trying to plug a hole in a boat with a cork. The larger the hole (the worse your nutrition is), the less the cork (nutritional supplements) will help.

The second most important nutritional supplement you can take is lots and lots of pure, clean water. I call water a supplement for the same reason. Too many people get most of their fluids from coffee, soft drinks, beer, and fake fruit drinks where the second ingredient on the label is sugar.

No Need

A person eating half a pound of sugar every day (the average American), getting 30% of his daily calories from junk-food (the average American), and 40% of his daily calories from fat (the average American…again), cannot possibly be getting enough vitamins, minerals, and other nutrients out of the "food" he or she is eating.

OK…you have changed your eating habits to include only wholesome, nutritious foods, and lots of pure, clean water…so now you have no need of nutritional supplements…right? Wrong!

A healthy, well-planned daily diet will still be much less effective than an integrated approach to nutrition. Adding basic nutritional supplements will make your nutrition program **much more effective**…and a Quality Exercise program will insure that the healthy food and supplements are being optimally utilized by your body. Once again…a **combination** of factors is the key to success.

I firmly believe that certain **basic** nutritional supplements should form an integral part of any complete, health-building nutrition plan…and the research backs me up here. For example, to get the necessary amounts of certain nutrients out of the typical American diet, you would have to eat more than 3000 calories per day. Hello excess body fat…and eventual obesity.

So which **basic** nutritional supplements am I talking about? It is an extensive list of six items.

1. A good multi-vitamin – high in the antioxidants
2. A good multi-mineral – containing enough calcium (1000-1200 mg) and magnesium (500-600 mg)
3. Extra vitamin E
4. Extra vitamin C
5. Flaxseed oil (Yes, I do know what it tastes like…but the countless health benefits are more than worth the two seconds of "special" taste in your mouth.)
6. A very high-quality whey protein powder

These are the six nutritional supplements that you should be using **FIRST**. Any other nutritional supplements you may want, or need, should be taken **in addition to these**. In fact, if you take a multi-vitamin/mineral supplement with enough minerals, enough vitamin E, and enough vitamin C already in it, you will only need three basic supplements: the multi-vitamin/mineral, the flaxseed oil, and the whey protein powder…and occasionally some extra vitamin C (read further).

Optionals

There are two other supplements that I also recommend, even though they are not **basic** nutritional supplements. These are creatine monohydrate and glutamine peptides. These will be discussed a little later.

Self - Medication

There are many good multi-vitamin/mineral products on the market. I want to emphasize here that I am talking about **multi**-vitamins and minerals. **Single** vitamins, minerals, amino acids, and herbs can have medicinal effects on your body. **Taking single vitamins, minerals, amino acids or herbs is self-medicating.** You wouldn't self-prescribe medicine for yourself (although some of you probably would…and probably do), so don't self-prescribe nutritional or herbal supplements either.

Some **single** vitamin, mineral, amino acid and herbal supplements can also interact with prescription and OTC (Over The Counter) medications to either increase…or decrease…the medicine's effectiveness.

Do you know which supplements can do this…with which medicines…and what their effects are, both positive and negative? If you are not an expert in this field of supplementation, leave **single** vitamin, mineral, amino acid and herbal supplements alone.

If you feel that you need a single vitamin, mineral, amino acid or herbal supplement, you should first do some serious studying of the subject so that you can ask knowledgeable questions and make intelligent decisions. Then you should seek out a qualified and competent professional to see if he/she agrees with your self-diagnosis. Otherwise, you are flying blind.

Gotcha

Now you should be wondering why, after all this hoopla about single vitamins, I still recommend **single** doses of vitamins E and C. Actually…I don't. I recommend **extra** vitamin E and C **in combination with** a good **multi**-vitamin/mineral product. The **extra** vitamin E is to bring the amount in the multi-vitamin/mineral up to my present recommended dosage of between 400 IUs and 600 IUs per day. My present recommended dosage of vitamin C is between 1000 and 1500 mg per day.

Some multi-vitamin/mineral products already contain these amounts of vitamins E and C, in which case no extra vitamin E and C would be necessary on a daily basis. In that case, I would only recommend **extra** vitamin C during special times of injury, illness or unusual stress.

Choose Wisely

Make sure that any vitamin E you take (also in your multi-vitamin) is **natural** vitamin E. Vitamin E is composed of eight different compounds, four called tocopherols, and four called tocotrienols. Natural vitamin E will have the prefix (d-) before the name. Synthetic vitamin E will have the prefix (dl-) before the name. When there is no prefix, always assume that it is synthetic vitamin E.

Many supplements use only the alpha form of vitamin E (d-alpha tocopherol), which is very good, but mixed tocopherols/tocotrienols are better for general health purposes, i.e., our purpose here. However, if your supplement contains only d-alpha tocopherol, don't worry about it.

Vitamin C is easier. It is also called ascorbic acid, and I am not yet convinced that natural or synthetic makes any great difference with vitamin C. What is important is that the vitamin C be time-released and that it also contain bioflavonoids, which work synergistically with vitamin C.

Nutrients and Hunger

A lack of **nutrients** causes hunger…and especially cravings. Your body cannot digest, absorb, or effectively use all the nutrients in the food you eat if sufficient vitamins and minerals are not present.

Your body needs nutrients…not just calories, so it will continue to be hungry until you have eaten enough food (too much) to finally supply your body with all the **nutrients** it needs. Hello over-fatness. This is one reason why junk-food and fast-food leaves you wanting more.

Never confuse hunger with appetite.

- Hunger is the **need** for nutrients and/or calories.

- Appetite is the **desire** for food.

Your first portion of a nutritious meal should satisfy your hunger. Anything after that (seconds, thirds, etc.) is purely appetite.

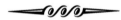

Energy

We cannot increase our energy. Energy is produced, not increased, so there is no (healthy) supplement which can increase energy. However, **we can increase our body's ability to produce energy.**

What and **how** we eat and drink determines our body's ability to produce energy. Needless to say, if we have even a minor shortage of any of several vitamins or minerals, our body's ability to produce energy will be compromised.

So, no (healthy) supplement can **give** you energy, but a good multi-vitamin/mineral will help your body to better **produce** energy…in the presence of high-quality, health-building food. Following the CTTC Nutrition Guidelines will greatly increase your body's ability to produce energy.

What Sucks the Energy out of Our Bodies?

- Fatty foods
- Sugar (including the simple sugars in foods and beverages)

- Drinking too much coffee (more than about 2 - 3 cups a day, depending on your size and sensitivity to caffeine)
- Drinking too much of other caffeine containing beverages, such as soft-drinks and some "energy" drinks
- Drinking excessive alcohol (more than one drink a day if you are a woman…or a small man… or two drinks a day if you are a man…or a very large woman)
- Not taking a good multi-vitamin/mineral regularly
- Not exercising regularly
- Not drinking after-exercise recovery shakes
- Not drinking enough pure, clean water
- Not exercising enough
- Exercising too much
- Not sleeping enough
- Sleeping too much
- Negative thinking
- Being around unhappy, negative people
- Too much stress (physical, mental, and/or emotional stress)
- Having a weak immune system

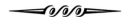

Protein Supplementation

For the purposes of health-building, maintenance of muscle, and control of body fat, I only recommend one type of supplementary protein. That protein is called whey protein, and it must be produced by a cross-, micro-, or ultra-filtering process, an ion-exchange process…or a combination of these. These processes do not use heat to produce the final product. This is extremely important, because processing with heat destroys the quality of whey protein. So if you are not 100% sure how a whey product has been produced, don't buy it.

High-quality whey protein is the ONLY type of protein that can strengthen your immune system.

Preliminary studies also indicate that high-quality whey protein **may** also play a role in promoting the use of body fat for energy. In other words, it **may** help you to lose excess body fat.

There are only three types of high-quality whey protein you should use.

- **Enzymatically Hydrolized Whey Protein Isolate:** This is the absolute best, highest quality protein there is at the moment. This is the protein you should use in your **After CTTC Workout Recovery Shake**. This recovery shake is the only time you actually need to use this superior quality of whey protein.

Enzymatically hydrolized whey protein isolate has the highest biological value of any protein on the face of the earth. Biological value (BV) measures how much of the protein you consume is actually absorbed and used by your body.

- **Whey Protein Isolate** (non-hydrolyzed) is the next highest quality protein available. Whey protein isolate is 90%, or more, pure protein.

- **Whey Protein Concentrate:** This is the protein you can use to sprinkle over your oatmeal or cereal at breakfast, or to increase the protein content of any meal…if necessary. This is also the type of protein that you should use in any **Between Meal Shake**. Whey protein concentrate is 80%, or more, pure protein.

Of course you can also use enzymatically hydrolyzed whey protein isolate (or non-hydrolyzed whey protein isolate) all the time but, since it is not necessary, I see that as a waste of money. Use whey protein concentrate for everything except your **After CTTC Workout Recovery Shake**, and spend the money you save on some good, health-building food.

Whey protein powders come in an amazing variety of flavors, so you are assured of finding one you like. The better ones also dissolve very easily, so you don't even really need a shaker anymore, although I still personally prefer using one.

Too Much of a Good Thing

"But Americans already have too much protein in their daily diets." Not true! Americans have too much **inferior-quality** protein in their diets. That is the real problem.

"Too much protein puts a strain on your kidneys." Do you have kidney disease? Do you have hepatitis? Then yes, you may have to restrict your intake of protein. Are you a diabetic? Then you will have to restrict your intake of sugars. Fortunately, I have none of these conditions so I concern myself with other, more important aspects of my health and nutrition. Besides, I am not talking about getting 400-500 grams of **extra** protein per day here.

If you are so worried about your kidneys, stop drinking alcohol. Alcohol definitely puts a strain on your kidneys (as well as your liver), but you still hear people discussing "too much protein" at cocktail parties. Go figure! People with normal functioning kidneys are not dropping dead from overdoses of high-quality protein. People are, however, dropping dead every day from overdoses of unhealthy foods.

The Mayo Clinic recently estimated the death toll from obesity-related causes to be 300,000 per year. The 65% (and more every day) of American adults who are over-fat should think of this in airplane terms again. This is the equivalent of sixteen large passenger airliners going down…**every week**. Let's see now…what should I be more concerned about, a few grams of superior-quality protein…

or joining the **more than 800 people** who are dropping dead...**every single day**...from obesity related causes. Hmmm...428 deaths from flying (world-wide)...versus 300,000 from eating yourself to death in America. Logically then, you should be most afraid of getting onto airplanes full of obese Americans.

Between Meal Meals

You have to **plan** your Between Meal Meals...and your normal meals...and your snacks. If you don't, you will wind up impulsively eating or drinking something you should not, and regretting it later. Hello more body fat.

Between Meal Protein Shakes

- Mix 15-20 grams of whey protein concentrate with one cup of skim milk. Use fifteen grams if you are smaller...twenty grams if you are larger. If you want more volume, add as much water as you want.

- If you want to use more milk, then mix 10-15 grams of whey protein concentrate with two cups of skim milk. Add water if you desire more volume. Do not use this shake if you are attempting to lose excess body fat. It contains too many carbohydrates.

- If you are attempting to gain muscular weight, still use skim milk but add berries, fruits and/or nuts to the shake. To do this, you will have to either use a blender or eat the added ingredients as you drink the shake.

"Sports" Bars

An occasional alternative to the **Between Meal Protein Shake** can be one of the many sports bars (a healthier kind of candy bar...not a bar where you drink beer and watch sports on TV) on the market. Just be very careful with your choice here.

The calories range from about 100 calories all the way up to about 500 calories per bar. The fat runs from about one gram to about ten grams, the carbohydrates from about fifteen grams up to about 100 grams, and the protein content ranges from a worthless one gram up to about thirty grams.

Choose a high protein (preferably whey), low fat sports bar, with low to medium carbohydrates. Avoid carbohydrate ingredients such as sucrose, dextrose, fructose, high-fructose corn syrup, and other simple sugars. Glucose polymers or slow-digesting maltodextrins are the best ingredients for supplements because they are slow-release carbohydrates.

Some of these bars taste like dry cardboard, but others are quite good. Since it is a matter of taste, you will just have to try a few until you find one or more that you like. There are currently more than 100 different sports bars on the market, so you can certainly find a couple that suit your taste and needs. Keep one with you for emergencies.

MRPs

Meal Replacement Powders (MRPs) are an even better choice for a between-real-food-meal. These come in individual one-serving packets and the good ones provide complete, high-quality nutrition in a glass. They are just so darn convenient, I just can't imagine **not** using them.

A good MRP dissolves instantly, tastes great, and is very affordable. Each serving contains from about forty to more than fifty grams of protein, which is really overkill, so I divide each packet into two servings. That still provides me with 20-25 grams of first class protein per serving, but cuts the cost in half...making MPRs an even better bargain.

Again, look for a product that is high protein, low fat, and low to medium carbohydrates. The guidelines for these carbohydrates are the same as those for the sports bars (see above). The protein should be primarily whey isolate, whey concentrate, a combination of the two, or at least with these two types of whey being the **primary** sources of protein in a blend of other quality (egg or milk) proteins. I personally stick with the higher quality whey products. The difference in price is negligible, especially when you use them as I suggest.

 As with the **Between Meal Protein Shake**, you can mix MRPs with water, skim milk, or a combination of water and skim milk, according to your personal taste and situation.

Emergency Food

Do you occasionally not have time to make, or eat, a nutritious breakfast? Are you sometimes too busy to have a good lunch? MRPs are one of the best substitutions you could find...infinitely better than coffee and a donut. In fact, you can carry MRPs with you as "emergency food" so you will not be "forced" to eat something you shouldn't because "there was just nothing else available." MRPs could literally save your butt...from getting bigger.

Take a Shake

All these shakes can be conveniently taken with you in a Tupperware® type shaker. I put the dry ingredients for my **After CTTC Workout Recovery Shake**, my **Between Meal Protein Shake** or half an MRP in the shaker before I leave home. When I need the shake, I just add plain water, shake it for a few seconds, and drink it. What could be easier? You could also put the ingredients into a smaller container and then just mix them in a large glass when you need one.

The <u>After</u> CTTC Workout Recovery Shake

Use **only** after each CTTC Workout. Mix the following three (or four) ingredients in a large amount of plain, cool water:

- An amount of **enzymatically hydrolized whey protein isolate** that comprises 20-25% of your total daily protein needs. So if you should be taking in a total of 120 grams of protein per day, this shake should contain approximately 25-30 grams (20-25% of 120) of protein.

- 25-50 grams of dextrose (glucose): 25 grams if you are small (LBW)…50 grams if you are big (LBW)…35-40 grams if you are somewhere in the middle (LBW). This is the **only** time your body actually needs…and can efficiently, effectively, and constructively use…simple sugars (dextrose-glucose, in this instance). At this time (after intense exercise), the simple sugars will go directly to replenishing the carbohydrates (muscle glycogen) in the muscles you have just exercised, instead of being converted to body fat. This will enhance and speed up your recovery processes. This is a very good thing.

- 3-5 grams of **creatine monohydrate**: three grams if you are small (LBW)…five grams if you are big (LBW)…four grams if you are somewhere in the middle (LBW).

Creatine: I absolutely recommend creatine monohydrate powder, unless you have some form of kidney disease. It is very affordable, and **it works**. It speeds up and improves recovery from exercise, it will make you stronger, and it helps redistribute the water in your body from places you don't want it (under your skin, for instance) to places you should want it (your muscles, which are, remember, 70% water). Creatine will give you fuller muscles, which, in turn, will make your body firmer and shapelier.

Optional: 1-2 teaspoons of **glutamine peptides** (an amino acid): one teaspoon if you are smaller (LBW); two teaspoons if you are bigger (LBW); in between if you are in between (LBW). I call this ingredient optional because it is quite expensive. However, the recovery and health-building benefits of glutamine are so amazing that, if you can afford it, I definitely recommend that you use it…unless you are suffering from liver or kidney disease.

The Before Sleeping Shake

- Mix 20-25 grams of **whey protein concentrate** and one teaspoon of **flaxseed oil**, in water (or take the flaxseed separately). Use twenty grams of **whey protein concentrate** if you are smaller (LBW); twenty-five grams if you are larger (LBW). This is the best time to take your flaxseed oil. If you are using more than one teaspoon, you can take the other 1-2 teaspoons with breakfast and/or lunch.

Exercise Nutrition for Building or Maintaining Muscle and Losing Body Fat

What you eat and drink (or don't) **before** you exercise will determine what your body will use for fuel (energy) **during** your exercise. It will determine whether you use protein (by cannibalizing your own muscles), carbohydrates (which your body uses first for fuel), or body fat (which I am sure you would prefer) as a source of energy during exercise.

What you eat and drink (or don't) **immediately after**…and approximately one hour after that…will determine how quickly and how completely your body will recover from the exercise…or not. In other words, it will greatly influence the results, either positively or negatively, that you will ultimately receive from all your hard work. It will also partially determine how long and how intensely the after-exercise fat-burning process will continue.

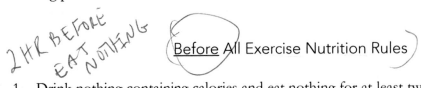

Before All Exercise Nutrition Rules

1. Drink nothing containing calories and eat nothing for at least two hours before your exercise session. **How** and **what** you have eaten for the past twenty-two hours will determine if you have enough energy for your exercise session, **not** something you eat an hour or two before you exercise. However, eating or drinking calories during these two hours **will** interfere with the fat-burning processes during your exercise.

2. 30-45 minutes before exercising, drink 10-15 grams of **whey protein** powder (any one of the 3 different kinds)**,** mixed in plain, cool water. This is the only exception to **Nutrition Rule Number 1** above. It has nothing to do with providing energy for your exercise session, but **may** enhance the fat-burning process during exercise.

During All Exercise Nutrition Rules

- Drink one cup of plain, cool water every fifteen minutes during your exercise. Drink more than this if you perspire a lot, or if it is very warm where you are exercising. You should sip this water continually during you exercise session. Don't just gulp down a whole cup of water every fifteen minutes.

After Aerobics Nutrition Rules

For Intense Aerobics Lasting Thirty Minutes or Longer

1. Thirty minutes after you finish your aerobic exercise, drink 25-30 grams of **whey protein** powder (any one of the three different kinds), mixed in plain, cool water. This will prolong the fat-burning process which the aerobic exercise has started. Whatever you do, **do not** eat or drink anything that contains any type of carbohydrates!

2. Wait another 30-45 minutes before you eat or drink anything (except more plain, cool water, of course). This will also prolong the fat-burning process which the aerobic exercise has started.

3. After these 30-45 minutes, eat a medium sized meal, consisting of a medium amount of high-quality protein (20-25 grams), low fat, a medium amount of fibrous carbohydrates, and a small amount of starchy carbohydrates.

These rules are for exercisers who are trying to lose excess body fat. If you do not have a problem with excess body fat, you should add from 50 to 100 grams of dextrose (glucose) to the above shake, depending on your LBW and the length of time that you exercise. Your after exercise meal should then also contain more starchy carbohydrates.

After a CTTC Workout Nutrition Rules

1. **Within** twenty minutes after you finish the ten-minute cool-down and stretching part of every CTTC Workout, drink an **After CTTC Workout Recovery Shake**.

2. Wait another 45-60 minutes before you eat or drink anything else (except more plain, cool water, of course). This is the perfect time to take a twenty-minute "recovery enhancing" nap, if possible.

3. After these 45-60 minutes, eat a medium sized meal (approximately 20-25% of your daily calories) consisting of a larger amount of high-quality protein (25–35 grams), a medium amount of fibrous carbohydrates and a medium amount of starchy carbohydrates.

A Healthy Guilt Complex

Never forget to drink your **After CTTC Workout Recovery Shake** within twenty minutes after you finish the ten-minute cool-down and stretching part of a **CTTC** Workout.

For some reason, it is difficult to convince most people of how **incredibly important** this is. I actually feel more guilty about forgetting my shake than I do about missing a workout. I can always make up the workout, but if I don't have my **After CTTC Workout Recovery Shake** then I know that a good part of the butt-busting work I just did in the gym was for nothing. The workout will not have contributed 100% to my progress because now my body does not have all the nutrients it needs…**when it needs them**…to completely and effectively recover from the exercise.

This is really dumb so I hope you will also develop this guilt complex. If it helps you to remember to always drink your **After CTTC Workout Recovery Shake**, then it will be one of the only healthy guilt complexes you can ever have. And **no, it is not possible** to get the same results using normal, healthy food. Normal food cannot get into your system and then to your muscles fast enough. So even if you decide to use **no other** recovery techniques, **use this one**. It is that important.

Why

A major portion of your after-exercise recovery begins (and even occurs) in the two-hour period **immediately following** your **CTTC** Workouts. This is why the **After CTTC Workout Recovery Shake** and your after-exercise meal 45-60 minutes later are so incredibly important. Never miss these two meals.

The same holds true for the **After Aerobics Exercise Recovery Shake**…and your after-aerobics meal…when you have done intense aerobics lasting thirty minutes or longer. Never miss these either or your exercise recovery (and progress) will suffer.

The Before Going to Bed Rule

On **CTTC** Workout days, drink a **Before Sleeping Shake** shortly before retiring for the night. This will provide your body with the nutrients it needs to **continue** recovering from the **CTTC** Workout, while you are sleeping. On days when you have only participated in aerobics or exercise activities, this shake will usually not be necessary, unless the aerobics or exercise activities were extreme (long or intense).

Overdose

Once again, I can hear the screams: "Too much protein!" So let's think this one over again…logically.

More than half of all Americans are over-fat. **Nine million Americans are morbidly obese**. Type II diabetes is rampant (twenty million and growing). Bones are shattering everywhere from the ten million Americans with osteoporosis (and another thirty-five million at risk). Alcoholism and prescription drug abuse are increasing at a staggering pace. Alcoholism is now the third leading cause of **preventable** death in America. A "balanced diet" belongs in the realm of science fiction. People are dying from relying too much on medicines…the list goes on and on…but we should be overly concerned about a few grams of superior-quality, immune-boosting protein? That really makes sense, doesn't it? I have already mentioned proper priorities in this book…and thinking logically…and just thinking…

In fact, since your body cannot store protein like it can store fats and carbohydrates, you must make sure that you provide your body with some high-quality protein at **every** meal. If you don't get enough high-quality protein every day, your progress (whether losing excess body fat, building muscle, or both) will come to a screeching halt. Get enough high-quality protein and you will maximize your results.

Back to Reality

One last thing about nutritional supplements, and nutrition in general: What I have written here about health-building nutrition and nutritional supplementation **is idealistic**. I am well aware of that fact. As I said earlier about exercise, we are not professional athletes or fitness fanatics. We are people living in the real world and, as such, we will not be able to follow all these guidelines all the time. However, the more closely and the more often you can follow these nutritional guidelines, the quicker and better your results will be.

This is about **you**. It is your body, your health, your self-image, your self-esteem, your self-confidence, your self-discipline, your body fat, your goals, and your choices. Faithfully following the **CTTC** Nutrition Program will be more difficult for some than for others. If you are married, have four kids and work full time, of course it will be more difficult for you to find time to plan and prepare your meals than it will be for someone living alone, with fewer responsibilities. That is **not** an acceptable excuse. That just means that you will have to plan and budget your time much **better** than they do.

Nutrition Goals

Your two main goals regarding health-building nutrition should be as follows:

1. Whenever it is possible, you should follow the **CTTC** Nutrition Program guidelines as closely as possible.

    In other words, **when your life allows it**, embrace the challenge of following the **CTTC** Nutrition Program to the letter. Use this time to get a little fanatic about your nutrition…no cheating…and watch your progress soar. Of course, this must be done hand in hand with the **CTTC** Exercise Program…or another Quality Exercise program.

2. When this is not possible, **always strive to limit the damage you do**.

    Many times it will not be possible to follow the **CTTC** Nutrition Program to the letter. That is OK. During these times you just have to make sure that you do not really go overboard or, what we in the business affectionately refer to as "pigging-out." This requires self-discipline! Read the sections on **The Set Point** and **The Line** in Chapter 4 again.

Fortunately, both **CTTC** programs build self-discipline as you go along, so when situations come up such as, "I just baked this chocolate cake…you simply must try a piece," you will be able to answer with, "OK, but just a little piece…no, no, half of that," instead of insulting your host by refusing to eat even a small piece.

If they continue to push, make some excuse such as having had a lot of trouble with your digestion lately. Whatever you do, do not say that you are attempting to lose excess body fat (or anything similar to that) unless you are in sympathetic company. Many others will take this as a personal challenge to get you to eat as much of the "forbidden fruit"…or chocolate cake in this instance…as possible. Don't provide them with any ammunition and your life will be much more pleasant.

Occasionally

I am human. I too enjoy pizza, ice cream, tortilla chips, French fries and other "nasties." I also drink soft drinks (but not those sweetened with sugar), beer, wine, and even hard liqueur. But I do these things **only occasionally**. By occasionally, I mean seldom to almost never…except for maybe the wine and beer…sometimes.

My wife and I don't eat out regularly so, when we do, it is a real treat for us, and then we want to eat something completely different from what we normally eat at home. These are the times we splurge a little. Then yes, I will have French fries with my meal (but not always). At an Italian restaurant I will order lasagna, perhaps, but never spaghetti, which my wife often makes at home. Then we may have ice cream for dessert…but also **only occasionally**.

Tortilla chips are a real treat for me, so I really enjoy them the few times I allow myself to eat them. Because it is also an **occasional** treat, if I can't have a **really good** pizza, then I would rather not have pizza at all. This way, we actually wind up eating French fries maybe ten times a year, pizza four or five times a year, and ice cream once every few weeks, but usually only in the summer. It just seems to taste better then.

I can still get away with eating or drinking more of these things (and more often) than my wife can. That's life! Since when has life been fair? Get used to it. The fact that she has to be more disciplined than I do actually works in my favor. Since I always support her, I wind up eating much less of the "bad" foods than I would if I were on my own. She is a great support system for me. So who is the stronger sex again?

Hitting the Bottle

We have bottles of alcoholic drinks (and I am **not** talking about fine wines here) that are years old. That is how often we imbibe. I have already admitted to liking a cold beer when it is hot outside in the summer, and we drink one, maximum two, glasses of wine (nearly always red wine) with our evening meal, a few times a week. However, when we are following **Nutrition Goal Number 1** above, we drink no alcohol whatsoever, not even a glass of wine with dinner. This is imperative! Alcohol will screw up your fat-burning processes faster than pure sugar will.

Those Poor People

Before you start feeling too sorry for us, I have to tell you that we eat **a lot** of food. It is health-building, it is nutrient dense, and it is gooooood! We can eat **a lot** of food because of **how** we exercise and **how** and **what** we eat.

I will even admit that we "pig-out" once in a great while. However, we never do this unless ' or very close to, our ideal weights. Our "pigging-out" lasts one day, or one short weekenu ... Then we go back to **Nutrition Goal Number 1** again for a few days. We feel good because we have "being bad" out of our systems again – we had a great time while it lasted, **and we have not done too much damage.** Now we can look forward to the next time.

Knowledge Is Power

We are both able to physically and psychologically handle an **occasional** alcoholic drink, an **occasional** pizza, an **occasional** ice cream and even an **occasional** weekend "pig-out," because we not only understand how food affects our bodies, but we also know that our **CTTC** Exercise Programs can easily take care of an **occasional** "indiscretion" in our daily nutrition.

However, if you cannot handle **occasional**, then you will have to leave **occasional** alone until you have progressed to a point where you **can** handle it…both physically and psychologically.

Back to Exercise

If you are following a Quality Exercise program, **you will be able to eat more,** and be less strict with your food choices, than if you follow a non-Quality Exercise program or a program that mainly emphasizes aerobics to control your body fat.

Enjoy life … eat, drink, and exercise … but do it right!

Re-read this chapter and write down all the things you are **not** doing correctly with your daily diet.

After you do that, go back to Chapter 4: **"Why Would Anyone in His Right Mind Want to Lose Weight?"** and do the same thing. Re-read the chapter and write down all the things that you **are** doing which are throwing your hormones out of whack and making a fat-storing machine out of your body.

Decide which of these things you are willing to change…and then **DO IT.**

You will now be programmed for **SUCCESS.**

But Which Supplements?

Since the supplement companies are constantly bringing new products onto the market, and they keep improving the quality of their products…or not, I do not list any specific products or companies here. For up-to-date information about specific products and companies which I do recommend, go to our website at:

www.CTTChealthpublishing.com

Simplifying Diets

OK, I admit it. This has all been a bit complicated, and most people don't like complicated. So I will simplify "dieting" for you here by making use of the well-known **KISS** (**K**eep **I**t **S**imple **S**tupid) system. Then, because very effective programs often consolidate their ideas into compact **12 Step Programs** (and I never argue with success)…I'll go with the flow and include one of those for you here as well…at no extra cost.

The CTTC "KISS" Diet Evaluation Procedure

Avoid all diets that recommend, refer to, or even hint at:

1. Losing **weight** without having to exercise intensely

2. "Wonder foods" that will miraculously "melt your fat away"

3. Promising incredibly rapid **weight** loss (more than two pounds per week…unless you are very obese)

4. Being able to eat as much of your favorite (in other words, unhealthy) foods as you want

5. Eating only specific nutrients (eating only carbohydrates, or only proteins, etc.)

6. Eating only "unlimited quantities" of specific foods (eating only grapefruit for four days, etc.)

7. "Magic" combinations of foods (eating only proteins and fats together…or eating all the carbohydrates in a meal before consuming any proteins, etc.)

8. Inflexible menus (greatly limited choices of foods…or eating very specific foods at particular times, etc.)

These people are selling you empty hopes and dreams…
NOT solutions to your problems.
Don't let them con you!

The CTTC Simplified Twelve-Step Stop-Start Program

Stop:

1. **Stop**…eating crap.

2. **Stop**…drinking crap.

3. **Stop**…blindly believing everything you read or hear about exercise.

4. **Stop**…relying only on traditional aerobics (T-aerobics) for losing your excess body fat.

5. **Stop**…looking for "magic" or "miracle" solutions to your problems, whatever they may be.

6. **Stop**…beating yourself up, both mentally and emotionally.

Start:

7. **Start**…eating health-building foods.

8. **Start**…drinking health-building beverages.

9. **Start**…reading, studying and learning about scientifically proven, efficient and effective exercise techniques and health-building nutrition.

10. **Start**…using a Quality Exercise and Nutrition program to lose your excess body fat, shape your body, and build your health.

11. **Start**…identifying your problems…and then designing logical, practical, intelligent, efficient and effective plans to solve them.

12. **Start**…believing in yourself.

Chapter 13

AT HOME AND ON THE ROAD

Some of you don't, won't, or can't exercise at a commercial gym. Don't worry. All is not lost. There are other ways to successfully exercise. The equipment you have at your disposal is much less important than **how** you use the equipment.

The most important thing is that you apply the **Principles of Quality Exercise**…which you have learned in this book…to whichever exercise, or form of exercise, you choose to do or are able to do.

The most effective solution to this problem is to set up a small gym right at home. This can be done very inexpensively and still be incredibly effective. All you need are the following:

The Essentials:

- A pair of adjustable dumbbells

- An adjustable barbell

- Assorted weights for the barbell and dumbbells

- An adjustable exercise bench

- A large full-length mirror so you can constantly check your exercise form (technique)

The Almost Essentials:

- A bar that is high enough and strong enough for you to do pull-ups. It can be self-made, but is not necessary if you have a Smith machine (see below).

- A pair of (parallel) bars that are high enough and strong enough for you to do dips. They can also be self-made.

- An exercise bicycle (or treadmill) for Cardio-aerobics (especially if you don't live where you can nearly always exercise outside). I personally prefer exercise bicycles because I find that they are generally better than other types of aerobic machines for combining T-aerobics and Cardio-aerobics. But if you prefer walking/jogging, go for the treadmill.

- A Smith machine, which is a barbell that slides up and down vertical poles and is equipped with safety hooks that enable you to stop the exercise and "hang up" the barbell at any time during an exercise. It makes certain exercises, such as squats, bench presses, deadlifts, etc., much safer, especially if you exercise alone. If you are a **serious** home exerciser, you definitely need either a Smith Machine or a "multi-exercise station" (see Extra Excellent Goodies below), in order to truly exercise efficiently and effectively.

Extra Excellent Goodies:

If you have the space, one of the "universal" type, multi-exercise stations, preferably with a weight stack where you can adjust the amount of weight with one simple movement of a pin, would also be a great investment in your exercise program, your body, and your health.

When choosing one of these machines, be sure to consult the **CTTC** Workouts to see which exercises are really important. Many of these machines include the more "trendy" exercises (such as a pec dek and/or some attachment for the abdominals) at the expense of the more basic and effective exercises (such as the bench press, pull-down, or leg press). The quality of these machines also ranges from excellent to actually being dangerous…and the price is not always a guarantee of quality.

Do your homework and be very choosy here. If possible, go to a sports store that specializes in this type of exercise equipment and explain to the sales person that you want to use it to **seriously** exercise, not just to go through the motions. I do not recommend buying any piece of serious exercise equipment from someone who does not themselves exercise. They cannot possibly know what is good and what is not good. The same goes for exercise bicycles, treadmills, or any other kind of sophisticated exercise equipment. There are some great machines out there now, so don't get scammed. If a salesperson is pushing you to buy something you are not quite sure about…run away! Also, don't get distracted by "cute" or hi-tech gadgets on the apparatus that are not necessary to your exercising…or would you buy a car just because it has a really nice CD player in it?

Take your time and shop around. Make a list of the most important exercises (use the **CTTC** Workouts as a guide) and make sure that you can do most of them on any machine you consider buying. Never buy any exercise machine without trying it out first. When you get down to a choice of a couple of different machines, make a list of pros and cons versus cost, compare them, and then go for the best machine for your money.

A good personal trainer can save you a lot of time and money here also. He or she can prevent you from making any major mistakes when purchasing exercise equipment. Find one you trust and make use of his/her knowledge and experience.

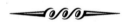

No Equipment Training

Now I am going to take away the last excuse you could possibly have for not exercising. Sorry about that. The following exercises can be done at home, at the office, in your hotel room or even outside. This is a short list of some of the very best exercises of this type that you can do. All of these exercises can be done alone.

For a better understanding of the correct exercise techniques, read the **"Explanation of the Exercises"** for similar exercises in the **CTTC** Workout chapters.

Back

- **Pull-ups** (palms of hands turned away from you): It is seldom that you cannot find a bar somewhere that can safely support your weight. I highly recommend those chinning bars that you can fix in nearly any doorway by turning them until the ends are securely pressed against the doorframe. Have one of these in a doorway in your home for pull-ups, and to just hang on for a few seconds, several times a day, to decompress your spine. It is one of the best things you can do for your back, your spine and your posture. You can also take one with you when you travel. Get one and use it. Your spine will thank you!

- **Chin-ups** (palms of hands turned towards you): You can do these with a shoulder-width grip to put the emphasis on your back muscles, or you can use a narrower grip to put more emphasis on your biceps.

  Another great piece of exercise equipment is an elastic band. You can use it not only for stretching, but also as an aid for doing pull-ups and chin-ups. I personally use a six-foot length of surgical tubing, but the commercial elastic exercise bands can also be used. Wrap both ends of the elastic around your chinning bar and grip the bar with your hands over the elastic. This will keep it from slipping. Now stand in the middle of the elastic with both feet. By adjusting the length of the elastic, or by bending your legs, you can get just enough help to allow you to do several pull-ups or chin-ups. Eventually you will be able to do these exercises without the help of the elastic.

- **Hanging Rows:** You can use your doorway chinning bar for this one too. Put your feet on a chair, table or some other stable object. When you are hanging with straight arms, your body should be as parallel with the floor as possible, facing toward the ceiling.

  You can use a wide grip, with palms facing away from you and elbows out, to emphasize the back of your shoulders and the area between your shoulder blades. To emphasize the rest of your back and involve more biceps in the exercise, use a shoulder-width grip with your palms facing you, and pull with your elbows going past (close to) the sides of your body. Pull up until your chest touches the bar. Lower and repeat.

If keeping your body parallel to the floor is too difficult, then use your elastic to help you, or keep your feet lower to begin with, and work your way up to parallel as you get stronger.

Chest

- **Pushups:** To emphasize your upper chest, put your feet up on a chair, a couch or a bed. Keep your hands wider than shoulder width and your elbows out.

  To emphasize the rest of your chest, keep your feet on the floor, your hands wider than shoulder width and your elbows out.

  To add more emphasis to your triceps, keep your hands at shoulder width and your elbows closer to the sides of your body. If you elevate your feet, you will also emphasize some upper chest with this position.

  You can make all three of these exercises more difficult by doing them between two chairs, which will enable you to go lower. I have a pair of mini-parallel bars (about eight inches high), which I carry with me for this purpose. They are more stable (safer) than chairs.

Shoulders

- **Handstand Pushups Against a Wall:** This is for the more athletic among you. You kick into a handstand against a wall, keeping your hands a little wider than shoulder width. Then you **slowly** lower yourself down as far as your strength level will allow, and push back up into a handstand again. As you get stronger, go lower. If you are really strong, you can use the mini-parallel bars described above.

- **Lateral Raises:** (See the description of this exercise in **The CTTC Workout #1, Friday.**) You can use any two objects that are equal in weight. Plastic water bottles are ideal for this. If you only have smaller water bottles and they are not heavy enough, put a few of them in two plastic bags and use the bags like dumbbells. Or you can buy plastic dumbbells which you fill up with water when you want to use them. You can also use your elastic band for this exercise.

- **Dumbbell Upright Rowing:** (See the description of this exercise in **The CTTC Workout #2, Friday.**) You can use the plastic water bottles, etc., mentioned in the preceding exercise.

- **Shoulder Presses with an Elastic Band:** Wrap each end of the elastic around each hand and stand with both feet in the middle of the elastic. Bring your hands to your shoulders and then press the elastic band to arms length over your head while moving your elbows out to the sides. Lower your hands to your shoulders again and repeat. You can use the plastic water bottles for this exercise too.

Waist

- **Crunches:** See the description of this exercise in **The CTTC Workout #1, Monday**.

- **Seated Trunk Twists:** See the description of this exercise in **The CTTC Workout #3, Friday**.

- **Reverse Leg Raises on a Table:** Lie face down on a strong table or desk with your legs and hips hanging over the edge. Hold on to the sides of the table or desk in order to keep your upper body from moving. Now **slowly** raise your legs behind you as high as you can while still keeping them straight. Hold this position for 5-10 seconds and then **slowly** return to the starting position. Repeat. Your hips (pelvis) should also rotate up and down when you raise and lower your legs.

- **Back Extensions on the Floor:** Lie face down on the floor with your arms extended straight in front of you. **Slowly** raise your head, arms, shoulders, and legs up as high as you can. Hold this position for 5-10 seconds and then **slowly** return to the starting position. Repeat.

Triceps

- **Dips Between Chairs:** Support yourself on your hands between two chair seats. Place your feet on the floor in front of you, on a third chair, on a couch or on a bed. **Slowly** bend your elbows and lower yourself between the two chair seats as far as your strength level will allow. Push back up to the starting position. Repeat.

- **Triceps Extensions with an Elastic Band:** Position yourself as if you had just done a "Shoulder Press With an Elastic Band." Beginning with both arms and the elastic band extended above your head, **slowly** lower your hands behind your head. Keep your elbows pointed towards the ceiling with your upper arms against the sides of your head. When your hands cannot be lowered any further, **slowly** extend them above your head again. Do not let your upper arms move. Repeat. Water bottles work here too.

- **Triceps Pushdowns with an Elastic Band:** Wrap the elastic band around your chinning bar and then do Triceps Pushdowns. (See the description of Triceps Pushdowns in **The CTTC Workout #1, Friday**.)

Biceps

- **Horizontal Curls:** Perform "Hanging Rows," palms facing you, but with your hands very close together.

- **Biceps Curls with an Elastic Band:** Wrap each end of the elastic around each hand and stand with both feet in the middle of the elastic. With your hands by your sides and your palms facing forward, slowly raise (curl) your hands forward and up until they are by your shoulders. Slowly lower them to the starting position again. Keep your upper arms tightly against your sides and do not let them move. Repeat. Water bottles work well here too.

Legs and Cardio-Aerobics

- **Deep Squats:** Holding onto the back of a chair, a desk, a doorknob or some other stable object to keep your balance, **slowly** squat down completely, keeping your back straight and looking forward and slightly up. **Slowly** come back to your starting position. Repeat.

- **Deep 1½ Squats:** This is an addition to the "Deep Squats" above. You squat down completely, but come only halfway up. Then you squat down completely again…then come all the way up. This is one repetition. Repeat.

- **Jump Squats:** Squat down halfway **slowly** (thighs parallel to the floor), then jump up as high as possible, remembering to push off from your toes as your body leaves the ground. Also, use your arms when jumping. When you come down, land on the balls of your feet and **slowly** absorb the impact until you are again in a half squat. Make sure that you do not go deeper than a half squat. Keep your upper body in the same position as for "Deep Squats." Repeat.

- **Jump Squats up Stairs:** These are the same as "Jump Squats," except that you jump up a flight of stairs, one step at a time. Then you turn around and jump back down the stairs, one step at a time. Repeat. You will have to concentrate when doing these or you will wind up eating a step. Be careful.

- **Running Stairs:** Of course you can also just run (or walk) up and down flights of stairs. If you want to increase the intensity, carry a water bottle in each hand. That will **definitely** take care of the intensity problem.

- **Interval Sprints:** If the weather permits, run sprints outside using the **CTTC** Cardio-Aerobics System which is explained in **The CTTC Workout #1, Monday**.

- **Lunges:** In a normal lunge, you take a big step forward with one foot. Your front leg bends until the knee reaches about a 90° angle while staying directly over your front foot. Then you push off with your front foot and bring it in line with your back foot again. You then repeat the exercise with your other foot.

- **Walking Lunges** are done the same way except that instead of bringing the front foot back, you bring the back foot forward into another lunge with the other leg. In other words, you will be walking, but taking very large, deep steps. This one is a killer.

Calves

- **Standing Calf Raises** (on a step): See the description of this exercise in **The CTTC Workout #1, Wednesday.**

- **One-Legged Calf Raises** (on a step): See the description of this exercise in **The CTTC Workout #2, Wednesday.**

- **Walking Calf Raises:** These are done just like the other calf raises, except that you are doing them as you walk. You rise up on the balls of your feet with each step, making sure that you keep your weight on the big toe side of your feet, and rising up as high as possible with each step. This will really put a bounce in your step. These can also be very effectively combined with "Interval Sprints." Do **Walking Calf Raises** during the minimum/medium (rest period) part of the sprints.

  Important: You **must** stretch your calves **every time** after you exercise them! This will increase their flexibility, help to prevent injuries to your calves, and help to prevent muscle soreness.

Only a Few

These are just a few of the exercises you can do at home, and on the road. There are many books on calisthenics and exercising with elastic bands. Read some of them for more ideas. With a little imagination, you can come up with some exercises of your own. This will also build your interest in exercising. Just remember to always apply the **Principles of Quality Exercise** which you have learned in this book to whichever exercise you design or choose to do, and you will be successful.

The Best Exercise Machine

Do you know what the very best exercise machine is for the upper body? It is a simple 15-20 foot climbing rope. No chrome, no digital panel showing your pulse rate etc., and it doesn't cost $1000.00. However, climbing a rope will work every muscle in your upper body, with the exception of those involved in overhead pressing movements. Add "Running Stairs" or "Interval Sprints," and a few "Handstand Pushups," and you have an excellent full-body workout, in a minimum amount of time, and for an absolutely dirt-cheap price.

Good…But Not Best

Keep in mind that exercising with elastic bands, springs, water bottles, etc. (or even using your own bodyweight) can never take the place of good old-fashioned weights. Weights are more versatile, more exact, more efficient, and will produce superior results, much faster.

Don't avoid challenges…embrace them!

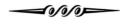

Chapter 14

JUST FOR THE LADIES

It should come as no surprise that most women begin exercising because they want to look better. They want to lose excess body fat and develop a firmer, shapelier body. Others begin exercising to improve sports performance, to please their husband or boyfriend (or both), to rehabilitate from an injury or an illness, to improve their self-image or maybe even because their doctor said they would die soon if they did not start exercising. I want to deal here with that very large group of women (no pun intended) who want to look better.

For the Last Time

The first item on my agenda is to, for the eleventh time, debunk the biggest farce that has ever been perpetrated on women about exercise. This is the age-old "If I exercise with weights I will develop big muscles" syndrome.

A Vision

What kind of a super denial trip is that? Picture this, ladies. You have a gym full of hormone-raged young guys who are trying everything humanly…and sometimes inhumanly…possible to put any small amount of noticeable muscle whatsoever on their scrawny frames. Their growth hormone output is at its peak and you can smell the testosterone in the air. They are lifting big weights and, after their workouts, will down huge protein shakes and eat like barbarians, trying to somehow build just a tiny bit more muscle.

Accidental Muscle

Now enters a person of the female persuasion, with narrow shoulders, flaring hips, breasts, and one-twentieth of the absolutely-necessary-for-building-large-muscles hormone, testosterone, in her system that these guys have. And what is she afraid of? She is afraid that she is going to somehow, **accidentally** build big muscles.

How ludicrous is that? I have been exercising with weights for more than fifty years now…my wife for more than twenty-five years…and neither of us has ever seen anyone…male **or** female…**accidentally** build large muscles. I very seriously doubt that you are going to be the first one.

Fear

"Yes, but female bodybuilders have big muscles." See, I can read your mind. I have two words for you: anabolic steroids. Unless you are planning to use anabolic steroids, your fear of building too much muscle is just another excuse (and a pretty lame one at that) to not begin a Quality Exercise program.

Bad Hair Day

It's like saying that you are afraid to go to school because you might wind up being another Einstein… and you don't like his hairstyle. The vast majority of women need to be much less worried about body-**building** and be much more concerned with "body-**reducing.**"

Too Muscular

Many women bodybuilders (and some other female athletes) look "too muscular" not so much because they have large muscles (many don't), but because they have body fat levels of around 15%, or even less, when they are in competition shape. Of course this is also the only time you see pictures of them…taken when they are pumped-up, oiled-up, tanned-up and with special lighting. This makes their muscles very visible and, even if they are not large, they will **appear** to be large under these very special conditions.

If you had a body fat level which my wife and I consider to be reasonable and attainable for most women (20-25%), you would still have to lose 25-40% of that body fat before you could even **begin** to look "too muscular." For most women, that would require months of extreme dieting and exercising. I know my wife doesn't worry about that…and I don't think you have to either.

Chances Are…

Of course there are some females with more than the average woman's share of muscle. You know some of these ladies too. In high school we called them "tomboys." They could run faster than many of the boys, were good athletes, and were quite strong even though they had never lifted a weight in their entire short lives. And more than likely, they also had higher **natural** levels of testosterone than the average teenage female.

Femininity

It is conceivable that these women, with good coaching, 4-5 days of hard training per week, a super nutrition program, and a heavy dose of fanaticism, could actually build enough muscle…even without using drugs…to be considered unfeminine by most people. However, as tomboys, it was usually their **attitude** that made some of them seem less feminine…**not** large muscles.

If you were one of these women, you would have known it long ago. The chances of the rest of you building large muscles are absolutely **zero,** especially by only using the three, thirty-minute weight workouts per week that are incorporated into the **CTTC** Exercise Program.

I'm Still Not Sure

If you are still worried that you might somehow **accidentally** turn into an ugly mass of monstrous muscle, then think about this. If you ever get to the point where you think that you are developing too much muscle...**do less!** That is the difficult and complicated solution to this "problem" that so many women seem to fear so greatly.

What is much more likely to happen is that you will become firmer and shapelier...all over...with strong, shapely legs (think of dancers' legs), upper arms that won't flap in the breeze, only one set of hips, and buns that will vibrate, instead of wobbling, when you walk. That doesn't sound very unfeminine to me.

Remember, even if you were to liposuction every ounce of excess body fat away, you would still have a flabby body...unless your underlying muscles are firm and healthy. The best, most efficient, effective and longest lasting way to do this is through Quality Exercise with weights.

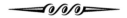

Different?

Should women exercise differently than men? For the most part, no. As you learned in the chapters on aerobics and fat-loss, muscle is absolutely indispensable for controlling our body fat and for creating a strong and shapely body. In this chapter you have learned (I hope) that building too much muscle, especially upper body muscle, is simply impossible for the vast majority of women. Therefore, exercising the back, chest, shoulders and abdominals should be basically the same for both men and women.

Because the arm muscles are very involved in most back and chest exercises, women do not usually need to do much direct exercise for their arms. That is one small difference.

Kicking Men's ...

Now, however, we do come to a major difference. Although women generally cannot match men for upper body strength, they are just as strong as men (or even stronger, pound for pound) when it comes to lower body strength. Women are genetically predisposed for this strength. It has to do with child-bearing and having to single-handedly shoulder the burden of their entire families (which sometimes includes a lazy, fat-ass husband) throughout life...or something like that.

Note from Anoushka

My husband, the big-shot professional acrobat and fitness expert, cannot even begin to keep up with me when it comes to exercising our legs. He blames it on his bad knees…but we both know the truth. He's just a sissy.

Want a Big Butt?

Because of this fact, it is much easier for women to build large muscles on their lower bodies than on their upper bodies. So what do these women, who are so afraid of building big muscles, do? They do little or no exercise for their upper bodies, where they **can't** build large muscles, and spend the vast majority of their time exercising their lower bodies, where they **can** build large muscles. Figure that one out.

Trivia

Here is a trivia question for you ladies. Which muscle in the female body can be built easiest and biggest…or biggest the easiest? Answer: The gluteus maximus…more commonly known as your butt…which is short for buttocks. By still believing in the fantasy that you can spot-reduce excess body fat by exercising a specific part of your body (see the first article in Chapter 20), many women are actually building bigger butts, instead of smaller ones.

Now maybe you are thinking, "But you said it is impossible to accidentally build too much muscle." It is, but **this is not accidental**. These women are working hard to build big butts, doing exercise after exercise specifically for that area. Many T-aerobics classes spend much of the time working this muscle. If these women are not also following Quality fat-loss Exercise and Nutrition programs, then the body fat on top of their ever-expanding gluteus maximus will remain…and their butts will look even bigger than before. Somehow, I don't think this is their intention.

Use It or Lose It

What do you do if you want a muscle to get smaller? You can either over-exercise it for hours every day, like marathoners do with their skinny legs…or you can exercise it as little as possible. Think what a broken arm or leg looks like after only 4-6 weeks of being immobilized in a cast. Not being a masochist at heart, I choose the "do as little as possible" approach.

Small and Tight

What do you do if you want a muscle to get bigger? You exercise it intensely. If you want a muscle to stay small, but tight, you do just enough Quality Exercise to keep that muscle healthy and firm, but not enough to make it grow. Intelligent and effective exercise is the answer, not dumb work.

So, for many women, all this exercise concentrated on their buns is building bigger butts, not smaller ones. This is why the **CTTC** Exercise Program uses **no direct exercises** for your buns. It uses only **indirect** exercises. These are enough to tighten and lift your booty, but not enough to make it bigger. The rest of the **CTTC** Exercise Program (combined with the **CTTC** Nutrition Program) will help you to get rid of the excess body fat covering your buns, thereby creating what most women actually want – a smaller, firmer behind.

This way, the **CTTC** Exercise Program, once again, saves you a lot of wasted time and energy which you can put to much better use somewhere else, such as with your kids, your job, your husband or boyfriend (or both)…or just enjoying life more!

Gynecology Chairs

AGREE

Now I am going to disillusion you again. Those adductor and abductor machines, which are so popular with the ladies, are another complete waste of time for spot-reducing excess body fat on your hips and thighs. These are the machines where you sit down and either squeeze your thighs together, or push them apart, by pressing against pads on the inside or outside of your knees. My wife calls them gynecology chairs. I refer you again to the first article in Chapter 20.

If you need to strengthen these **small** muscles for a specific sport, or to recover from an injury, or for some other specific reason, then they are wonderful machines. But for losing body fat or for shaping your thighs, squats and leg presses, using various foot positions, will give you much better results in a fraction of the time. These exercises use the **large** muscles of the hips and legs, thereby creating shape and using **lots** of (fat) calories in the process. And once again ladies…**spot-reducing is a myth**. I'm sorry!

And if you still don't believe me, prove it to yourself once and for all. Do only one of these exercises for several months and if at the end of your little experiment you have legs which are fat-free on one side but still over-fat on the other, please write me…and the exercise physiology departments at every university…and "Ripley's Believe it or Not"…and the Tooth Fairy, Santa Claus, etc., etc.

The adductor chair (where you squeeze your thighs together) is, however, a great way to stretch your inner thighs after exercising your legs. You sit in it and let the pads gently stretch your legs apart for 30-60 seconds. Repeat this several times while you relax. Great stuff.

Size…Not Weight

I have to make something very clear here, again, for those of you who still have losing **weight** imprinted on your brains. Muscle is more dense than fat (by about four times). Therefore, a pound of fat takes up about four times more space than a pound of muscle does. This means that if you lose ten pounds of fat and gain ten pounds of muscle, you will **weigh** exactly the same on a scale. However, you will have lost a lot of **size**. You will be much smaller!

Key

The difference in size and shape between a 5'4", 120 pound woman who has 40% body fat, and a 5'4", 120 pound woman who has 20% body fat, is enormous…pun again definitely intended. The woman with 20% body fat will be slender and shapely, while the woman with 40% body fat is chronically obese, **both at 5'4" and 120 pounds**. This is why it is so important to keep accurate records of your measurements and take photographs at regular intervals. Forget about **weight** and concentrate on **shape** and measurements.

Quality Muscle = better shape!

Empowerment

Empowerment is a point that is hardly ever brought up by instructors or other proponents of women exercising with weights. Maybe they just never thought about it, but I find it one of the most important and most satisfying results that women receive from this kind of exercise.

Women who begin Quality Exercise with weights are invariably surprised at how conquering "heavy" weights and becoming stronger gives them so much self-confidence, creates a better self-image and makes them mentally stronger as well. It empowers them!

Combining Quality Exercise with weights and some type of martial arts training will enhance these benefits even more. This combination will do wonders for creating strong, confident women (young or older), who will be much less influenced by advertising, fads, fashion, peer pressure, and what "other people" think of them. They will become strong, confident, self-thinking independent women with lots of self-esteem, a healthy self-image and a healthy body-image too…and isn't that what true women's liberation is all about?

Magic

Building a shapelier body requires most women to use a little magic. Women who are born with the genes to become tall, long-legged, with not-too-narrow shoulders, small waists, and narrow enough hips…are limited editions. Most of the rest need to create an illusion.

Just as wearing horizontal stripes will make you look shorter and wider, and vertical stripes will make you look taller and thinner, developing (or not developing) specific parts of your body will also create an optical illusion. For instance, very thin, toothpick legs, with no shape to them will make even a small butt stick out and look bigger than it actually is. Having well developed, shapely legs (like dancers) will actually make your buns look smaller.

Illusion is a girl's best friend. It is one of your best weapons, so use it wisely when shaping your body. **Develop** those areas that contribute to a better shape and **reduce** those areas that detract from a better shape. Just losing **weight** is a simplistic wish…and will ultimately produce inferior results. It is exactly like sculpting a statue of a beautiful woman:

- First take a large block of stone.
- Now chip away everything that doesn't look like a beautiful woman. Simple, isn't it?

Sigfried and Roy

They are beginners. Women have been masters of illusion for centuries…using make-up, wigs, eyelashes, high heels, silk stockings, padded panties, compress girdles, "falsies," shoulder pads and push-up bras, to name just a few. However, when you have to squeeze into your summer clothes and bikinis, the illusion can instantly disappear…unless you have taken the time and effort to create a longer lasting illusion: your very own **hardbody**.

Decorating

One sure way to destroy any illusion is to put a younger, tighter face (lift) on top of a saggy, run-down body. It's like hanging new curtains in a condemned house. They won't make the house look better. The stark contrast will only make the house look even more pathetic. Fix up the house first, and then hang new curtains. That works.

For the same reason, why on earth would you work your butt off (literally), building and maintaining a strong, shapely, and healthy body, and then not have a face to match it? I am all for a little help in the face department when it is needed, but only if you take good care of your body…and your health…**first**.

While we are on the subject, I feel the same about breast enhancement, whether that be enlargement, reduction or a little anti-gravity work. As with faces, there is a limit to how much exercise alone can help in these areas. Therefore, I feel a little outside help here is also completely appropriate, but once again, only if you are taking good care of the rest of your body as well. After all, if you had a **pretty** face but bad teeth, wouldn't you want to get your teeth fixed?

Note from Anoushka

Being only forty-four years young, I have not yet undergone either of these procedures. Thanks to Quality Exercise and health-building nutrition (and living with an extremely knowledgeable personal trainer for the last twenty-plus years), I do not need them…yet. However, when the time comes, I will only hesitate long enough to find a truly qualified, competent and experienced doctor to perform the procedure(s).

Stay Realistic

My bottom line (no pun intended this time) on cosmetic surgery: It remains a personal choice. Just make sure you are doing it for the right reasons, not to fulfill some unrealistic expectation(s). Cosmetic surgery will **not** transform you into a different person; it will only make you a more (physically) attractive you. You need to like **you** first.

Supplements and Surgery

A recent article in the official medical journal of The American Society of Plastic Surgeons reports that cosmetic surgery patients who used nutritional supplements recuperated **17% faster** than those who did not use supplements. This is another example of why I do not separate all these different aspects of health and well-being. You simply can't separate them and still be optimally effective.

"Magic bullet" solutions are always much less effective than an integrated approach to any problem. This is why, when someone asks me a question about their nutrition, I ask them how their exercise program is going. Likewise, when asked about an exercise program, I first ask them what they are doing nutritionally. A **combination** of factors is **always** much more effective!

Billion $ Cellulite

There is a lot of controversy about this subject, which is why a lot of people are making megabucks selling anti-cellulite products. However, there are a few points which stand out above the controversy.

1. Chemically and physiologically, what is called cellulite is no different from your normal, everyday, run-of-the-mill, body fat.

2. Cellulite seems to occur mainly in places on the body which have poor blood circulation… particularly the upper legs, hips, and butt areas.

3. Cellulite occurs predominantly in females.

I want to emphasize here that the following is only a theory of mine…an educated guess, based on a combination of scientific facts and logic. You decide if it makes sense…or not.

a. We know that the upper legs, hips, and butt are areas where many women gain excess body fat most easily.

b. We know that excess body fat hinders blood circulation.

c. We know that cellulite tends to occur in areas that have poor blood circulation.

When you lose excess body fat, circulation in these areas will automatically improve. Add the correct type of exercise to further increase blood circulation in these areas and you should be well on your way to preventing, eliminating, or reducing cellulite.

But what causes that lumpy, orange peel appearance that we call cellulite? Once again, this is just a theory of mine. You decide again if it makes sense…or not.

I believe this has mostly to do with the health and condition of your skin, not because cellulite is a different kind of fat. If the walls of your cells (both skin cells and fat cells) are not healthy, strong, and elastic, they cannot properly restrain the pressures exerted on them and will then be pushed into irregular, bulging shapes, not unlike a bump (weak spot) on an inner-tube.

Poor blood circulation adds to this problem. The cells cannot efficiently rid themselves of their waste products, thereby further diminishing the health of these cells.

What to Do

One of the basic principles of the **CTTC** Exercise Program is to improve blood circulation to all parts of the body, simply because good circulation is vital to both body fat loss and to your general health. That it might also be part of a cellulite solution would just be another freebee of the program, much like how developing full, supple, shapely muscles will also help to smooth your skin from the inside out.

If your skin is not properly hydrated (moisturized), it will lose its elasticity. Anything that will help to moisturize your skin will help to keep your skin healthy. Comparative research has shown that many low to moderately priced moisturizers work just as well, or even better than many of the expensive brand names, so don't be brainwashed into thinking that expensive is always best. The most important thing is to use them liberally and often. Also, don't use petroleum based products, usually indicated by the word "petrolatum" in the list of ingredients. Of course, drying your skin out with overexposure to the sun's rays…or tanning beds…is never a good idea.

The Cheapest Solution

The all-time best way to keep your skin moisturized is to do it from the inside out. Drinking lots of pure, clean water will do more than anything else to keep your skin healthy and elastic.

More Logic

Good nutrition is another important factor in keeping these cells healthy. Your skin is constantly renewing itself. You acquire millions of new skin cells every day. It is only logical that if these new skin cells do not have high-quality building materials (health-building, nutritious food and sufficient vitamins and minerals) to form themselves, your body is not going to be able to produce strong, healthy, elastic skin.

Vitamins and minerals are of utmost importance here, and they also work best from the inside out. Don't just smear them on the outside (vitamin creams, etc.). A good, high-quality multi-vitamin/ mineral will go a long way towards improving and maintaining the health of your skin. This has already been discussed in the chapter on nutrition, Chapter 12.

My wife has been a practicing sports massage therapist for nearly twenty years. She can usually give an amazingly accurate analysis of a client's eating habits simply from the condition of their skin. That should tell you something!

Another Win-Win

I think you will have to agree that this all sounds quite logical. The nice thing about my theories is that all of these things are also good for your general health and well being, so you can't lose. This is another win-win situation!

Now Is the Time

Begin incorporating the **CTTC** Exercise and Nutrition Programs into your life today and amaze yourself with the changes you can make in your body, in your health and in the quality of your life!

While We Are on the Subject of "Just for the Ladies"

Peer Pressure

I constantly hear that there is so much pressure on women to be thin. As a "real man" (although my wife would certainly dispute that description), I refuse to take the rap for this "pressure" anymore. Most men actually don't prefer really thin women. If you ladies would take a peek into a few men's magazines, you will find that there are no "skinny" models in most of them. You find really skinny models in **women's** magazines, not men's magazines. **Women** made Twiggy into a superstar... not men!

I also personally don't consider "skinny" or really thin women to be very attractive. Many of them just look emaciated and unhealthy, and I don't think you will find those two words in the dictionary as synonyms for pretty or beautiful, much less sexy.

Look at it this way. If you put a 140 pound "hardbody" fitness model on one side, a 130 pound Playboy Playmate on the other side, and a 100 pound fashion model in the middle (all of the same height, of course), I will guarantee you that the vast majority of men will have one eye looking to the left, and the other eye looking to the right. Only a very small minority of them will notice anything in the middle, and that's a fact!

So, ladies, guess where all this "pressure" is coming from? You are thinking this way and trying to get really thin…**for other women**…not for most of us men! If you are over-fat, you should be much more concerned about becoming one of the **half a million** American women who die every year – **1,350 every day** – from cardiovascular diseases, which is more than the next six causes of death combined. In airplane terms again, four large airliners going down **every day**.

A recent survey in Holland found that **only 6% of men actually prefer thin women**, and 1% even prefer over-fat women. 59% had no preference regarding the figure of a potential partner. That leaves 34% with no opinion whatsoever…which means that 34% of Dutch men would make perfect partners for you ladies. What woman wouldn't give her best pair of shoes for a husband who has no opinion whatsoever?

I am not saying that you should not be thin…or even really thin…if that is what you want **for yourself**…and as long as you are healthy. It remains, after all, a matter of personal taste. Just be sure that you are doing this for yourself and not for someone else. Nobody is putting this pressure on you…you are putting it on yourself…or you are allowing the pressure to be put on you. It is a choice – **your choice** – so stand up and be a real (independent) woman.

My wife often says the same thing to me. "Stand up and be a real…whatever." She also threatened to divorce me for chronic neglect…or something like that. I don't know…I wasn't really listening.

Bottom line: Real men love a woman for **who** she is…**not** for how skinny she is!

Be Yourself … Do It for Yourself … Whatever It May Be!

Chapter 15

HAD I KNOWN I WAS GOING TO LIVE THIS LONG, I WOULD HAVE TAKEN MUCH BETTER CARE OF MYSELF

Boy, have we ever screwed this one up over the last few decades. Somewhere along the way, **not** being healthy has become accepted as being "normal."

> It never ceases to amaze me that people who do absolutely nothing for their health are always surprised when they get sick. They should actually be surprised that they have occasional periods of being "not too sick." – R.E. Dickson

No Time

Most people "just don't have time to exercise" for a couple of hours a week in order to build and maintain their health, but always seem to find time for other, unimportant things. They can't afford a couple of dollars a day for some effective, health-building nutritional supplements, but always seem to have $5.00 for a designer cup of coffee, or money for a Gargantuan Gulp and a double McCoronary with fries. But when they **permanently** lose their health, they are suddenly willing to sacrifice **everything**, and pay any amount to get it back. All of a sudden, their priorities in life assume the correct order again. Sadly, by that time it is often already too late.

I'm OK…Really

One international organization defines health as "the absence of disease." In other words, if you are not yet quite sick enough to need a doctor or a hospital, you must be healthy enough. Apparently it is acceptable if you are not strong enough to carry your own groceries, or if you can't play with your kids for a short time without becoming exhausted. Catching a cold several times every year is not questioned, and being too stiff or too over-fat to bend over and pick something up off the floor is considered humorous instead of sad. Not being able to mentally and emotionally handle the challenges of daily life has now become a part of daily life…even for children. How pathetic is that?

Yup, we have really lowered the bar on what we consider to be health. However, there is a very big difference between being "truly healthy" and just being "not very sick."

Where Did I Go Wrong?

Bad health can actually begin in the womb if your mother smoked, drank alcohol, used over-the-counter, prescription, or street drugs, or followed a diet which did not provide all the necessary vitamins, minerals and other nutrients. Bad genes from either parent add to the problem, and not exercising from a young age practically insures a life of less-than-optimum health. Or you can **choose** to take personal responsibility for, and control of, your own health.

> "Health is much too important to leave to the doctors." – Dick Holzaepfel

But My Doctor Said

How many times have you heard someone who doesn't exercise and is over-fat say something like, "My doctor checked me out last week and he said that I am in excellent health. I feel great." Obviously, neither he/she nor his/her doctor has a clue as to what good health, much less excellent health, means. It is always interesting to hear these doctors' explanations when one of their patients drops dead from a heart attack shortly after they have declared them to be "in excellent health."

It is also always interesting to see just how "healthy" the doctor himself really is. An over-fat, non-exercising doctor, nurse or dietitian giving out advice about exercise, nutrition, losing excess body fat or building health doesn't have a whole lot of credibility with me. A doctor, nutritionist or other healthcare professional who is him/herself unhealthy is very probably not going to put you on the right path to "true health." Think about it. If a doctor doesn't even care about his own health, how much is he going to care about yours?

If you have never enjoyed excellent health, how can you possibly know what "feeling great" really feels like? I have personally never heard anyone who has gone from obese to a healthy bodyweight say, "Gosh, I wish I were really fat again. I felt so much better then…and I was much happier too."

Better Living Through Chemistry

NOT ME

People seem to have convinced themselves that no matter what they do to themselves, the doctors and/or some miracle drug will be able to completely patch them up again. And they expect it to be done quickly, painlessly and with as little inconvenience to themselves as possible.

Houses don't have bathrooms anymore. They have become mini-pharmacies, stocked with a plethora of pills, drinks, syrups, salves, sprays, powders, suppositories, patches and creams, mostly developed to alleviate only the symptoms and make you **feel** better, not make you **be** better. But as long as you **feel** OK, you must **be** OK, right? Wrong! Spend your money on things that will build your health (like a gym membership), instead of on things that say **"For Fast Relief"** on the package.

No child is badly raised or just plain lazy anymore. Now they all have some trendy affliction and the solution is to drug them…oops, sorry…to medicate them into acceptable behavior until some magical time when they can be taken off the drugs…sorry, medications…and then they will miraculously be "healthy." As if missing all those years of problem solving, social interaction and normal consciousness will somehow have no negative effect on their personalities and ability to successfully manage their adult lives.

And if it does have a negative effect, we can just put them on another…uh…medication and say that they need this one because they had difficult childhoods. Why not? Mommy has pills to take care of her stresses during the day and pills to go to sleep at night. Daddy may use something to keep himself "sharp" at work and both may have a couple of drinks just to "relax" sometime during the day. In fact, more than five million American women have a serious problem with alcohol, so "relaxing" should not be one of their problems anymore. Unfortunately for the kids involved, many of these women are also mommies.

More than 40% of Americans take at least one prescription drug. More than 80% take at least one medication regularly. Nearly 17% of Americans take at least three different prescription drugs and 30% take five or more medications regularly. Most of these drugs and medications are for **preventable** conditions. Medicine use has **doubled** between 1999 and 2006. Shouldn't that ring some alarm bells?

Respectable Junkies

These things have become so much a part of our modern, unhealthy lifestyle that more than twelve million "normal" American adults and 2½ million teenagers are drug addicts…oh, excuse me…they are "abusers of prescription medications." We certainly don't want to call the problem by its real name. We might hurt someone's feelings. In fact, these two groups constitute the fastest growing drug problem in America (150% increase in only the past five years) and their drugs of choice are pain pills and tranquilizers. Now we have a situation where stoned-out-of-their-brains parents are trying to tell their kids how dangerous drugs are. "OK, Mom. Can I have a couple of yours instead? Yours are from the doctor, so they can't be bad for you."

Good versus Bad

Never forget: As a parent, you are **constantly** setting examples for your kids. The only choice you have is whether you are setting **good** examples or **bad** examples.

Don't Worry…Be Happy

There were more than 157,000,000 prescriptions written for anti-depressants in 2003. 11,000,000 of these were written for children. Use of these drugs for children has increased 500% in the past 10 years. More than 1% of kids **under five years old** are also now "under treatment" with anti-psychosis drugs. This is macabre. At the time of this writing, the new concern is a "minor" side effect that prescription anti-depressants seem to have on some of these younger patients. The side effect appears to be suicide. Well, at least they will not be depressed anymore.

Has anyone stopped for a moment to consider the possibility that a society that needs to write more than 30,000 anti-depressant prescriptions…**per day**…for children who are apparently so mentally unstable that they need to be drugged all the time…should **not** be considered a normal situation, and that maybe…just maybe…there is something else going on here which would not require constantly drugging most of these kids into la-la land? Yes, I know…anti-depressants are **sometimes** necessary… but for millions of children? Give me a break!

Hospitals Are Full of Sick People

If you get sick or injured, you just check into the nearest hospital and the people there heal you or put you back together. No big deal, right? Well, you might want to consider the following.

- Adverse reactions to FDA approved drugs contribute to the deaths of approximately 130,000 hospital patients every year. In 1994, this was the fifth leading cause of death in America.

- 7,000 hospital patients die from medical errors every year.

- 12,000 hospital patients die from unnecessary surgeries every year.

- 20,000 hospital patients die from other hospital errors every year.

- 100,000 hospital patients die every year from the 2,000,000 infections that patients get while they are in the hospital.

Not Very Healthy

Add all these numbers together and you can see that for more than a quarter of a million people each year, a hospital stay will not be a very healthy experience. By the way, these figures come from articles in *The Journal of the American Medical Association*, not from some radical, anti-hospital group.

Cures That Kill

Hey…it's not over yet. According to The National Academy of Sciences, for one, 100,000 more people die from other medical mistakes each year in America. That brings the total to about 350,000 deaths every year from doctors and medicines which are supposed to give us back our health…not kill us. That is more yearly deaths than from car accidents, AIDS, and guns combined.

Another recent report in *The Journal of the American Medical Association* put the figure at more than 750,000 people who die each year as a result of a system which has changed from being a health-care system to a disease-management system.

Think about this for a moment. Even at the lower figure of 350,000, that is **nearly 1,000 deaths every single day of the year**. Once again, this is the equivalent of three large passenger airliners going down each and every day of the year. And some of you are afraid of flying? You should be much more afraid of getting sick or injured and winding up in a hospital.

Can you imagine the furor we would have from consumer advocate groups and the FAA if three large passenger planes started going down every day? Doesn't it seem curious that this is **not** the case with our disease-management system? Nobody seems to care. Well, you had better learn to care about your own health because, based on results, many of those whose job it is to care aren't doing the best work possible.

As of this writing, an arthritis prescription drug has just been pulled off the market after five years, but not before it caused an estimated 160,000 heart attacks and strokes, resulting in the premature deaths of an estimated 30,000 people. Another drug has caused serious heart problems in 90,000-140,000 patients, causing death in 44% of them, according to The American Heart Association. A couple of other drugs have now also quickly been pulled off the market.

You're Not Out of the Woods Yet

Don't think that this doesn't apply to you simply because you rarely take prescription medicines. The number of people who die each year from adverse reactions to common, everyday, over-the-counter (OTC) medicines such as aspirin and acetaminophen, to name just two, is also shocking. About forty-four people die every single day of the year from OTC's. **16,000 deaths a year** should also make you think twice before popping that FDA approved, totally safe, with no side effects, OTC...or giving it to your children.

Every year Americans have 700,000 adverse reactions to drugs which result in a visit to an Emergency Room.

No Such Thing

Anything and **everything** you put into your body has a "side effect" of some kind...whether it is a good effect or a bad effect. Illegal drugs, prescription drugs, OTC drugs, any medicine, and even food...all have an effect. Some have large effects and others have smaller effects, but **everything** has a physiological effect of some kind on your body...even plain water.

> There is no such thing as a medicine that is 100% safe...with no side effects! It just doesn't exist.

It's All in Your Head

What you **think** also results in physiological reactions in your body, which is why words and thoughts produce happiness, sadness, fear, anger, laughter, depression, etc., just as drugs can. This is why words and thoughts can do so much harm…or so much good. Hey…could **positive thinking** then be part of the solution to many of these problems? Nah…it's just too logical to be of any use.

In Our Best Interests

At least we can rest easy in the knowledge that our representatives in government, in all their infinite wisdom, are busy trying to improve this situation with the OTCs…or at least to better inform the American public about the possible dangers of OTCs. Well, I am sure they will eventually get around to that just as soon as they take care of regulating (and even banning some of) our **basic** nutritional supplements. **Basic** nutritional supplements should obviously take priority because they have been conclusively linked to…ZERO deaths per year…zilch! Null, nada, nix, none! No deaths…but how many times have you been warned about an overdose of multi-vitamin/minerals? Now, in contrast, how many times have you been warned about the possibility of dying from taking an aspirin? We should be much more concerned about overdoses of **ignorance**…not **basic** nutritional supplements.

Hi, I'm from the government and I'm here to help you!

If Americans are not careful, we will wind up with the same situation they now have in Europe where the governments have over-regulated nutritional supplements to the point where it is nearly impossible to find a decent multi-vitamin/mineral. In some European countries you need a prescription from a doctor in order to buy **basic** nutritional supplements, even though most doctors have **no** training and **minimal** knowledge in this field.

You can, however, still freely buy a "magic" necklace which a TV infomercial claims can heal virtually any human affliction, especially those which doctors and modern medicine have not been able to successfully treat. This is definitely an overdose of ignorance…but it is still legal…and freely available.

It's Not Magic

I am not trying to do a hatchet job on all medicines, doctors and hospitals here. All three are absolutely essential and they have saved my life (literally) more than once. The vast majority of doctors and other medical professionals are conscientious, highly skilled and very professional, but they are not magicians. Mistakes are made. For instance, it has been estimated that around 20% of senior citizens are being prescribed drugs that are potentially dangerous for them, without their doctors even realizing the danger. Why? Because doctors are not pharmacists. They only have time to learn a little bit about the most prescribed basic medicines.

A New Way of Thinking

I only want to make you aware of the risks that are out there and the importance of actively taking care of your own health so that you will need these wonderful people and services as seldom as possible. **The first responsibility for your own health is yours,** not your doctor's, and any doctor worth his salt will back me up here. We have to change the way we think about our health and the medical community. We need to rely more on ourselves and less on doctors and medicines. You should not assume that anything that may happen to you can be fixed with a trip to your doctor, a few pills, or a spare part put in at your local hospital. True health just isn't that simple.

> Quality Exercise combined with health-building nutrition should be your body's number one medicine!

For instance, if you have high blood pressure and you have not tried bringing it under control (under a doctor's supervision) with Quality Exercise and Nutrition...**before** you reach for a blood pressure medicine...then you are only prolonging your health problems instead of actively doing something to solve them.

Choices

The two largest causes of **preventable** death are still smoking and obesity, and both are lifestyle choices!

Congratulations America! I have just heard a report stating that obesity has finally overtaken smoking as the number one cause of preventable death in America. Well done. Let's celebrate with something to eat. And while we're at it...let's supersize that!

Get a Life...With Some Health

Most people live in a state of denial when it comes to their health, but one fact is undeniable. **Each person has a point of no return relative to his or her health.** If you allow yourself to cross this point of no return, you can never, ever completely regain your health again! **After passing this point, the damage is irreversible.** Doctors and medicines can only try to slow the degeneration and/or ease the symptoms, but your health will be gone **FOREVER**.

Emphysema, Type II diabetes, osteoporosis, other degenerative bone and joint diseases and, of course, cardiovascular diseases (which kill eighteen million worldwide each year) are just a few of the things which can rob you of your health...and I cannot emphasize this enough... **PERMANENTLY.** The truly sad thing about this is that most of these situations are preventable, if you take action soon enough.

A Long Road

Non-smoking, Quality Exercise, and a health-building nutrition plan can prevent (or help to prevent) most diseases and can also cure many…unless you procrastinate too long. Once you have allowed your health to deteriorate to a point where you are no longer physically capable of exercising at a high level (Quality Exercise), the road back is very long and very difficult. Just ask anyone who has had to rehabilitate themselves after a serious injury. The road back to good health from a debilitating disease is even more difficult…if at all possible.

Incredibly Selfish

Please don't let this happen to you. It is not fair to yourself. It is certainly not fair to the people who will eventually have to take care of you. And it is absolutely not fair to your loved ones, whom you will leave behind much too early…or do you think that you would be doing them a favor?

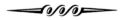

True Health

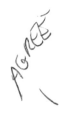

So what is true health? My definition of true health consists of eight different factors. The better these factors are integrated with each other, the more optimum your total health will be. Remember, your health is **your** personal responsibility, not your doctor's or your HMO's or anyone else's. Of course these and others play an important role, but **no one can give you good health**. You have to make it happen.

1. **Strength:** You should be strong enough to safely and easily take care of things that come up in your daily life. For example, women should be able to safely and easily lift relatively heavy objects (kids, groceries, etc.), move furniture, handle their own luggage when traveling, etc. Both men and women should be strong enough to handle most situations which could come up in their work or at home. This is what I call **functional strength**. It enables you to function effectively and efficiently, and not be dependant on other people for most situations in your daily life. Strength empowers you. It enables you to live more independently. Read this again ladies!

    However, say you live on an upper floor of an apartment building, or were staying in a hotel, and a fire broke out. Could you climb out the window and down a rope to safety? Could your children do it? Could you climb down the rope with one of your kids on your back? What if you fell off your roof or a balcony and were hanging from your hands. Are you strong enough to pull yourself back up to safety, or would you have to just pray that help arrives before your grip fails?

Sadly, shortly after writing the above paragraph, this very thing happened close to where we live. There was a fire on the fourth floor of a luxury hotel. Four hotel guests were cut off from all fire escapes and the fire department had not yet arrived. The only way out for them was to tie bed sheets together and climb down from their fourth floor balcony. Three of them were strong enough and survived. The fourth one was over-fat, not strong enough to hold on, and fell to his death. These things do happen more often than you think.

I call this **survival strength** and it has literally saved my life several times already. Strength is not only your first line of safety for surviving all kinds of accidents. It is also your first line of defense against many forms of criminality. A strong and confident looking person is never a criminal's first choice as a victim. They prefer weak, unsure looking people.

2. **Cardiovascular Condition:** This is the same situation in a different form. Just being able to function effectively in your daily life is one thing (playing physical games with your kids, for example), but could you run ½ mile or more to save the life of a loved one without dropping dead from a heart attack before you get there? These things are like having insurance. If the need ever arises and you don't already have the insurance, it is too late.

Strength and cardiovascular conditioning should be tailored to each individual's lifestyle. The **minimum** level should be that which provides the best quality of life for each individual. The upper level should be determined by survival. Firefighters, police officers, members of other emergency services, mountain climbers, extreme sporters and other people who live extraordinary lifestyles need much higher levels of strength and cardiovascular conditioning than do weekend warrior office workers.

3. **A Strong Immune System:** Unfortunately, this is a very rare commodity nowadays, even though the great Louis Pasteur gave us the right answer more than 100 years ago when he said: "The key to medicine (health) is host resistance (a strong immune system)." We didn't listen.

We don't allow our own immune systems to do their work anymore. At the first sign of a symptom, we immediately start popping pills, breaking fevers and stuffing ourselves with antibiotics. Most people and most medical professionals too, have forgotten that a strong immune system has to be **built** and constantly **maintained**.

More than 2000 years ago, Hippocrates said, "Let thy food be thy medicine." We didn't listen to him either.

Bacteria can be killed with antibiotics…well, not all of them anymore. Thanks in great part to overuse and misuse of antibiotics over the years, some bacteria are now completely resistant to all antibiotics. When you hear about a normally healthy young person dying from some type of bacterial disease, there is a good chance that one of these resistant bacteria was the cause. Sweet dreams!

So Key

Antibiotics, however, do not work on viruses at all. **Viruses can only be killed by your own immune system.** If your immune system is weak, the virus will win.

Biological Freaks

Yes, some people seem to have been born indestructible. How many times have I had to hear about some guy who smokes two packs and drinks a fifth of whisky every day, lives to be 100 years old, and was never sick a day in his life? Unfortunately, circumstances have long ago proven that I certainly do not belong to this tiny, elite group of biological freaks, so I am forced to follow a different path. Call me a pessimist, but I am not willing to bet my future health and happiness on the miniscule chance that I do belong to this exclusive club. I also do not base my financial future on my winning the lottery. I just don't like the odds on either one of these bets, and the consequences of being wrong don't excite me too much either!

It is possible to build a stronger immune system, just as it is possible to weaken your present immune system. Once again, it is not so much **what** you do, but **how** you do it that makes all the difference. The **CTTC** Exercise and Nutrition Programs are specifically designed to strengthen your immune system, not weaken it. Check the following list and see where you stand.

Positive influences on your immune system	Negative influences on your immune system
• Having a positive mental attitude • Being happy and laughing often • Being socially active • Having happy, positive thinking friends • Avoiding negative people • Getting enough quality sleep • Quality Exercise • Having more quality muscle tissue • Losing excess body fat • Raising body temperature by exercising, saunas, steam baths, etc., to induce profuse sweating • Using stress management techniques • Regularly having a good sports massage • Drinking high-quality after-exercise recovery shakes • Having a diet of high-quality, health-building foods • Eating some high-quality protein at every meal • Having enough essential fatty acids in your diet, especially the Omega 3s • Having enough fibrous carbohydrates in your diet • Having enough fiber (25-35 grams) in your diet • Drinking green tea • High-quality whey protein supplements • High-quality multi-vitamin/mineral supplements – high in the antioxidants • Vitamin C supplementation • Glutamine peptide supplementation • Allowing your immune system to do the job it has been designed to do.	• Having a negative mental attitude • Being unhappy • Being lonely • Negative thinking people • Not getting enough quality sleep • Too much stress • Not exercising at all • Exercising too intensely, too often, or too long • Being over-fat • Not actively promoting after-exercise recovery • Long periods of cold temperatures • Having an unhealthy diet • Having a high-fat diet • Having a diet high in **simple** carbohydrates • Consuming saturated fats and trans-fatty acids • Not having enough high-quality proteins in your diet • Not keeping cortisol under control • Attempting to lose body fat too quickly • Misuse of medicines • Overuse of medicines

4. **Flexibility:** At first glance, this would not seem to be that important to good health, but think about it again. If your joints have begun seizing up and your muscles are so stiff that you don't have full ranges of motion anymore, you are handicapped to some degree. You will also be more likely to sustain a serious injury if you fall or have to make a sudden movement.

Believe me, stretched or torn ligaments, tendons or muscles are no laughing matter. They are extremely painful and they take a long, long time to heal.

You are as old as your spine. Someone with a stiff spinal column is already an old person physically, no matter what their chronological age. Just ask anyone who has ever injured their lower back. You go from a young, vital being to a 100-year-old cripple in one shot of blinding pain. If you follow the **CTTC** Exercise Program correctly, using good form on the exercises and stretching, both between sets and after exercising, you will not only maintain your flexibility, but probably even improve it significantly.

5. **Mental and Emotional Stability:** This could be the most important of all the eight factors because, without this one, attainment of the other seven health factors will be much more difficult, if not impossible.

Success begins in the mind. Self-esteem, self-confidence, self-discipline, a healthy body-image, realistic and attainable goals, and the right priorities in life are all essential to success. But you have to begin with an honest self-image. You must first acknowledge and accept your weaknesses. Only then can you begin to develop a plan to improve them. Denial gets you nowhere. I know – I tried denial for a few unhappy years myself. It just doesn't work.

A bright future is based on accepting your past. You can't go forward in life until you have accepted, and then let go of your past failures and heartaches.

Develop the ability to accept your mistakes and failures…and then learn from them. Many times you can learn more from your mistakes and failures than you can from your successes. What did you do wrong and why did you do it? How can you avoid making the same mistake(s) in the future? **When you do lose…don't lose the lesson!** Turn the negative into a positive. Eliminate the things in your life that are making you fail.

Life is a process of learning by studying, analyzing, and trial and error. Not trying is just not acceptable!

Please notice that I keep saying **develop**. These things don't just happen. You have to exercise your mind to strengthen and develop it, just as you do your body. These qualities, when properly developed, will positively influence your business life, your social and family life, as well as your personal relationships with other people. If you do this…and can also manage stress…you can be in control of your life. That would certainly be a nice change for a lot of people.

The **CTTC** Exercise Program will help you to develop or improve all of the above traits, and is a great stress-buster as well. I do advise adding another form of stress management to your life, simply because stress management is so important to both your mental and physical health. My personal preference is **Transcendental Meditation**, which my publicist and I have practiced since the mid 1960s…without becoming fanatic, long-haired, commune-living, funny-dressing, commie freaks…although I was one of the very few short-haired hippies during the 60s. I have just always had trouble conforming.

Stress weakens your immune system, causes and/or accelerates many diseases, and speeds up the aging process! Therefore, I strongly recommend learning a form of meditation which suits you personally.

When you compare yourself to others…You Lose!

Being truly healthy has another mental component which everyone should incorporate into their lives. Don't compare yourself to people who are less healthy, less happy…or less anything…than you. "I may be fat, but at least I don't look like he/she does." This is just another form of lying to yourself.

Instead, always compare yourself to the best that **you** could possibly be. After all, you are the one who will benefit from positive changes and you should be doing it for yourself anyway.

People often say that I look good for my age. First I thank them. Then I gently correct them by saying that actually, the way I look and feel should be considered normal for my age. Most other people my age, or any age for that matter, have just not taken good care of themselves, so they don't look or feel as good as "normal" **should** look and feel.

Average is not necessarily "normal." Average is just that…average. I have personally always thought of "normal" as continually striving to better oneself. Concern yourself **less** with what other people think about you. What they think is **not** important. Concern yourself **more** with what you think about yourself. That **is** important.

> No one can make you feel inferior…without your permission!

This is a good place to clear up another incorrect interpretation of a word which has caused untold misery by its use. Will-power should actually be called wish-power. **Will-power does not exist.** It is only a word that is used by people who have not developed enough self-discipline. They are not the same things.

> Unsuccessful people try to rely on will-power.
> Successful people use self-discipline!

6. **Balance:** By balance, I do not mean going through life with a chip on both shoulders. Simply stated, balance means not expecting too much of yourself but, at the same time, not expecting too little of yourself either. It means being interested in most things and being passionate about at least one thing in your life…but not being fanatic about anything!

Hopefully you also earn your living by doing something you really enjoy. This is of monumental importance if you want to lead a truly happy life. Anybody can work for a living. **The real trick is to plan your life so that you can earn a living from one of your interests or passions.**

The important point here is to do something useful with your life. It doesn't have to be anything earth-shattering. Just discover what your natural talents are and then do something constructive and meaningful with them. By doing something worthwhile with your life, you will earn, and deserve, true respect, both from yourself as well as from others. Whatever you do, don't forget to enjoy life!

You only have one life, so don't waste it. This is the only chance you will ever have to do all the things you want to do. **Don't count years…count happy memories!**

> If you suspect that you may be wasting your life…you probably are!

Do good things for yourself and your loved ones, and do good things for others. It took me a really long time to learn this one…and because of that I am still apologizing to people.

Live your life so that, at the end, everyone around you is crying, but you are still smiling.

7. **Happiness and a Good Sense of Humor:** I have this on my list of true health factors because I just don't know any truly happy people who don't also have a good sense of humor.

> A person with no sense of humor has no understanding of life!

Is humor that important? Well, the Academy Awards people obviously don't think so. They give an Oscar for "Most Fashionable Shoe Style in a Foreign, Animated, Black & White, Documentary Short Film"…but have no category for comedy…even though they always need a comic to present their awards show. Sorry, but as a professional comic myself, I just had to get that off my chest and…as an acrobat…ditto for the stuntmen. No Academy Award for them either…only for the "action movie stars" who wouldn't be "action heroes" without the stunt-studs…and studesses! 'Nuff said.

The fact is, happy people have stronger immune systems, get sick less often and recover faster from illnesses and injuries than unhappy people do. In addition to that, **happiness is the number one predictor of longevity!** So, if you want to live longer, healthier, and happier… stop taking life so seriously and start laughing more.

Learn how to play again! Growing old is inevitable…growing up is optional. You don't stop laughing because you get old…you get old because you stop laughing!

Happiness also seems to be quite a good alternative to depression…so I don't see how you can have true health without being truly happy.

Can you develop a sense of humor? I definitely think so. Once again, the key word is develop. Spend more time with funny, happy, optimistic people and stay away from sour, unhappy pessimists. Watch more good comedy movies and good comedy TV sitcoms. Watch fewer heavy dramas and depressing documentaries. I videotape our favorite comedy sitcoms, and then my wife and I begin each day by having our first cup of coffee in bed while watching one or two of them. It's a great way to start every day with a laugh.

> Happy people don't always have the best of everything.
> They just strive to make the best of everything that comes their way!

If laughing is too strenuous for you in the beginning…then start with a small smile and gradually work your way up to a chuckle.

8. **Prevention:** Prevention is everything when it comes to health, so know your numbers. The numbers I am talking about are:

- Blood pressure
- Total cholesterol
- HDL cholesterol
- LDL cholesterol
- Ratio between HDL and LDL cholesterol
- Triglycerides
- Blood sugar and morning insulin levels (both are predictors of diabetes)
- Homocysteines – high levels increase the risk of heart disease, strokes, Alzheimer's disease, cancer, osteoporosis, miscarriages, neural-tube defects, and will accelerate memory loss and the aging process.
- Uric acid levels (can indicate potential problems with gout and/or kidney stones)
- Resting pulse rate

By the way, if you really want to increase your levels of insulin, cholesterol, triglycerides and uric acid (and this would be a really bad thing)…and lower your "good" cholesterol (HDL)…eat and drink lots of **simple** carbohydrates…often. If you still feel too healthy, combine these simple carbohydrates with lots of unhealthy fats. Then bend over and kiss your sweet health goodbye.

As we age, a couple of other tests need to be added to this list. These include a **PSA** test for men and **PAP** smears and **mammograms** for the ladies as well as everyone's personal favorite – a **colonoscopy** after we hit age fifty. Of course there are many other important diagnostic tests, but I will leave those up to your health care professionals. These are the basic tests that can often indicate whether further tests are warranted or not.

One of the most exciting new developments in preventive medicine is the **64 - CT Heart Scan**. This new diagnostic tool can discover potential heart problems in time to correct them with Quality Exercise and Quality Nutrition instead of with life-threatening surgery, dangerous drugs or…the ultimate cure…death. Check it out.

You will need to have all these (except your blood pressure and resting pulse rate) regularly checked by health care professionals. You can keep an eye on your blood pressure by checking it on the machines found at many pharmacies and drug stores. Home blood pressure meters are also quite inexpensive now. These will also give you an accurate reading of your resting pulse rate, which should be taken first thing in the morning, before you even get out of bed.

A healthy male, in relatively good cardiovascular condition, should have a resting pulse of between 65 and 72 beats per minute. A healthy female, in relatively good cardiovascular condition, should have a resting pulse of between 70 and 80 beats per minute. As your fitness improves, your resting pulse rate can drop to as low as 50 beats per minute or less for men, and 60 beats per minute or less for women. This means that your heart is working more efficiently and pumping more blood with fewer beats. This is a good thing.

Snap, Crackle, Pop

I am also a firm believer that regular chiropractic adjustments and sports massages are very important to total health and injury prevention. My wife is a certified Sports Massage Therapist and I know for an absolute fact that she prolonged my career as a professional acrobat by at least ten years. She is also greatly responsible for my being able to rehabilitate my torn chest muscle (pec) in record time, and for keeping the disc problems in my lower back manageable over the years.

Jock Docs

I personally prefer medical professionals who are, or have been, athletes, and who still exercise. They undoubtedly have personal experience with injuries and they will understand that I am motivated and will strive for a full recovery from whatever brought me to them in the first place. I am not just interested in relief from symptoms. There is a big difference.

Since most people are really only interested in relief from unpleasant symptoms, that is how many doctors treat them. Over time, their patients have taught them to react this way.

Be Natural

Although it may seem contrary to popular belief, the natural order of things – "normality" if you will – is not only for a person to be physically **and** mentally strong, but also to be healthy and happy. Any deviance from this should be considered abnormal and serious steps should be taken to alleviate the problem(s). A Quality Exercise program should both increase health **and** improve quality of life. The **CTTC** Exercise and Nutrition Programs have both been designed with these ideals in mind.

Unfortunately, the most difficult product in the world to sell is **prevention**.

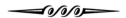

Tough Luck

OK, you do everything right and you still lose your health. Hey, it happens. Non-smokers get lung cancer, runners drop dead from heart attacks, happy people get depressed, and then there is always the unexpected accident. There are no guarantees, but **not** doing your best to become, and then stay healthy and happy, should **not** be an option.

Just as youth is wasted on the young (my publicist and myself are a couple of the rare exceptions to this rule), old age also seems to come at a bad time.

While many people don't have goals in life, I even have a goal in death! I don't want to rust away, or rot away. My goal is to die healthy! I will do what I can to keep myself in good mental and physical health, for as long as possible, so that I can fully enjoy as much of life as I am able to, for as long as I am able to. The two most effective tools I have to accomplish this are Quality Exercise and sensible nutrition. With some hard work and a little luck, I will die after enjoying a really terrific last day. Wouldn't that be a wonderful way to go! We actually have a couple of entertainer friends who have managed to do this.

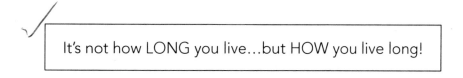

It's not how LONG you live...but HOW you live long!

A Last Thought

When I was earning my masters degree in public/therapeutic recreation, I worked with people, young and old, with every type of physical and/or mental disability imaginable. As an entertainer, I often do shows for these groups of people. Every time I perform for them, it reminds me once again of how truly fortunate I have been. I am especially moved because the wonderful life I have been able to lead so far has been possible largely due to my good health and strong body.

A very satisfying childhood (mainly because of sports), an absolutely incredible college experience (mainly because of gymnastics), which even included an education (although it isn't always apparent), and a successful and very fulfilling career in show business (thanks again to my physical abilities), have all been possible only because I made (and kept) myself strong and healthy.

I simply cannot imagine anyone who has been fortunate enough to have been born with a healthy mind in a healthy body, allowing either of these to deteriorate to the point of becoming a disabled person…by choice!

It's an Insult

I may be out of line here, but it's my opinion…and it's my book…so: **You do not have the right to do this!**

- If you claim to be a religious person, then you do not have the right to do this to yourself because it has to be a personal affront to the Higher Being (whoever that may be for you) who blessed you at birth with the precious gift of a healthy mind in a healthy body!

  I truly believe that He/She would be much more pleased if we would show our respect by taking better care of these two wonderful gifts, instead of attempting to impress Him/Her with big, expensive buildings, fancy clothes and elaborate ceremonies…but then, those things aren't really for His/Her benefit anyway…are they?

  The eighteenth century German poet and philosopher Novalis summed it up nicely when he said, "There is but one temple in the universe, and that is the body of man." Good advice… just make sure that you build your body into a small temple…not a massive cathedral.

- If you claim to be family oriented, or a social person, you most certainly do not have the right to do this to your children, your loved ones, and the people around you who are then forced to adapt their lives to accommodate your voluntary disabilities. Social activities then have to be planned around what you are still able to do with your voluntary disabilities. Maybe you don't mind when friends and family members feel obligated to come to you because you are too over-fat or unhealthy to go visit them anymore, but then you should also not feel neglected when these visits become fewer and fewer as time passes.

  These people also have families, so when it comes to the point where your grown kids are forced to decide whether it is worth it to spend a few thousand dollars to fly their whole families from California back to Chicago to visit grandma (instead of a couple of hundred dollars to fly grandma to California…but grandma doesn't fit into an airplane seat anymore), well…what would you choose to do in this same situation…and what could you afford to do? The next questions are: How many times would you be willing to do it…or be able to afford to do it?

Or think about this one: You always hear parents say how they are willing to die for their children. Don't you think your children would prefer that you live for them, and be healthy… for them if not for yourself?

- You also do not have the right to do this to yourself because it is a monumental insult to all persons on Earth who were not fortunate enough to be born with a healthy mind in a healthy body, and who have to struggle every day of their lives with a handicap which they did not **choose** to have!

- Lastly, you do not have the right to do this because it shows a lack of respect for yourself…and for others.

Disclaimer

I am not trying to be mean-spirited here. I am attempting to get you to think about what you are doing, as well as the consequences of what you are doing, not only to yourself, but also those who love you and those around you. If this speaks to you, then get off your butt and get busy working to regain the most precious possession anyone could ever have – excellent health!

> When you have good health, you have everything.
> Without good health, you have nothing.

Spread the Word

If you have a friend or loved one who needs this advice, then loan them this book or, better yet (especially for me), buy them their own copy as a present. Think of it as giving the person a second chance at the precious gift of health!

A REMINDER FOR THOSE OF YOU WHO ARE OVER-FAT

If you do not smoke, losing excess body fat is the single most important thing you can do to improve your health!

Losing excess body fat reduces most of the risk factors for dozens of diseases...all at once!

Using Quality Nutrition will further reduce all these risk factors, and will further enhance your health!

Adding Quality Exercise will not only continue to reduce these risk factors, and still further enhance your health, but will also provide you with a stronger and shapelier body and a better quality of life! For what more could you ask?

If you take care of your HEALTH ... the FAT will take care of itself.

Chapter 16

WORTH THEIR WEIGHT IN FAT

This book can put you on the right track to creating a stronger, healthier and shapelier body, but no book, DVD or video can ever replace the advice of a qualified and competent personal trainer.

The **CTTC** Exercise and Nutrition Programs will bring you to a very high level of fitness and well-being, and this book will provide you with the knowledge you need to ask intelligent questions and make better choices concerning exercise and nutrition. However, when you reach a level where you feel that the desired shape of your body (or any other fitness goal) has been mostly achieved, you will probably want to specialize even more.

This is where exercise really becomes interesting. You may want a little more roundness to your deltoids (shoulder muscles), or your calves could be a little shapelier. This is when you begin to really sculpt your body the way you want to have it...within reason, of course.

The Next Step

I will be writing follow-up **CTTC** Exercise Programs which will bring you even further along by addressing specific problems and specializing on specific body parts. If you want to progress even more than this, you will occasionally need the services of a **qualified** and **competent** personal trainer. He or she can ensure that you enjoy results exceeding those you will have already achieved with this **CTTC** Exercise and Nutrition Program.

DIY Surgery

This is comparable to trying to take responsibility for all aspects of your health. You can (and should) learn as much as possible about taking care of your own health...from books, the internet, and other sources...but if you needed something more specific done...such as an operation...would you read a book about it and then try to operate on yourself? If you answered yes to this question, I would love to meet you in person. The rest of us would seek out someone more qualified to do the procedure...like a surgeon. Do the same with your fitness needs. Seek out someone who is qualified and competent.

Where Are They?

The problem is finding a **qualified** and **competent** personal trainer out of the thousands on the market. This chapter will help you to make an educated, informed choice if you do decide to go the personal trainer route. It will also help you to better evaluate the advice you may be getting from the instructors at your gym, or from anyone else for that matter.

Basically, there are <u>five categories</u> of trainers:

 1. **Unqualified, uncertified, and incompetent:** Need I say more?

2. **Certified...but unqualified:** This person has completed a certification program, but lacks some of the attributes...such as experience, or the ability to accurately analyze exercises and problems...which are necessary to be truly **qualified** for what they are doing. For instance, some gyms still have aerobics teachers giving instruction in the weight room...even when they do not exercise with weights themselves.

    Just spending a lot of time in the gym doesn't necessarily mean that someone is qualified either. I have driven trucks, busses, vans, cars, and motorcycles for hundreds of thousands of miles on 4 continents, but I assure you that you do not want me working on your car. I have spent countless thousands of hours driving these vehicles over the past 40+ years...but I know absolutely nothing about fixing them. I leave that to people who are qualified.

3. **Qualified** (whether certified or not), **but not really competent:** They have the knowledge and the experience, but they may be unorganized, always show up late for their appointments, or not be able to motivate you. They may not be able to effectively adapt their methods or their personalities to their clients. In other words, they just may not be effective as teachers.

4. **Qualified and competent, but not certified:** This category does actually exist. In fact, some of those in this category are the ones who set up the present certification programs. Of course they are now certified...at least by their own organizations. I have nothing against certification. It helps to insure **minimum** standards in any profession, but fitness certification is like any other type of schooling. It should teach you that there are things that you don't even know that you don't know about the subject...and where you need to go to continue to learn more.

    Passing the test for a driver's license does not instantly make the person a good driver. Some get better with experience...and some remain bad drivers for their entire lives. Even doctors have to spend years as interns and residents because they just can't learn it all from the books and courses in medical school. They also need years of hands-on experience. Remember too that if you have a class of 100 students and 20 of them fail...student number 80 still gets exactly the same diploma as the best student. They are now both certified, but which one do you think is more qualified?

 5. **Qualified, competent, and certified:** You can't go wrong with one of these.

Horror Stories

Those are some of the reasons why good, competent, qualified trainers are difficult to find. I have exercised in gyms...big and small...all over the world and could write another book just of horror stories I have personally witnessed.

I saw an older man seriously injure his knees on the very first exercise of his very first day in the gym. The instructor was certified, but certainly not qualified or competent.

I recently saw a 350-pound man doing one-arm triceps extensions, with a couple of minutes rest between sets. The instructor who set up this "fat-loss" exercise program is not only certified but is also a licensed physiotherapist. However, he himself does not exercise with weights, so he has zero experience, which is why he had this man doing an exercise that is totally worthless for someone who is morbidly obese and attempting to lose excess body fat.

Of course, after only a few weeks this well-meaning man gave up. He stopped coming to the gym because he saw absolutely no results from his "certified" fat-loss exercise program. What a shame.

I have seen people performing exercises with such bad form that it was difficult to see exactly which exercise they were actually attempting to do. I once saw a certified instructor whose triceps (the muscles on the back of your upper arms) got sore from doing a basic exercise…for his **back** muscles. It even took me a while to figure that one out.

Being able to accurately analyze exercise movements **is an absolute prerequisite** to being a competent trainer.

Gymnastics to the Rescue

Both as a gymnast and later as a gymnastics coach, I was always fascinated with analyzing the various tricks. I was not just interested in doing them, but also in knowing the exact how and why of the tricks. That way, I could not only learn them better myself, but also better teach them to others. It was a pleasure for me to spend hours carefully figuring out all the angles and the tiniest movements of each trick. My knowledge of anatomy, kinesiology, and biomechanics was not only indispensable for doing this, but I also got a giant dose of practical application from the experience. This training also carried over to exercise, enabling me to much more easily and precisely analyze the many different movements involved in moving a weight…and I still love it!

Hands-on Experience

The answers to most exercise questions…or problems…have come from hands-on experience, not from doctors, dietitians or exercise physiologists sitting at their computers at some university. Their input is extremely valuable, but without practical experience, their information cannot be put to its best use.

Obsolete

In addition to having the knowledge, a qualified and competent personal trainer should have the ability to clearly and effectively transfer that knowledge to you. Choose a trainer who not only guides you through your program, but also **teaches** you. A competent personal trainer's goal should be to eventually make himself obsolete by teaching his clients enough that they can continue to **successfully** exercise, without his constant guidance. For a control session, new or specialized programs or to solve special problems, of course you should always ask for your personal trainer's expert advice again.

A good, qualified, and competent personal trainer should also possess the following qualities:

- A positive attitude
- Enthusiasm
- Friendliness
- Patience
- Understanding
- He or she should preferably also be a happy person, with a good sense of humor. I sincerely believe that a person with no sense of humor can have no real understanding of life.

The bottom line here is that if you don't feel comfortable with a particular trainer, then he or she is probably not the best trainer for you!

Born Beautiful

Here is another thing to consider when evaluating a trainer. The biggest guy or the thinnest girl in the gym is not necessarily the best trainer. In many cases that 6'2", 200 lb., twenty-five-year-old Adonis was once a 6', 180 lb., eighteen-year-old Adonis. That not-an-ounce-of-fat-on-her-body aerobics instructor may have been fat-free long before she ever took her first aerobics class. She might have initially begun taking aerobics classes just because it was fun or fashionable, for her health, or even just because the instructor was cute, and then later she decided to become an instructor. Of course, this is not always the case. It is just another point to consider in your search.

In Your Shoes

There are others who have had to study and work really hard in order to shape their bodies the way they wanted them. That is why, generally speaking, these **may** be the better trainers. They have themselves successfully done what you are attempting to do.

A trainer who has him/herself lost 20, 30, 40, or more pounds of excess body fat through Quality Exercise and an intelligent nutrition plan…and has kept it off…knows something about losing excess body fat. A skinny aerobics instructor whose pre-workout meals consist of candy bars and energy drinks **may** not be able to empathize with your problem very well.

Likewise, a naturally muscular guy **may** not understand that building muscle can be difficult for others, because it is so easy for him.

I once had a gymnastics coach who was himself a national champion. However, because he was a natural at gymnastics, he never had to analyze what he was doing in order to learn it. He just did it. He had no idea of how he actually did tricks and, as a result, he had no idea how to teach them either. Fortunately, we had so much talent on our team that we were able to teach each other…so we did…and quite successfully I might add, even though he was the "certified" coach.

Whatzizname

Arnold Whatzizname was a great bodybuilder, but he was never a ninety-seven-pound weakling. He can just look at a weight and he grows. OK, I exaggerate here slightly. Of course he worked incredibly hard (and intelligently) to get where he did, but he is also so naturally gifted that most of us mere mortals, even after years of exercise, cannot hope to even reach the point where he started out.

There is, however, another bodybuilder by the name of Frank Zane who had to struggle for every ounce of muscle he gained. He learned everything he could about nutrition and building shapely muscle, and became one of the most knowledgeable people in the sport on these subjects. He never became massive, but he did sculpt such an aesthetically beautiful body that he won the coveted Mr. Olympia title three consecutive times, defeating competitors fifty pounds bigger than himself. In fact, he is one of the very few persons to ever defeat Arnold Whatzizname in competition. Frank Zane knows the difference between quantity and quality.

Half a Man

Another bodybuilder by the name of Bruce Randall more than halved his bodyweight, from 401 pounds to 189 pounds, in only eight months, and subsequently won the Mr. Universe contest.

Now, which of these three great athletes do you think would better understand your particular problems and could better help you to shape and sculpt your body?

The Bottom Line

A qualified and competent personal trainer can save you literally years of wasted time and effort. They are truly "worth their weight in fat"…**your fat**…so when you do find a good one, listen, learn, and treat him or her well.

Remember, one of the differences between a wise person and a fool is that a wise person learns from **other** people's mistakes! That lesson also took me a lot longer than it should have.

Knowledge + Experience = Success...YOUR Success!

Chapter 17

WHO AM I, AND WHY SHOULD YOU LISTEN TO ME INSTEAD OF TO ALL THE OTHER "EXPERTS"?

There are two answers to this question.

Answer #1 – You shouldn't listen to me. At least you shouldn't listen only to me.

The greatest practical philosopher (someone who offers ideas which can actually help you, instead of only spouting idealistic drivel) I have ever known is my former gymnastic coach at the University of Iowa, Dick Holzaepfel. When I began to have doubts about my lifelong plan to study medicine, he said to me, "Health is much too important to leave to the doctors." Of course I was too young, too dumb and too full of myself to have any idea of what he was talking about at the time. Fortunately, I did not remain young and I eventually figured it out.

What he was futilely making an attempt to tell me was that you should never blindly accept one person's, or one group's ideas about anything. Nobody has **all** the answers. You should, however, carefully examine **every** idea to see if it has any merit or not.

He also told me that "Ignorance is bliss."…and then added that I was one of the happiest people he had ever met. I am still working on that one.

When I told him that I had gotten a student job as a garbage collector, his only comment was, "If you stand around long enough, your place in life will eventually catch up with you." Now that is practical philosophy at its best.

Read, Listen, Learn

If you really want to find the truth and make intelligent, informed decisions about anything, you will have to read, study, question, listen and learn from all possible sources. This is notably true in the medical world. And you should definitely be suspicious of any doctor who is offended by your wanting a second opinion, or that you have been studying your particular ailment or treatment so that you can ask intelligent questions.

It is also true when it comes to your exercise and nutrition. If you ask your instructor a reasonable question and he or she can't give you a logical and satisfactory answer, or is too unsure of him/herself to say, "I don't know, but I will find out," I would start having my doubts about him or her. No one has **all** the answers and with better and better research, **the answers keep changing**. So if someone claims to "know it all," then that is exactly what he or she is – a know-it-all. Seek your information elsewhere!

Of course, you have to have a certain amount of knowledge on the subject yourself in order to be able to ask reasonable, intelligent questions, which is why you need to read, study, question, listen and learn.

> How can you possibly hope to succeed at something you know little or nothing about?

Back to School

If you are genuinely serious about building a strong, shapely, healthy body and getting and keeping your body fat under control, you will have to study and ask questions. Read books on the subject, including this one of course, and start forming your own ideas and opinions. But form them from scientific research done on healthy individuals and athletes, not research done on rats or unhealthy people, unless you happen to be one of these...or aspire to be one of these.

Great Abs

Don't get your health and fitness advice from gossip magazines, or from "fitness" magazines whose articles and advertisements are mostly for clothes, cosmetics and other lifestyle products.

Their main concern is to sell you another magazine next month by coming up with yet another new workout to melt that fat off of your waist. And you should be asking yourself: "Why didn't the other six or seven "ultimate abs" workouts in previous editions of the magazine do the trick?" Read the articles and if something interests you, look for books or scientific articles which will give you more detailed, less biased information on the subject.

> The more you know about a subject, the easier and more quickly you will be able to achieve goals related to that subject.

Answer #2 – Because I Am Qualified and Competent

You don't know me. I have never been on Oprah, Dr. Phil or ESPN. The study and practice of health, exercise, and nutrition has always been a passion of mine, but only occasionally a commercial interest. My objectives and priorities regarding fitness and health have also changed several times during the fifty-plus years of my involvement in these fields, which gives me an even broader understanding of the different processes involved here.

Not a Freak

I am definitely not one of those goody-goody, never smoked, never touched alcohol, don't like junk-food, just love to punish my body with exercise for hours every day, can't wait to wake up and run five miles in -10° weather, exercise freaks.

At certain times in my life I have consumed too much alcohol. (Hey, I went to college…and still like to party occasionally.) I have smoked cigarettes (for twenty-five years…I stopped twenty years ago.) I have lived on fast-food (I already said that I went to college), and although I always loved practicing my chosen sports, I have always hated to exercise. And no, sports and Quality Exercise are **not** the same things.

I think this history gives me a unique insight, as well as a more realistic outlook, when it comes to exercise and nutrition for average (read: non-fanatic) exercisers and other people like me who just don't like to exercise.

Been There…Done That

I started out weak and skinny, trying to gain strength and muscular weight. Later in life, due to bad choices on my part, I allowed myself to become over-fat and out of shape. I then had to struggle to lose my excess body fat and regain my health. I have been successful at both. More importantly, for four decades I have helped countless other people to do the same, not for monetary gain, but simply because I enjoy helping people and sharing my knowledge.

In addition to the many gymnasts I have helped to coach over the years, I have worked with people young and old, male and female, and in many other sports and occupations.

Many of the athletes I have worked with were involved in sports that use weight classes, or where bodyweight plays a major role. This meant that I was not only responsible for keeping them at their competition weights, but also insuring that they were always able to compete at the highest level of their abilities. These athletes have to maintain minimum body fat levels combined with maximum strength levels, and also avoid getting sick, all at the same time. This is definitely not an easy task.

In order to be able to do this, I have to really understand how different types of exercise and different kinds of foods truly affect the human body. This type of personal training is very complicated and time consuming, but I enjoy it immensely. It involves doing a lot of research and analysis, and I learn something new every time I do it.

Total Loss

From a skinny, weak, wannabe athlete, I transformed myself into an Olympic-caliber gymnast, known for my strength. As I write this (2006) I am fifty-nine years young. Two years ago, I decided to finally retire from my profession of the last thirty-plus years as a professional acrobat. From my gymnastic and acrobatic careers, plus the occasional automobile or motorcycle accident, I have one leg and one arm shorter than the others, an elbow and a knee that don't quite straighten anymore, scoliosis, and chronic neck and low back problems. I have bad knees, neither of which can bend all the way anymore, and one shoulder that isn't too good either. I have torn one pec (a chest muscle) completely in half, have partially torn one bicep and one hamstring as well. I have dislocated both elbows and a collarbone, broken several ribs and had a beauty of a compound fracture of one of my femurs (thighbone). I stopped counting strains, sprains, or injuries to fingers and toes long ago.

With this kind of list, I have had to learn how to train safely, efficiently, and effectively. I would never have made it this long as a professional acrobat if I didn't know how to keep my body strong, flexible, and healthy. I can help you to do the same. So if you, or someone you know, are using an old injury or a sore back, etc, as an excuse to give up exercise, or not to start exercising at all, read the above paragraph again.

No Excuse

Other excuses I often hear are, "I can't afford to join a gym," or, "There is not a good gym in my area," or, "I don't have room to train at home." Sorry, but I just don't buy it. I have exercised in good and bad gyms all over the world. I have exercised inside and outside, in hotel rooms and small apartments. I exercised in a six foot by six foot storage compartment on a circus train in Africa for an entire year, and I have even built my own gyms in small trucks a couple of times when there was no other possibility for me to exercise.

I have exercised with primitive equipment and with modern equipment. I have bought equipment, borrowed equipment, and built my own equipment in order to continue exercising. Once again, if you are genuinely serious about creating a strong, shapely, and healthy body, you will find a way. It may not be easy and the conditions may not be optimum, but those are just bad excuses that unsuccessful people like to use.

Reality Check

If I could manage to exercise under the circumstances I have mentioned above, then you can certainly find a way. Lack of time is also not a valid excuse. If you can't take three hours out of an entire week for your own health and well-being, then your life is really out of control and you need to take a reality check of your priorities. Three hours is less than two percent of your week. Don't try to tell me that you use more than 98% of your time efficiently. I won't buy that either.

> If you have no time to exercise,
> you'd better reserve lots of time for disease. – Dr. Colgan

A Lifetime Passion

I have been fascinated with strength and health since I was a young boy, because I had neither in abundance. Strength manifested itself with an interest in exercising with weights, and my interest in health became a lifelong study of the medical sciences. I originally wanted to become a doctor and was accepted to the University of Iowa on the honors program in pre-medicine. I have studied anatomy, kinesiology, physiology of exercise, biomechanics, nutrition for health purposes, and performance nutrition…and I continue to do so. I spend a fortune on books, reading everything I can get my hands on concerning exercise, nutrition, fat-loss and health. My attitude has always been that if I can learn just one thing, or get just one new idea from a book, then it was worth reading the entire book.

This viewpoint, combined with my education, sports background and five decades of personal experience, enables me to quickly and accurately determine what has possibilities, what is pseudo-science and what is just pure crap.

In addition to my extensive studies, over the past forty-five-plus years I have personally tried almost every exercise, nutrition, and fat-loss system which has shown any possible merit whatsoever…and even some that didn't.

Of course there are other people out there who have also exercised for many years and also have excellent academic credentials, but there are four additional reasons why I am very good at this.

What's the Difference?

1. I have always been really enthusiastic about helping people. I love it. Helping other people to succeed gives me a real kick, as well as inspiring me to do better myself.

2. I am…and have always been…lazy. However, I am "functionally lazy." I am an achiever, but I want to achieve with the least possible effort on my part. For instance, I didn't enjoy studying most subjects in school, so I learned how to speed-read. That cut my study time in half, which made studying those subjects almost bearable. I consider my laziness as resting **before** I get tired. That sounds so much better than being just plain lazy.

3. Of course, being lazy, I hate to exercise. I exercise for only three reasons: so I don't feel like, function like, or look like people who don't engage in Quality Exercise.

4. Last, but hardly least, I love to eat. Unlike many people, I do not have an irrational fear of "strange" foods, so I have eaten lots of different foods in lots of different countries. And there are only a couple of foods that I have ever tried that I didn't like. On top of that, my wife is a fabulous cook, which makes **not** overindulging nearly impossible.

Dangerous Combination

You will have to agree that hating to exercise, loving to eat and having a wife who is a great cook is a very dangerous combination if you also want to be the proud owner of a strong, healthy, shapely body of the low-fat variety. Therefore, my only recourse has been to learn as much as I can about exercise and nutrition so I can **eat as much as possible** and **exercise as little as possible**, without becoming a blimp. That is exactly what I have done and, with this book, I can help you to do the same.

I Could Be Wrong

Keep in mind that you don't have to believe everything I say in this book. In fact, you don't have to believe anything I say in this book. After more than thirty years in show business, believe me, I can handle rejection. Heck, some very close family members still don't exercise at all, and when we had our nutritional supplement company, some of them continued to buy worthless multi-vitamin/minerals from the supermarket, even though they could buy excellent ones from us at cost price! Go figure.

Some of them still don't use nutritional supplements, not even a multi-vitamin/mineral. Go figure.

One of them is a fanatic amateur athlete who, even though he knows that I have advised world champions, has **never** asked me a single question about training, nutrition or nutritional supplements for his sport. Go figure.

A female family member, who is about 5'2" and 190 pounds, recently bought a completely worthless "miracle exercise machine" from a TV infomercial without asking our advice beforehand. What she got was a plastic stick with a length of rubber tubing attached to it and a few lines of "instructions"… for about $85.00! Go figure.

But I am not alone. The mother of friends of ours bought a second-hand car (which turned out to be a lemon) without first asking the advice of her two sons, who are both excellent car mechanics! Go figure.

It's All Up to You

So…who you listen to, what you accept as quality advice, and how hard you are willing to work, is completely and 100% up to you. Just don't con yourself, and do your very best not to let anyone else con you either. Strive to analyze things logically and intelligently before making a decision and always use common sense.

Whatever you finally choose to do, I sincerely hope that you will be successful in achieving your health and exercise goals. It could be, literally, a matter of life or death…**YOURS.**

TESTIMONIALS

I am not going to bore you with pages and pages of testimonials from every person I have ever worked with. So here is what a few people from different backgrounds have to say about how I was able to help them. In the end, you will have to decide if I know what I am talking about, or not.

A Medical Doctor

To the Reader,

I happily write this testimonial for Bobby Dickson, with whom I have been acquainted for more than twenty years. I met Bobby and Anoushka when I first started my fitness training at the same gym where they train.

During this time, Bobby has been very helpful to me, especially in getting my training programs "tuned to my personal possibilities," and supplying me with nutritional guidance in which he is very well informed from his gymnastic background, from his education, and from his studies as a Personal Fitness Trainer.

Not only is his knowledge extensive, but also his communicative faculties are so well developed that he is a great tutor, able to effectively give information and guidance to people of all abilities and from all layers of the population.

His insights into sports nutrition are of such a standard that I recommended him to the sports physiologist in the hospital where I work, as well as to the sports surgeon of our medical team, who is also the Chief Surgeon for the Philips football (soccer) team of Eindhoven – one of the top professional soccer teams in the world.

His book is filled with practical information and I would enthusiastically recommend anyone to try his programs!

Dr. Jan J. H. Pallada, MD
St. Anna Hospital
Geldrop, The Netherlands

A Fitness Professional

To the Reader,

When Bobby Dickson told me that he was writing a book about exercise and nutrition, it seemed very logical to me because I often refer to him as a "walking encyclopedia."

I met Bobby about eight years ago via associates of mine at the fitness center where I was employed full-time (I have since moved and am currently employed full-time at a fitness center in another part of Holland). I got to know Bobby very quickly. Always on the ball, he is constantly asking why you are doing what you are doing, and is always questioning your existing opinions, "new" trends, and old-fashioned ideas, with arguments that make you stop and think.

As an experienced old-timer in this field, he has seen many trends come and go, but he keeps returning to the basics to make it clear to you what it is really all about. No matter which viewpoint concerning training or nutrition we spoke about, it became obvious that commercial interests often weighed heavier than the interests of the unknowing sports person who, on the basis of these commercial interests, sometimes gets a distorted picture of his training. You cannot open a magazine anymore without finding some nutrition and/or exercise tips in it. As a professional you can sometimes hardly see the forest for the trees, much less as a layman!

When speaking with Bobby, he always appeals to your own professional knowledge. Often, some deep digging is necessary! Being conscious not to sound like a know-it-all, he enjoys sharing his experience with the serious listener. When asked for advice about an (for him) unknown subject, he will first study it before giving an answer, and he also asks others to do the same – a very good (personal) trainer who is critical and honest.

For me personally, he has often functioned as a very reliable reference book and it will be fantastic when this knowledge is available to everyone in book form!

Bobby, I wish you much success with your book!

Gabriëlle Welmers
Groningen, Holland
Certified Aerobics and Fitness Instructor
Certified Sports Massage Therapist

A Professional Acrobat

To the Reader,

My name is Istvan Deltai and I am a professional acrobat and handbalancer. In 2000 I performed in a show with Bobby and Anoushka for the first time. It was immediately obvious that all three of us were exercisers, so one of the first things we did was to seek out the best local gym for our training.

I had already been seriously training with weights for many years, and considered myself to be very well informed about this type of exercise. We trained together for a few weeks and Bobby occasionally offered small pieces of advice on how to perform certain exercises I was doing. They were mostly very small changes in body or hand positions, but the difference they made in the "feel" of the exercises was incredible.

At that time I weighed 76 kg (167 lbs.) with very low body fat, and had been trying for a long time to get my muscular weight up to my goal of 80 kg (176 lbs.), without success. One day I mentioned this to Bobby and he said that if I would trust him 100% and do exactly what he said to do, he could guarantee that I would weigh at least 80 kg, with no gain in body fat, in less than two weeks.

I did not believe this for one second, but I had seen how well his other suggestions had worked and thought, "What have I got to lose? It is only for a couple of weeks and then I can go back to my normal training again." Besides, I was very curious how Bobby thought he could accomplish something in less than two weeks that I had not been able to do with many months of intense training.

To make a long story short, Bobby wrote a personal exercise program for me, made some small changes to my diet, and told me which nutritional supplements I needed to take. In less than two weeks, I weighed 80+ kg, just like he promised. I was astounded, to say the least.

Bobby's exercise program seemed very strange to me and went against many concepts that I had previously learned as "absolute rules" of strength training. I never believed that the small changes he made in my diet could be so important and I had also never used supplements because I always thought they were just a scam.

It is five years later, and I now weigh 85 kg. (187 lbs.). That is 9 kg (20 lbs.) of solid muscle that I have added to my body since Bobby first helped me. I still use the concepts he taught me, and even go back to his original program a couple of times a year, because it still works.

As I said, some of Bobby's ideas may sound very strange, but I know they work. That is why I am very happy to recommend Bobby's book to everyone.

Istvan Deltai
Budapest, Hungary
Professional acrobat and handbalancer

A Policeman-Athlete

To the Reader,

My name is Rob Haans. I have been practicing judo and jiu-jitsu almost all my life. I have been a member of the Dutch National Jiu-Jitsu Team for about nine years, and during that period I have won both National and International tournaments. I am also a professional fitness instructor.

There are probably as many theories about training as there are instructors and because of that, it is sometimes hard for the inexperienced athlete to know what is good or not.

When I first met Bobby, I had just finished my own education as a fitness instructor. The funny thing was that almost everything Bobby told me that day was new to me. It was also different from all the other things I had heard or tried before, and I thought that was really fascinating.

My biggest problem has always been my struggle with my bodyweight. By then I was competing in the under 78 kilogram (171.6 lbs) weight class, but I always had to lose 4 or 5 kilograms (9-11 lbs) to reach this weight, and I could feel that I was always missing some energy on the day of the tournament.

The first thing Bobby told me was that I had to go up a weight class and that we could make sure that, with his training and nutrition programs, I would get the necessary kilos of muscle mass in about a year or two. I believed him right away, not only because I knew he had been training some of the world's top athletes, but also because I trusted him as a person, even though we had never met before. By that I mean that I really got the feeling that Bobby was doing this because he likes to help people (in this case, me), instead of being like so many other trainers who just like to tell other people how good they are. Sometimes in life we are just lucky to meet the right persons, and I knew this was one of my lucky days.

Within two years I had gained 10 kilograms (22 lbs). I went from 77 kilograms (169.4 lbs) to 87 kilograms (191.4 lbs). I had no problems to reach my competition weight of 85 kilograms (187.0 lbs) and I have never felt more full of energy in my whole life! Things went really well for me during this period. I won the European Championships in 1999, the World Championships in 2000, and the World Games in 2001 – all three of the major tournaments in my sport.

The two most important things I learned from Bobby's training methods were "how to train smart instead of only training hard" and "how to be ready on the right day"! And those two things are, if you ask me, the key elements in any competitive sport.

I cannot begin to say how much Bobby's help meant to me, and I strongly advise everybody to try his programs!

Rob Haans
Certified Fitness Instructor
Copenhagen, Denmark
3rd Dan Black Belt in Judo
5th Dan Black Belt in Jiu-Jitsu
Former hand-to-hand combat instructor for the Royal Dutch Police Units
Dutch National Jiu-Jitsu Champion
European Jiu-Jitsu Champion
World Jiu-Jitsu Champion
World Games Jiu-Jitsu Champion

Author's Note: Rob married Vibeke (a three-time World Jiu-Jitsu Champion...so far...she still competes) and they are now raising their family in Denmark. However, since the World Jiu-Jitsu Championships were to be held in Holland in late 2006, Rob decided to make a comeback after a four year layoff. He asked me to help him prepare for it and I very happily agreed to do so. Rob is a great athlete, an exemplary Champion, and a really nice guy to boot. That's a combination you don't see often enough in the sports world, unfortunately, and that makes him a winner even when he loses...which is very seldom.

Update: November, 2006: Rob Haans easily regained his title as World Champion. Rob is now the only man to ever win Jiu-Jitsu World Championships in two different weight classes. Once a Champion, always a Champion!

More World Champions

- Saskia Habraken
  Multiple times World Kickboxing Champion

Saskia tore a ligament in her ankle. During her long recovery, she added forty pounds of excess body fat. Her comeback match was against the European Champion and Saskia had waited much too long to begin losing the forty pounds. First she went to a dietitian, who put her on a really stupid low-calorie diet and used no nutritional supplements. After Saskia literally passed out a few times during training, she came to me.

Under my supervision, she not only lost the forty pounds in time for her comeback, but the European Champion was literally "saved by the bell" in the first round, and barely made it out of her corner before she was KO'ed in the second round. The martial arts magazines said that they had **never** seen Saskia so strong, and in such good condition.

- Daniella Sommers
  World Kickboxing Champion
  World Full Contact Karate Champion
  Multiple times World Boxing Champion

I had already been working with Daniella for some time when she called me two weeks before her second world boxing title defense. She was in bed with a severe case of the flu. I designed a nutrition program, heavily based on nutritional supplements, to boost her immune system and maintain her strength. Two weeks later she successfully defended her world championship title. She said that she felt so strong and energetic that she could have immediately fought again.

A Professional Athlete

- Peter Aerts
  Multiple times Super Heavyweight World Muay Thai Champion
  Multiple times Super Heavyweight World Kickboxing Champion
  Multiple times winner of the King of Kings (K-1) Tournament

Peter mysteriously began losing weight while competing at a K-1 Tournament in Japan. In a few short weeks he lost forty pounds, nearly 19% of his total bodyweight. He was put in a special clinic, but the doctors could not find out what was wrong. Trainers and the martial arts magazines said that this was the end of his career.

I had already been taking care of Peter's performance nutrition, but now I had to design an extremely radical nutrition program for him because his body would just not accept normal food at that point.

Four months later, Peter successfully defended his Super Heavyweight World Muay Thai title.

Shortly thereafter, Peter invited my wife and me to be his guests at the world's largest martial arts exposition in Essen, Germany. At the evening show, Peter was interviewed in the middle of the huge sports arena. He then proceeded to tell this vast crowd of (mostly) coaches and martial artists that he would not be standing there as the current World Champion if it were not for the help he received from Bobby Dickson. Well…I am not at all embarrassed to tell you that, at that point, the lump in my throat was at least as big as the ice-cube in my Scotch-on-the-rocks. I was very moved by his gratitude.

I then put together another nutrition program designed to build more power. Not long after that, Peter won the King of Kings (K-1) Tournament in Japan again…this time with a knockout in 115 seconds of the first round. His pre-illness competition weight was 215 pounds. His weight for this tournament was almost 235 muscular pounds, a gain of 9% over his previous competition weight, and an amazing 34% gain in solid bodyweight from the low point during his illness.

A Young Athlete

In contrast to working with mature World Champions, one of my younger subjects was Jeffrey Zweeger. Jeffrey was a typical eight-year-old, going to school and playing with friends. In addition, he was taking music, dance, and karate lessons, and was beginning to enter age-group judo competitions.

Jeffrey began literally falling asleep in school and was sometimes too tired to do his homework in the evening. His activities suffered as well as his grades. The conventional solution to this problem would have been to treat the symptoms by cutting back on the activities which he not only enjoyed so much, but which also contributed so much to his total development as a person.

I chose to adapt his nutrition to suit his activity level, and to keep the adaptations doable for an eight-year-old boy. Jeffrey reacted very quickly to my program. His much improved recuperation from exercise was immediately noticeable. He became stronger and faster. There was a marked improvement in his overall physical development, especially when compared to his peers at the judo school. He began doing his homework again, paying attention in class, and his grades started climbing. A couple of years later, Jeffrey's grades were excellent, he was in superior health, and he was winning international age-group judo tournaments. Needless to say, his father is still one of my staunchest supporters.

What a novel idea – that the fuel you put into a child's body will not only influence their physical development, but also the way their little brains function. It's just too logical to be true!

One Who Knows Me Well

To the reader,

Bobby is a coach in every positive aspect of that word. He knows how to teach, to nurture, to encourage, and how to incorporate his vast knowledge of the human body and the human mind.

I remember vividly the role he played at The National Summer Palaestrum (a summer gymnastics camp) where – even then (in the middle 1960s) – he knew exactly how the kids could lose the extra pounds they were gaining from all that wonderful and abundant food.

He was soooooo far ahead of his time with his low fat, high-quality protein, moderate complex carb approach, as he has been with many of his other ideas.

For a guy who finds humor and ridicule in so much of life, he is also one of the most caring people I know.

Lucy Koviak, BS, MS
Former gymnast, former girlfriend (forty-plus years ago), and life-long friend
High School teacher for the past eighteen years

Chapter 18

MORE ABOUT THE AUTHOR

The Right Stuff

Unlike Arnold Whatzizname…I *was* the proverbial ninety-seven-pound weakling. As a young boy I was much too weak for my chosen sport of gymnastics. At that time – the 1950s – exercising with weights was absolutely taboo for athletes in most sports. Most coaches would tell you that exercising with weights would make you slow and "muscle-bound." However, when I looked around, the strongest athletes all exercised with weights. It just didn't make sense to me, even as young as I was, so I ignored all the "experts" of the day and started on my own quest for strength, success in my chosen sport, and maybe, with a little luck, some shapely muscle as well.

Unfortunately, I didn't ignore my tennis instructor when he told me that holding the big, heavy wooden tennis racket (the only kind in those days) with both of my small hands was wrong. It felt right to me because I could hit the ball better and with more control…but he was the teacher, so he must be right…yes? In this case…no! I wonder what he thinks about playing tennis with two hands now? By the way, I never became a really good tennis player.

On the other hand, I did ignore everyone who told me that you have to use either an interlocking or an overlapping grip in order to play golf well. Again…because it felt right for me…I used (and still do) a baseball grip…and I went on to win age-group golf tournaments, in spite of their dire predictions.

I only mention these things to emphasize how important it is to choose the right people to believe, and also how important it is to believe in yourself and your own instincts.

A Great Legacy

The small amount of knowledge and useful information that was available at that time came mostly from the fledgling bodybuilding community, not from the "scientific community." What a great legacy for these pioneers of physical culture, that an amazing number of assumptions and theories…born out of pure experience in those early days…are still valid, or have been only slightly refined during the past fifty-plus years.

Interestingly, many of these men and women are still exercising with the old tried and true (but now improved) methods, still look great, and are still living happy, active and productive lives. They are living proof that these methods are timeless…and definitely the way to go!

In contrast, we will see if pole-dance aerobics, belly-dance aerobics (How many thin belly-dancers have you ever seen?), Special Forces Commando Full-Body Underwater Booty Survival Workouts, strip aerobics (my personal favorite), Magic Ultimate Ab Machines, etc., etc., are still around after the initial novelty wears off.

Olympic Beer Gut

Using this little bit of knowledge…and a lot of trial and error…I eventually built myself up to a respectably muscular 142 pounds, at a height of 5'6". After my college competitive gymnastic days were over, I beered myself up from my competition weight of 137 pounds to an impressive (?) 162 pounds – a gain of 25 pounds of not-so-pretty blubber – which is really a lot on a 5'6" frame.

Then I decided to give the Olympic team another try. I put my knowledge back to work, designed an exercise and nutrition program for myself and, at the 1972 final Olympic trials several months later, I competed at a weight of 117 pounds – a loss of 45 pounds, or more than 38% of my total bodyweight. Some of that weight was also muscle, but that was calculated. I wanted to be as light as possible, without losing any strength. I succeeded here as well because I was the strongest I had ever been in my entire life.

Just to test my personal limits, I later built myself up to 175 rock-hard, muscular, fat-free pounds. So, with knowledge, a good plan and hard work, I have been able to manipulate my own *muscular* bodyweight by 58 pounds during my adult life. That doesn't just happen by accident.

Practice What You Preach

I do not teach traditional aerobics and I do not offer advice about steps, Tai-Bo, jazz-dance, Boot Camp…or any of the other forms of aerobic exercise…because I am not certified, qualified or competent to do so. I only say that these are wonderful "exercise activities" which can be *valuable additions* to a Quality Exercise program.

However, aerobics for losing excess body fat is a completely different matter. Here I *do* know what I am talking about, and ditto for teaching efficient and effective cardiovascular conditioning for health purposes.

Once again, most people are just wasting way too much time and energy by relying on these more traditional forms of aerobics to gain control of, and then manage their body fat…or to get in, and then stay in good cardiovascular condition.

Sad Sign of the Times

It is a sad sign of our times that I have to say here that I lost my body fat *without* the use of stupid diets or diet pills, and I built the muscle *without* using steroids or any other type of muscle enhancing pharmaceuticals.

Where to Start

An inquisitive mind, knowledge, logic, common sense and hard work were, and remain, my only tools. They can work just as well for you, and the CTTC Exercise and Nutrition Programs are a great place to get started.

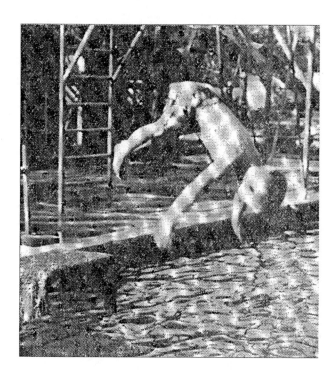

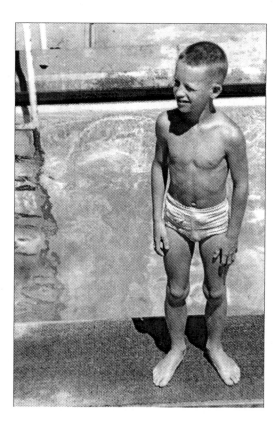

The Early Years

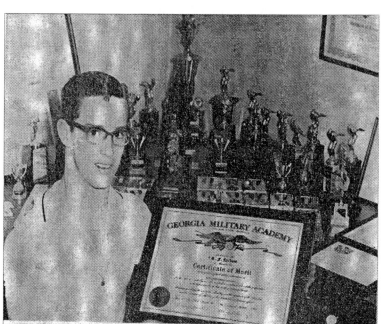

YOUNG WINNER—Robert Dickson, 15-year-old diver and gymnast, exhibits part of the more than 180 medals, certificates, trophies and ribbons he has won for his athletic abilities. The Portales youth holds a laminated plaque naming him the outstanding gymnast at Georgia Military Academy, where he will be a junior this fall.

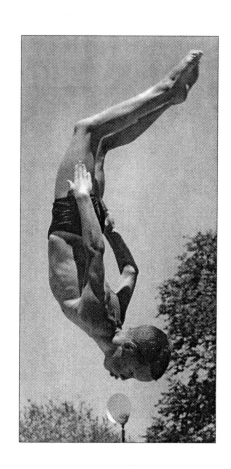

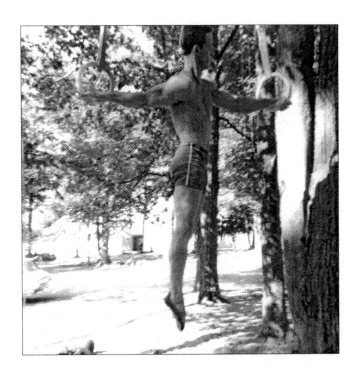

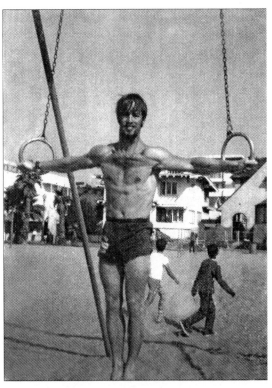

Well on My Way

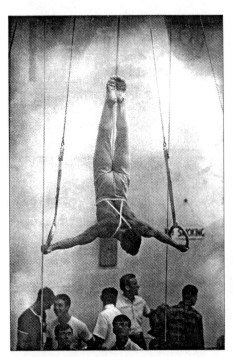

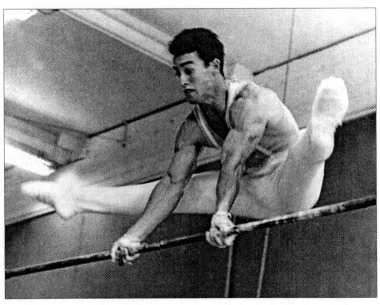

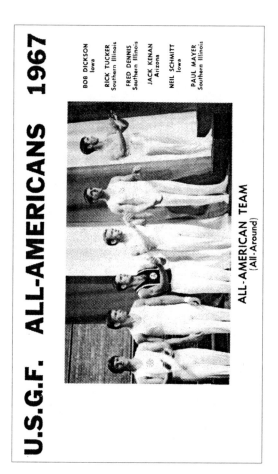

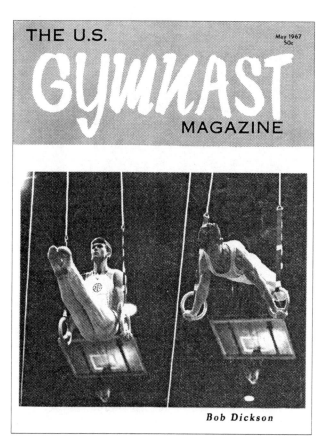

The Realization of Goals

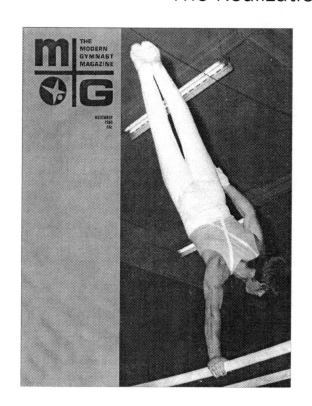

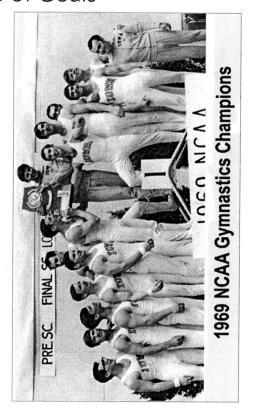

Another Goal Achieved

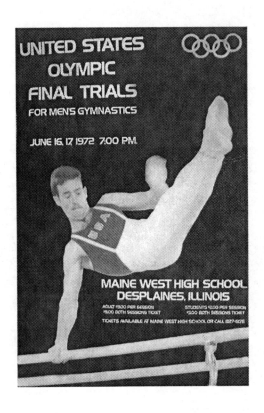
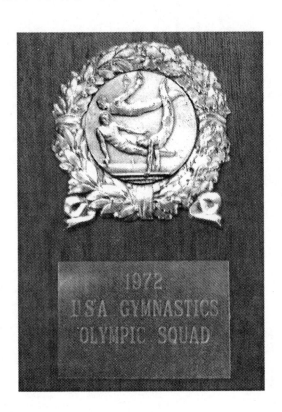

A Passion Past

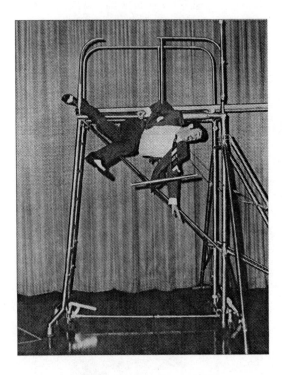
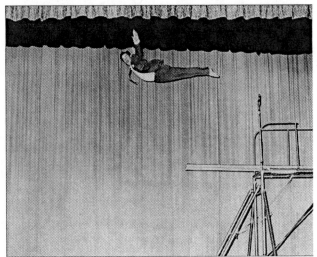

Another Passion Found

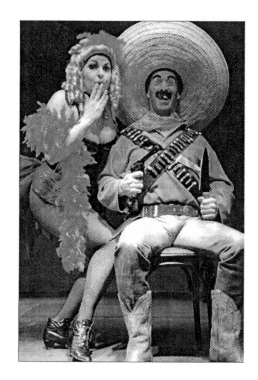
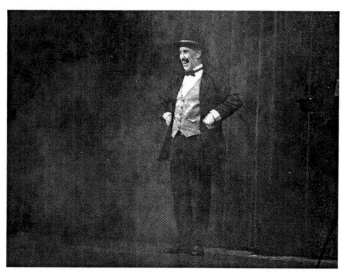

A Lifelong Passion

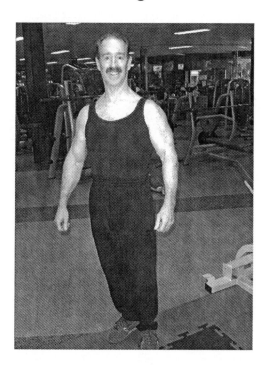

The author…60 years young!

(The poor guy had to follow his own CTTC system to get in shape for this photo.)

Curriculum Vita

Robert E. Dickson
Height: 5' 6"
Weight: 150 lbs.
Born: 1947

Education

Georgia Military Academy, Atlanta, Georgia – (High School)

- One of the highest ranking cadet officers
- Vice President of the Senior Class
- Vice President of the Honor Council
- Voted Most Popular by fellow classmates
- Co-Captain of the gymnastic team

University of Iowa, Iowa City, Iowa

- Accepted in the Honors Program for pre-medicine
- Bachelor of Science in Physical Education
- Teacher Certification from the College of Education

Indiana State University, Terre Haute, Indiana

- Master of Science in Public Recreation
- Emphasis on Therapeutic Recreation

Sports Accomplishments and Honors

Swimming and Diving

- Won first medal at age 4 for springboard diving
- From age 4 until age 13, won numerous age-group and Jr. Olympic championships in swimming
- From age 4 until age 15 (when I retired), was undefeated in springboard diving

- Won the New Mexico State High School Diving Championship as an 8th grader. However, I was disqualified before the finals because, as an 8th grader, I was not yet "officially" in high school. Strangely enough, the high school coaches didn't object to an 8th grader entering the competition until they realized that I was going to win. Go figure! As a consolation, I was allowed to dive in the finals (exhibition only, but with scores) and won...scoring 100 points more than the "official" winner...as well as breaking the old state high school record by 60 points. Afterwards, I was the only one smiling.
- Won the New Mexico State High School Diving Championship again (officially this time) as a 9th grader...just to make a point

Gymnastics

- From age 8 until age 14, won many age-group gymnastic championships, predominantly in trampoline and tumbling
- New Mexico State High School All-Around Gymnastics Champion as a 9th grader
- 2 times Georgia State High School All-Around Gymnastics Champion, winning all 6 events the second time
- Co-Captain of the Georgia Military Academy gymnastic team
- Voted Most Outstanding Gymnast, every year, by fellow teammates at Georgia Military Academy
- Voted Most Promising High School Gymnast by university gymnastic coaches
- Member (alternate) of USA versus Mexico gymnastic team at age 17
- Entered University of Iowa on a full athletic scholarship for gymnastics
- 1967 Big 10 Gymnastic Team Champions
- 3rd place (team) at the 1967 NCAA National Gymnastic Championships
- 1968 Big 10 Gymnastic Team Champions
- 3rd place (team) at the 1968 NCAA National Gymnastic Championships
- 1969 NCAA National Gymnastic Team Champions
- Co-Captain of the 1968 Big Ten Championship gymnastic team (with Neil Schmitt)
- Co-Captain of the 1969 NCAA National Championship gymnastic team (with Rich Scorza)
- AAU All-American
- USGF All-American
- NCAA All-American
- Nominee for the George Nissen Award (the "Heisman Trophy" of gymnastics)
- Member of numerous All-Star gymnastic teams
- Invited participant at the first World Cup of Gymnastics
- Member of the 1968 United States Olympic Gymnastic Training Squad
- Member (alternate) of the 1972 United States Olympic Gymnastic Team

The 1967 Iowa gymnastic team was the first gymnastic team to win a Big Ten Championship for the University of Iowa since 1937.

The 1969 NCAA National Championship gymnastic team was the first NCAA national championship team, **in any sport,** since the University of Iowa began participating in intercollegiate sports in the 1880's.

The 1969 NCAA National Championship gymnastic team is, as of this writing, still the **only** national championship gymnastic team in the history of gymnastics (since 1917) at the University of Iowa.

As of this writing, the University of Iowa has had only eight championship gymnastic teams in its 90-year history of gymnastics. The 1967-1969 teams still remain the most successful gymnastic teams **ever** at Iowa. At the time, they also represented the best consecutive 3-year performance at the national level for any previous Iowa teams, **regardless of sport**. I have the distinct privilege of having been co-captain of two of these teams. I am also one of only three gymnasts (with Keith McCanless and Don Hatch) to enjoy the honor of having competed on all three of these record-setting gymnastic teams.

Gymnastic Coaching Experience

- Certified to teach beginning trampoline at 10 years of age
- Instructor at several private gymnastic clubs
- Instructor at dozens of national gymnastic clinics
- Instructor at 2 different international summer gymnastic camps
- Organized and directed a gymnastic program for the Muscatine YMCA, Iowa
- Assisted with the men's gymnastic program at the University of Iowa
- Organized and directed a gymnastic program for 6-16 year olds at Indiana State University
- Men's Program Director at the Indiana Summer Gymnastic Camp
- Assistant men's gymnastic coach at Indiana State University
- Helped to coach many All-Americans and NCAA National Champions in gymnastics

Personal Training Experience

I was successfully using weights to build strength for my chosen sports some twenty years before "resistance exercise" even began to become accepted by most coaches and other "experts" of the time. I was also successfully using special diets and crude nutritional supplements more than forty years ago. These two factors were instrumental in my transformation from a somewhat talented, but physically weak, athlete into an Olympian known for my strength.

I began seriously helping other people with exercise when I was about seventeen years old. In addition to the many gymnasts I helped to coach over the years, I have also worked with athletes in many other sports, plus acrobats, trapeze artists, dancers, martial artists, members of the police, SWAT team, and military commando forces, fitness professionals, physical therapists, doctors, All-Americans, National Champions, European Champions, World Champions…and many "normal" people as well.

In the 1990s, my wife and I were asked to organize a nutritional supplement department for a Dutch sporting goods store, which we did. During this time, we did hundreds of nutritional analyses for athletes and serious exercisers in the area. As word got around that someone was giving advice that was based on results, instead of just trying to sell products, people began coming from all over Holland and Belgium for our help. This eventually evolved into our beginning an import-export business in superior-quality nutritional supplements. During this time I also formulated a couple of nutritional supplement products specifically for our athletes.

At this point, elite athletes also began coming to us for guidance. Since Holland is very strong in competitive martial arts, many of these elite athletes were martial artists. Eventually we were advising, training, and providing performance nutrition products to elite athletes from five different countries. We never approached any athlete ourselves. They all came to us of their own initiative after hearing from their fellow athletes just how successful our advice and products had been for them.

Publications

I have written articles on performance nutrition for Belgian, Dutch, German, and American martial arts magazines and I have also contributed to a German book on the health and fitness possibilities of exercising on a mini-trampoline.

The second book in the CTTC series is *The CTTC Simplified Quick-Start Fat Loss Program*, which is written for people who are not interested in all the detailed information contained in this book.

The third book in the CTTC series will be *The CTTC Fountain of Youth Program*, which is designed to slow the aging process and ensure Senior Citizens of a much higher quality of life during their Golden Years.

Other follow-up books in the CTTC series are also in the planning stages.

Current Occupations

For more than thirty years I performed a comedy acrobatic act, which I learned from the great **Larry Griswold,** also a former University of Iowa gymnast. I finally retired as a professional acrobat in 2004. I now perform visual comedy acts with my companion, best friend and personal sports massage therapist for the past twenty-two years, my wife Anoushka. I still do some personal training, and I occasionally do some writing as well.

Chapter 19

Acknowledgments, or...Who is responsible for all this?

From the Beginning

I suppose I should start at the very beginning here, and that would be by thanking my parents for instilling in me a healthy interest in sports and exercise, at a very early age. They also always supported me 100% in my various sports endeavors, taking me to competitions all over the south-western United States, sending me to summer gymnastics camps, and even allowing me to attend a high school far away from home because it offered a sport program (gymnastics) which was not available where we lived. All this cost them not only a lot of money, but also an awful lot of time, for which I am sure they could have found much better use. Thanks for always backing me up!

Life's Lessons

Many people have influenced my life, some because they were such good examples and others because they weren't. One of the most influential people in the positive category is one of my former gymnastics coaches at the University of Iowa, Dick Holzaepfel.

This man certainly knows how to earn and deserve respect. Demanding never really worked too well with me, not then and not now. He not only still has one of the best win-loss records of any gymnastics coach in America, but is also one of the best-loved coaches around. He understands, and always taught, what competitive sports **should** really be about. He certainly put it into perspective for me. For coach Holzaepfel, teaching us the importance of priorities in life, and to **enjoy** our sport, was always more important than just winning...but we mostly won anyway... because that was fun too!

We learned that defeating a weaker opponent is **not** winning and that eliminating a better opponent by manipulating the rules also does **not** make you a winner. He taught me that **being the best you possibly can be makes you a winner**, every time! We learned when winning is important, and when it should be lower on the ladder of priorities, which it sometimes is...as strange as that may sound to some people.

One of the most valuable things he taught me was that your success does **not** depend on the materials, equipment or circumstances you have to work with, but on **what you do with them**. That was a particularly hard lesson for me, which involved my feeling about two inches tall and having tears in my eyes at the end of it all...but he never had to repeat it with me. Lesson definitely learned, and greatly appreciated. Thanks.

I could go on and on, but I'm sure my wife doesn't want to read any more Holzaepfel stories here. She's heard all of them a hundred times over the past twenty-plus years. Suffice to say that this man still practices what he preaches. After being widowed for several years from his lovely first wife Betty, he married another wonderful woman, Jean, at the young-old age of eighty-one. Good on ya!

So what has Holzaepfel got to do with this book? If I hadn't had the good fortune to have encountered him when I did, I'm absolutely sure that my life would have taken a much different direction, and I would not be writing this now. I owe this man a great debt of gratitude as well as a lot of my happiness in life. Thanks again, Coach!

In this same category belongs another of my University of Iowa gymnastic coaches, Sam Bailie. I went through three coaches in four years at Iowa, which is an indication of what was involved in my learning just the basic Life Lessons. Sam also learned some of Life's Lessons when he took over the head coaching job at Iowa. This particular group of gymnasts was certainly a job, and definitely a Life Lesson for him, but he loved every minute of it. If you don't believe me, you can ask him yourself. Every Friday is visiting day at the Shady Pines Happy Farm.

Sam and his much-better-everything, Topsi, became good friends and from them I learned that it is OK to be adventurous and try new things. They further confirmed my already deeply ingrained conviction **not** to listen to people who tell you that you can't do something. They are always moving around, taking chances, seeking out new experiences, grabbing at opportunities and just enjoying life in general, which they continue to do with outstanding success. Thanks for positively influencing my life in ways you still probably don't even realize, and keep up the good work!

Friends May Come and Friends May Go…

Next on this list has to be my partner-in-crime, fellow life-reveler, former rival, fellow gymnast, former scourge of the University of Michigan Athletic Department, and now also my publicist – my life-long friend, Charles Froeming. Charlie is the one who called me three years ago and asked me why I hadn't put my exercise and nutrition knowledge down in a book. If he hadn't done that, I might have put off writing this for another fifteen years. He said that if I wrote it, he would take care of the rest. Well, I'll drink to that! Here it is Chuck! Have fun!

Very Special

A special tribute goes to a **very** special someone: Sandy Froeming, Charlie's wife of thirty-seven years and my secret girlfriend for almost as long. Sandy died tragically in a car accident shortly before I finished this book.

Sandy is the perfect example of a truly wonderful, caring human being. For the many, many people who had the very good fortune to know Sandy, she remains an inspiration for us to strive to live our own lives just a little bit better in the future. Sandy and Anoushka designed the prototype cover for this book before Sandy left us. Anoushka and I love her dearly, and a little piece of our lives is now missing without her.

My Better Half

Ah, yes. Behind every successful man is a great woman…and she is usually kicking him in the butt to get him to do something. Well, let me tell you, I have one of the very best butt-kickers around and, yes ladies, I realize and greatly appreciate my good fortune.

Anoushka has really had to put up with a lot on this project, as she has had to do with many of my other sometimes loony schemes during the twenty-plus years that we have been together. She's always helpful, always supportive, always loving, always there.

I will not go into all the morbid details of what she has been through during the many months this project has taken so far, from my getting up at all hours of the night to insert another thought or idea into the book, to her sleeping curled up in a corner because our bed was still covered with open books at 3:00 AM while I researched material for this one. I could go on and on.

Without Anoushka's loving help and support, these pages would never have seen the light of day, that's for sure, and a heckuvalot of other good things in my life would also not have taken place. I cannot imagine my life without her and I cannot possibly thank her enough for all that she does for me and all that she means to me! I could go on, but my mascara is starting to run. Love ya, Nush!

My Lab Animals

Next on my list are all the people who have taken a chance, first by listening to my sometimes insane sounding ideas, and then by actually allowing me to experiment on them…sorry…allowing me to advise them. All have been rewarded with augmented success, and many have also become good friends.

Another special thanks goes to those who have very kindly written testimonials for me. For believing in me, and for the many nice things you wrote about me, your checks are in the mail…I mean…I thank each one of you very much.

Oprah

Now I want to thank Oprah Winfrey…three times. First for educating millions of her fans to the fact that Quality Exercise is hard work, secondly for setting such a good example herself, and thirdly for "discovering" Dr. Phil McGraw.

Dr. Phil

I want to thank Dr. Phil for making honesty acceptable again, and for convincing millions of people that it is in their own power to change any and all aspects of their lives for the better.

BDP (Before **D**r. **P**hil), it was always somebody else's fault if any part(s) of your life was really screwed up, and you could do very little about it yourself. Fortunately, Dr. Phil is helping to remedy that gross misconception.

I have always used a somewhat confrontational, get-in-your-face (but always with humor), make-you-think-for yourself, teaching method. Before Dr. Phil, many people had a problem readily accepting this approach. So thanks Doc. You have made my life a lot easier, and much more productive too.

Without these two fundamental changes in attitude, I would never have begun this book. Now, thanks to Oprah and Dr. Phil, at least some people are ready to hear, and possibly even accept, the truth as I see it concerning Quality Exercise as well as practical eating, living, and health-building habits.

Inspiration and Knowledge

This section involves a lot of people and I know that I am going to forget someone who really deserves to be mentioned here. I apologize now already, but no lapse of my memory can diminish, in any way, the importance of anyone who has contributed to either of these two very important aspects of my life.

I agree wholeheartedly with Rudyard Kipling, who said: "I not only use all the brains that I have, but also all that I can borrow." Like many other people, if I only used what I have, I would really be in big trouble.

The Sources

I was astounded when I first saw pictures of bodybuilders in a magazine at a friend's house. The magazine belonged to my friend's big brother, who was already exercising with weights at that time, the mid 1950s. I don't remember who any of those bodybuilders were because that wasn't what was important to me. What was important to me was the realization that it is possible to radically change your body. This was a very big deal to a really small, weak and skinny young boy…me!

The only magazines available at the time were *Mr. America* (and later *Muscle/Power*) from Joe Weider's organization, *Strength and Health* (and later *Muscular Development*) from the Bob Hoffman organization, and *Iron Man* from Perry Rader. Good books on the subject were nonexistent, so I began getting my first exercise information from these five sources. This turned out to be a blessing in disguise because each of these three organizations had a different, but overlapping outlook on the subjects of exercise, health, and nutrition.

Weider was (and still is) the most commercial, but had the best bodybuilders, and great inspirational photos. Hoffman was a weightlifter, so much of his information concerned building strength. Most of the people in his magazines were World and Olympic Champion weightlifters, but some were also bodybuilders, such as the great John Grimek, the only man to ever win the AAU Mr. America title twice. In my humble opinion, Perry Rader's magazine had the best overall information as well as the most interesting and informative articles of all these magazines at the time.

So right from the beginning of my "exercise career," I had a very diverse look at all the different aspects of exercise. This "basic education" has served me well over the past fifty-plus years. Later I became acquainted with another magazine, *MuscleMag International,* from Robert Kennedy (not the late-Senator), which gave me still another view of the subject. Mr. Kennedy went on to become one of the most prolific writers of bodybuilding books in the world. His books are excellent (so buy them) and his photos are awe-inspiring.

You must remember that, in those early days, bodybuilding was much more about a healthy lifestyle than it is today. It wasn't even called bodybuilding then. It was referred to as "physical culture" and they organized "physique" contests. There were champions like the great Bill Pearl, who entered the Mr. Universe contest once every five years or so, over a twenty-year competitive career, and won each time. Mr. Pearl was then, and still is a vegetarian, still gets up at 4:00 AM or so to exercise and still looks fabulous. People like Bill Pearl have always personified a healthy and aesthetic bodybuilding lifestyle to me, not the pharmaceutical freaks you see in the "sport" today.

As a young boy, I even wrote to this gentle giant of a man and asked what he thought I should do to gain strength for my sports. At the time I did not realize how busy a World Champion is, or that they made money by selling this information as courses (personal training by mail). Well, this multi-Mr. Universe sent me several pages of personalized, typewritten information (there were no computer printouts in those days) on exercise and nutrition, wished me luck with my sports ambitions…and never mentioned money. Later I realized what a wonderful gesture this was, and I learned a great lesson in altruism. Many years later, I got the chance to thank him in person at a fitness convention. Bill Pearl is a class act, and a wonderful example of a true champion. His books are terrific as well. Buy them and learn!

From another health-conscious bodybuilder by the name of Frank Zane I learned not only how important nutrition and nutritional supplements are, but also how **attention to detail is essential to excellence**, and how it is absolutely necessary if you want to reach your exercise goals as quickly and as efficiently as possible. This has saved me thousands of hours in the gym over the years. I thank him immensely for that.

I expanded my knowledge of nutrition and nutritional supplementation by also studying the ideas put forth by advocates of "natural foods" and "health foods." These included Jethro Kloss, Frances Lappe, J.I. Rodale and *Prevention Magazine*, Adelle Davis, and Dr. Earl Mindell, among others. As with all sources of information, they all have so-so, good, and better ideas, depending on the reader's interests or needs. I learned a great deal from each of them, and continue to do so. More great books to read and learn from!

Onward and Upward

Later, information about nutrition and exercise took a quantum leap when researchers finally started looking at the effects nutrition and exercise have on **healthy** people, and especially athletes. For the first time, we were able to see how exercise and nutrition actually affect healthy bodies instead of how they affect mice, people laying in hospital beds, or persons in rehabilitation programs. This made it possible to factually differentiate between "any" exercise and Quality Exercise, which I explain throughout this book.

Some of the best information in this area has come from people such as Dr. Kennith Cooper of The Cooper Clinic and The Cooper Institute for Aerobics Research, and Dr. Michael Colgan of The Colgan Institute of Nutritional Science. Even these two pioneers of exercise science differed somewhat in their opinions in the beginning. Dr. Cooper was very big on aerobics, while Dr. Colgan's interests also included Quality Resistance Exercise, i.e., exercising with weights.

Later, Dr. Cooper also came to the conclusion that aerobics alone is not the cure-all to health and fitness, so now he also advocates **combining** aerobics with resistance exercise.

Another prolific writer, with more than sixty books in the areas of weight training, fitness, bodybuilding, powerlifting, and nutrition, is Dr. Frederick Hatfield. Dr. Hatfield has the ability to take all the medical and scientific information and translate it into an easily understood, logical and practical format. Dr. Hatfield is a multiple World Champion in powerlifting, so he also practices what he preaches. Some of his ideas also differ from other experts so, as you can see, there is no "one size fits all" when it comes to health, fitness, and nutrition. Over the years, I have really learned a lot from Dr. Hatfield and his excellent publications. Buy them and study them!

Different opinions are good. They make you think about what you are doing, and what you are believing. One of the legendary "old-timers," whose opinions were respected (by some) from the time he established one of the very first gyms in the Los Angeles area in 1946, until his (healthy) death a few years ago, was the very outspoken Vince Gironda, affectionately known as "The Iron Guru."

Many people belittled Vince Gironda in the beginning, but they eventually learned to never summarily dismiss his "wacky" ideas, because, time after time, his "nutty" opinions were proven to be correct after all. It just took fifteen or twenty years for everyone else to figure it out.

Vince may have been a tad bit eccentric, but when Hollywood celebrities had to quickly get into shape for a movie, you would always find them at Vince's Gym…and they would be in shape for the movie… on time. Do you want some name-dropping of Gironda clients? How about Clint Eastwood, Burt Reynolds, Arnold Whatzizname, and even Cher, to name just a few. Great booklets, and a controversial book (of course) which will make you stop and think.

From Mr. Gironda I learned to carefully look into **every** idea, no matter how much it might differ from those being currently accepted…or especially because it **does** differ from those ideas being currently accepted.

Teachers give direction to the future course of your life.
Choose yours wisely.

Skeptics

Any new idea meets this same kind of skepticism, especially any new idea that goes against the current, accepted way of doing something. The skepticism usually persists until the new idea eventually becomes the current, accepted way of doing something, or until enough of the currently accepted authorities die.

This process is one of the ways I know if I am on the right track or not. If I (or anyone else) am onto something good, many of the "currently accepted authorities" (and the sheep of the world) will react as follows:

1. First they will ignore you.
2. Then they will make fun of you.
3. Next, they will attack you.
4. And finally…they will begin to copy you.

If you are copied widely enough, you become one of the next "currently accepted authorities." Then the process begins all over again. One of the secrets to becoming successful at something before most other people do is to seek out and find these pioneers of ideas before they become "currently accepted authorities."

Others who fit into this category and from whose books and articles I have gleaned enormous amounts of inspiration, information and ideas over the years are: Chris Aceto, Clarence Bass, Jerry Brainum, Dr. William Brink, Dr. Rick Evans, Charles Glass, Dr. Robert Haas, Ron Harris, Steve Holman, Dr. Robert Lefavi, Nelson Montana, John Parrillo, Charles Poliquin, Bill Reynolds, John Romano, Bill Starr, Dennis Weis, Dr. Jerry Wright, Dr. Michael Yessis, and Greg Zulak. I thank you all immensely.

Mental Health

I blame "my mental condition" (I call it that precisely because it leaves lots of room for interpretation) on people whose philosophy of life, the different ways they have expressed it, and the way they have lived their own lives, have had a great influence on my way of thinking, as well as on the way I have chosen to live my own life. The most influential of these people are: Benjamin Franklin, Oscar Wilde, Will Rogers, Dick Holzaepfel, and George Carlin. Now you know why I call it "my mental condition." You see, nothing is really my fault…I just do what the voices tell me to do!

So these are the people who have most influenced my ideas, beliefs and philosophies about lifestyle, exercise and nutrition, building my health and keeping my health. There are many others, of course, but these are the ones who made writing this book possible – them and my own fifty-plus years of personal experience with sports, nutrition, exercise, and living a happy, fun, productive, and fulfilling life. I thank all of you from the bottom of my heart.

Bull Schmitt

A huge expression of thanks goes to my fellow teammate and former roommate at the University of Iowa, and another fellow life-reveler (fortunately, I have several, in case any of them burn out), Neil Schmitt. I have always admired Neil, not only for his amazing gymnastic prowess, but also because he has always listened to his inner voice. Neil learned to manage his life at a much earlier age than most of the rest of us and he always walked his own path, at his own pace.

This was a very fortunate thing for me because, many times, Neil would drag me screaming down his path, thereby preventing me from doing something really stupid. He always took part in the fun, but he also always knew when it was getting out of hand, whereas I seem to have a genetic defect in this area. Needless to say, Neil has probably saved my life more than once. He is a true friend.

Neil has continued this (apparently life-long) self-appointed job of attempting to keep me on the straight and narrow, this time by keeping me focused on the truly important aspects of this book and gently guiding me with his exceptional insight. Without his help, this book would just be many pages of somewhat unconnected thoughts. Thanks, Big Guy!

Last One...I Promise

Finally, I owe an enormous debt of gratitude to Judy Gedney. As a former University of Iowa gymnast and long-time friend, I sent her one of the very first drafts of this book to review. The fact that she was a professor of biomechanics (and taught weight-training/strength enhancement) at Western Illinois University for thirty-eight years, is a co-founder of The World Drug-Free Powerlifting Federation, Inc., as well as The American Drug-Free Powerlifting Federation, and is still a competing powerlifter at the world championship level, may also form a tiny part of the reason that I value her opinions so much.

Judy not only reviewed my book, but took it upon herself to also technically edit it. Her input has been priceless and her encouragement has been invaluable to my self-confidence in this undertaking. Thanks, Judy. I owe you really big-time for this one! The chocolate is on the way!

I Lied...

A very last, but certainly not least, debt of gratitude goes to Karen McChrystal who did the final editing, revised the cover, and got the book into the form you now hold in your grubby little hands. In other words, I wrote the book and she handled all the difficult stuff. Thank you so much for your encouragement, your professionalism and your incredible patience. I hate to think what this book would look like without your expertise.

To all of you...live well.

Chapter 20

22 POPULAR MYTHS AND FAIRY TALES

Myth Number 1

Spot reducing is impossible.

It is a myth that you **cannot** "spot reduce," which means losing excess body fat from one specific part of your body.

There are, in fact, three successful methods for spot reducing. One is liposuction. The other two are by amputating some part of your body, or by contracting a flesh-eating bacterial infection on the part of your body that you want to spot reduce. These are the only three methods I know of that actually work.

It is, however, a myth that you can spot reduce by doing some particular exercise for a specific body part. Doing hundreds of reps and dozens of different exercises for your abdominals will not get rid of the excess body fat around your waist. And ladies, I'm equally sorry to break the bad news to you, but those dinky little exercises they like to have you do for your hips, butt, and thighs are also a total waste of time for losing excess body fat from those areas too.

You can't exercise body fat off like that. You also can't roll it off, massage it off, sauna it off, steam it off, cream it off, vibrate it off, magnetize it off, jiggle it off, wrap it off, yoga it off, meditate it off or positive think excess body fat off of one specific part of your body. No machine can do it, no special piece of equipment can do it, no miracle program can do it, no pill can do it, no patch can do it, and no trainer can do it for you either. It can't be done, period! Learn to live with it.

Think about this logically. If it were possible to spot reduce, then football linemen would have lovely thin legs under their rather large bellies. Their legs certainly get enough exercise to spot reduce them. Over-fat tennis players would have one fat-free, well-toned arm hanging from a much fatter body. Truck drivers would all have cute little butts from sitting on a vibrating seat for hours every day…and a whole lot of people would have fat-free jaws…for obvious reasons.

More logic: If it were possible to **gain** body fat wherever you wanted, you would never see guys with skinny legs and a beer-gut...or women with a thin upper body but huge hips. These people would simply distribute their body fat more evenly...or buy a "miracle machine" to do it for them. Everyone's body puts on body fat more in some places and less in other places. So if you can't put body fat on where you want it, you can't take it off only where you want to either.

When your body loses fat, it loses it from all over...**not** just from one specific place. And, as I said in the previous paragraph, everyone will also **lose** body fat from one place on their body faster than from another place. However, this has **nothing** whatsoever to do with exercising that particular part of their body. They will lose body fat from that place more rapidly no matter which exercises they do (assuming that they **are** losing body fat, of course).

The opposite is also true. There are other places on your body where you will lose body fat more slowly. I can do lower back exercises all day long, but the last excess body fat that I lose will still always be that little roll on my lower back. So when I feel the fat roll on my lower back becoming less and less, I know that I am finally getting close to the end of another fat loss adventure...no matter what exercises I did to get there.

One of the funniest images to ever work its way into my twisted little mind is that of all the over-fat people who have bought one of the hundred different "miracle ab machines," walking around with fat legs, arms, chests, backs, butts and heads...but with tiny waists and rippling abdominal muscles. Do you get the real picture now? Spot-reduction is a **myth**. It's not going to happen. Forget about it.

Myth Number 2

Strength training is dangerous for kids.

What do you think babies are doing when they hang onto your fingers and you pick them up off the ground? How about pulling themselves up and climbing out of their crib or playpen? If they get hurt, it will be from a fall, not from the strenuous climb. As they get older, children play sports, climb trees, chase each other and ride their bicycles like maniacs. These are all **uncontrolled** strength activities. Is it not logical that **controlled** strength training would be safer than that?

If they want to exercise with weights, of course they should be old enough (to be determined by a qualified and competent trainer), and have qualified, competent guidance. However, exercises using only bodyweight (such as climbing a rope, crunches, chins and pull-ups, back extensions, pushups, sprinting, or learning to do a handstand)...presented in a fun way...is not only safe, but will build strength, aerobic fitness, self-confidence, self-esteem and a healthy self-image. It will also create a wonderful foundation for future health and happiness for both boys **and** girls. For instance, pushup and crunch contests at home with mom and dad would be terrific...and it certainly wouldn't do mom and dad any harm either.

Myth Number 3

Traditional aerobic exercise is the best way to lose excess body fat and keep it off.

An emphatic **NO**! See Chapter 3.

Myth Number 4

You can get an effective, full-body workout in ten to fifteen minutes (or even less), a couple of times a week.

Boy do I wish this were true. I would be the first one to jump on this program. Unfortunately, it is just another wish. With no warm-up, no cool down, and minimum rest periods, you could only effectively do about six to ten sets of exercises in ten or fifteen minutes…maximum. This is enough to effectively exercise only one large group or two small groups of muscles…if you used very heavy weights and very short rest periods. But then you would still have to exercise at least three to four days a week in order to effectively work all five major muscle groups even one time a week. And remember, this does not include warm-ups, cool downs, or any cardio work.

I have, on occasion, exercised with weights for fifteen to twenty minutes a day, five or six days a week, when I had very little time due to work or other commitments. At those times however, I had my own gym in my home or apartment, so I could still get in a good workout. It was even possible to include some Cardio-aerobics. This is simply not possible by exercising only a couple of times a week, for a few minutes each time. Dream on!

The **CTTC** Exercise Program has been designed to be as efficient and timesaving as possible, while still providing you with an effective, quality, full-body workout, which also includes an efficient, health-building aerobics program. As your Quality Exercise program (with weights) becomes even more specific to your needs, it will become even shorter in duration, but there are limits to how little you can do and still realize quality results.

Actually, I will admit that it is possible to get a reasonably good, full-body workout in fifteen to twenty minutes, two to three times a week, which even includes some aerobic conditioning as well. You will read about it in Chapter 13.

Myth Number 5

You need to exercise for 1½ - 2 hours a day, 5 - 6 days a week to achieve good results.

First of all, you can either exercise for a long time, or you can exercise intensely, but you cannot exercise intensely for a long time.

If you don't believe this, then try running all-out 100-yard dashes with 1½-minute rest periods in between, and see how long you can hold out. If you could run six 100-yard dashes, each lasting twenty seconds, then you would have actually exercised for a total of only two minutes. The whole thing, including rest periods, would last for less than ten minutes, but I don't think you would be looking forward to a further one hour and fifty minutes of exercise. The longer you exercise, the lower the intensity of the exercise **has** to be.

The **CTTC** Workouts are not maximum intensity and they should last only about one hour, (including the warm-up and cool-down), but you will know that you have truly exercised when you have finished one. Then, the next time someone tells you that they exercise for two hours, you will have to laugh.

To answer the second part of this myth: Under normal circumstances, we mortals should never exercise with weights and/or intense aerobics for more than four days a week, and never more than two days in a row. Exercise (intensely) more than this and you will enter "the realm of diminishing returns." This means that you will be exercising more, with very minor results as your reward. This is the domain of professional and elite athletes again. For the rest of us, it is a waste of time and energy that could be much better spent enjoying life.

Or, if you exercise like this long enough and often enough, you will overtrain, and you will then enjoy **negative** results (including sickness and/or injury) for all your extra efforts. Neither one of these is good.

Myth Number 6

Doing lots of reps with light weights is the best way to "tone up."

First of all, what exactly is "toning up"? I hear this term all the time, but very few people are able to explain to me what it means. Toning up actually refers to improving the "tonus"…or quality…of your muscles. Tonus is the degree of tension a muscle keeps when it is in a relaxed state. The more tension (tonus) a muscle has, the firmer it is when you are standing relaxed. I very affectionately refer to ladies with a high degree of tonus as "hardbodies." Get it ladies? **Quality muscle = a firm body.**

Toning up is used instead of the correct term, "improving muscle quality," because the word "muscle" still has a negative connotation for many people…especially women. They associate the word with looking like Arnold Whatzizname, but tonus has nothing to do with the **size** of a muscle. It refers to the **quality** of a muscle, no matter what the size.

Doing lots of repetitions with light weights is **not** an efficient way to create quality muscle (tone up). It does not work the muscles hard enough. Using different amounts of weight for different numbers of reps, in a carefully planned exercise program, is a much better, faster, longer lasting and more effective way of creating quality muscle (toning up). The **CTTC** Exercise Program does this. Try it. You will be very pleased with your new **quality** (toned) **muscle** and how much better it makes you look…and **feel**…pun most definitely intended!

Myth Number 7

You have to exercise with "heavy" weights to build a strong, athletic body.

This is more a question for the guys (bigger muscles)…but the term **"heavy"** weights also applies to the ladies. YES, you do need to exercise with **heavy** weights to build larger muscles. However (ladies), you also need to use **heavy** weights to efficiently "tone up." Now the question is: **What is heavy?**

A **heavy** weight is any amount of weight that makes a particular muscle, or group of muscles, **work hard**. 100 pounds for one repetition on the bench press might be "light" for some exercisers, but the same 100 pounds for twenty-five reps will become very **heavy** as you go along. Five pounds can be **heavy** for a small stabilizer muscle.

Using correct exercise form, full ranges of motion, shorter rest periods between sets, and correct exercise tempos all make "light" weights **feel** much **heavier**.

If an exercise calls for twelve repetitions and you can only make eleven, you used a **heavy** weight. If an exercise calls for twelve repetitions and you stop at twelve, but you could have done more, you used a "light" weight. Muscles can't read. They can only **feel** if a task is easy (light), or if it is difficult (**heavy**).

Lifting **really heavy** weights is necessary if you want to become a weightlifter. Exercising with really heavy weights is **not** necessary for building a strong, athletic, or "toned" body. In the long run, your joints will thank you, because **really heavy** lifting can be very hard on your joints, especially as you get older. It is better to make the weights **feel heavy** instead.

Myth Number 8

Women should train differently than men.

For the most part…**no!** See Chapter 14.

Myth Number 9

Doing high reps with "light" weights builds definition.
Doing low reps with "heavy" weights builds mass.

Using a **combination** of lower, medium, and higher reps is necessary to effectively and efficiently develop either mass or definition. However, the number of reps is not the most important factor here. Your nutrition and aerobic programs play much larger roles in determining whether you create mass, definition, both…or neither.

Myth Number 10

Exercising with machines is better than exercising with free weights.

Any exercise is better than not exercising at all. Exercise machines are better than exercise gadgets. Exercising with free weights is better than exercising with exercise machines…most of the time. A **combination** of free weights and well-designed exercise machines, with an **emphasis** on free weights, is best. There is much more information on this subject in Chapter 7.

Myth Number 11

Certain exercises can change the shape of a muscle.

The only way to change the actual shape of a muscle is to tear it. I know this works because I have done it a couple of times. However, exercise cannot change the basic shape of any muscle. Muscle shape is genetically pre-determined. However, there are muscles which have two or more sections to them, such as biceps (two sections), triceps (three sections), and quadriceps (four sections). By changing hand or foot positions, arm or leg positions, the angle or direction of resistance, or the amount of weight used, you can **sometimes** emphasize one section of these muscles over the other section(s), thereby affecting the eventual appearance of the muscle **group**. The individual sections of a muscle group, however, cannot change their shapes, except for becoming larger or smaller.

Myth Number 12

With the right kind of exercise, you can change your basic body shape.

Sorry again, but if you are pear shaped, you can become a smaller pear, a bigger pear, or even less of a pear…but your basic pear shape will remain. The same is true for all other basic shapes. If you were born with wide hips and narrow shoulders, or short legs and a long torso…you will die with these as well. You can make tremendous improvements by creating illusions with Quality Exercise, but your basic shape will remain.

Myth Number 13

Exercising with weights will make you "muscle-bound."

Absolutely…**if you exercise incorrectly**, use weights that are too heavy for you, and if you do not use full ranges of motion…you will lose some of your flexibility. You will also lose your flexibility if you do not exercise at all, so I don't understand why non-exercisers are so afraid of losing flexibility. If you exercise **correctly**, most people will actually become **more** flexible, not less. Proper stretching is also a part of exercising **correctly**. Only people who are naturally very flexible anyway will, most likely, **not** increase their flexibility with exercise.

I used to carry a picture of the great John Grimek with me as proof of this. John Grimek was the only man to win the Mr. America title twice (in the 1940s). He was undefeated in bodybuilding contests, and was also an Olympic weightlifter. He is a legend in both sports. The picture I had was of him holding 250 pounds or so above his head…while in a full split with his legs. He could also bend over with straight legs and almost touch the floor…**with his elbows**! Gymnasts are also very muscular, but still extremely flexible. So much for "muscle-bound."

Myth Number 14

If you exercise like the bodybuilders say they do in the magazines, you will look like them.

First of all, not many of us…men or women…would **want** to look like most of the present bodybuilders. Secondly, all the bodybuilding magazines have to fill up their pages with something, month after month. This is no easy task, and they have to make it interesting as well. The fact is that most of the exercise articles are simply excuses to have a nice photo shoot with the bodybuilders, and many of the articles about nutrition are there to sell the magazine's own line of nutritional supplements, if they have one. The way competitive bodybuilders train has practically nothing in common with how we mere mortals need to exercise and, without the drugs, you can forget any similarity in exercise methods. Besides, these guys are genetic freaks. We couldn't look like them even **with** the drugs.

This is not to say that you can't learn anything from the magazines. Some are better than others, but you can learn from all of them. You can get new ideas, test your old ideas, learn to better analyze exercises and exercise programs, and learn a great deal about proper nutrition. Books and magazines can make you think and be more critical about what people write and say about exercise and nutrition. That is always a good thing.

After learning **The Principles of Quality Exercise** presented in this book, you will be much better able to separate fact from fantasy, bad from good, good from better, and better from best when it comes to health, fitness, and nutrition.

And I will say this: Even discounting the drugs, **nobody**…and I do mean nobody…knows more about losing body fat than bodybuilders. They successfully lower their body fat to amazingly low levels for competitions, time and time again. And many of the Golden Oldies of the bodybuilding community look better at sixty-plus, and even seventy-plus years old, than most other people ever did at any time during their lives. Practically everything I have learned about successfully losing excess body fat, I learned from bodybuilding, **not** from nutritionists or dieticians.

> Learn from people who have already been successful at what you are seeking to accomplish!

Myth Number 15

If you stop exercising, your muscles will turn to fat.

I only have three things to say about this one.

First: If it is possible to completely change the molecular structure of something (muscle to fat) by doing nothing (not exercising), then I am going to stop working for a living and just wait for all my worthless stuff to turn into valuable things. And then I will be stinking rich, because I really have a lot of worthless crap.

Secondly: If people with muscles become over-fat by their muscles turning into excess body fat, then from where do over-fat people who never had much muscle in the first place get their excess body fat? I could be wrong here, but I have a sneaky suspicion that they both acquire their excess body fat in the same ways. Yum, yum!

Thirdly: Why would you ever stop doing some type of exercise anyway? So you can become over-fat and unhealthy? Are you going to stop bathing and brushing your teeth as well?

Myth Number 16

The Balanced Diet

I love this one. This is the "magic bullet" solution that you will still get from lots of doctors, nutritionists, dieticians, and other "experts" out there who obviously know next to nothing about controlling body fat. "You need to eat a **balanced** diet." Heck, I can also offer advice like this. Are you sick? My advice to you is: "Get well." That wasn't too difficult, was it? Now go do it, on your own and with no information to help you succeed.

In a study done in The Netherlands, where the availability of fast-food is still much less than in America (but catching up fast, with very visible results), average people were asked if they ate a healthy, varied (**balanced**) diet. More than 80% answered yes to the question. However, when the diets of these 80% were actually analyzed, **less than 2%** met the **minimum** RDA's for nutrients. That's the truth about **The Mythical Balanced Diet**.

What the devil is a **balanced diet** anyway? Balanced what? Does a 200-pound man need to eat 200 pounds of food? Is the **balance** the same for a marathoner as it is for an office worker, or do we all have to decide for ourselves what **balanced** is? How do we do that if we are not experts in the field of nutrition? Even if we are nutrition experts, who has time to plan, prepare and eat a **balanced diet** every day? And if it is so easy, why are there still so many over-fat doctors, nurses, nutritionists and dieticians running around?

This is not a vicious criticism of health professionals. This is just not their area of expertise. Doctors study diseases. They don't have time to study health, much less nutrition. Building health is an entirely different field of study than diagnosing and treating diseases.

Nutritionists and dieticians mostly study nutrition for sick people. They also don't have much time left over for studying health-building nutrition, much less performance nutrition for exercisers and athletes. Thank goodness this is changing and we are now slowly beginning to get more **health professionals** instead of only **disease professionals.**

I will make a deal with the doctors and dieticians. I will not operate on people or write diets for specific diseases, and they should, in turn, not give advice about things that they are not qualified and competent to do so. Of course everyone has to tell you to ask your doctor. That is to cover their butts against lawsuits. I also have to say that in this book for the same reason...in fact, I will say it again here. Always ask your doctor before undertaking (or is that a bad choice of a word?) any new exercise or nutrition program.

Very simply, a **balanced diet** doesn't exist in our rat-race world. **The best we can do is to strive to eat reasonably well...as often as is humanly possible.** This simply means cutting **most** of the garbage out of our daily diets, **most of the time,** and choosing higher quality foods, **more often,** as is explained in Chapter 12 of this book. Good luck.

Most people are not aware that in 1998 **the RDA Committee of the US Academy of Sciences** at long last caved in to the overwhelming amount of positive scientific research and finally had to admit that **the average American diet does not contain enough vitamins and minerals.** It took them almost sixty years to admit it, but their recommendation now is for **most** Americans to take **basic** nutritional supplements.

Myth Number 17

You become over-fat by eating too much fat.

Not completely true. **Certain kinds of fats will actually help you to lose excess body fat.** You will find the real reasons for becoming over-fat in Chapter 4.

Myth Number 18

Eating or drinking carbs just before and/or during exercise will give you extra energy for your workouts.

It depends. The energy you need to successfully complete a one-hour exercise program (such as the **CTTC** Exercise Program) is determined **firstly** by how and what you have eaten during the past 24–48 hours, and **lastly** by what you have eaten 2–3 hours before you exercise. If you need a pre-exercise energy drink to get through a one-hour exercise program, there is something seriously wrong with your daily nutrition program.

A pre-exercise energy drink containing carbohydrates will **negatively** affect your body's ability to use body fat during and after exercise, so if you are exercising to lose body fat, drinking one of these would be a **huge** mistake.

Note: Contrary to what most people think, this advice **also** applies to endurance athletes. They should **not** consume (high-glycemic) carbohydrates for 1½ - 2 hours before an endurance event. They should, however, consume (simple) carbohydrates **during** an endurance event. A nutrition program for an endurance athlete is a whole different ballgame.

Myth Number 19

There are certain nutritional supplements that work almost as well as anabolic steroids.

No, some actually work better…for filling the bank accounts of the supplement companies that make these claims for their products, that is!

How stupid is this? Imagine that you are a professional athlete, or an Olympic hopeful. There are legal and affordable nutritional supplements that work **almost** as well as illegal and expensive anabolic steroids, but you still choose to risk your athletic career…and possibly going to jail…by using the illegal anabolic steroids (or any other banned drugs for that matter). That really makes sense, doesn't it?

If you really believe this marketing crap, then please contact me, because I have a great used car and some prime swampland for sale. Sorry…the Eiffel Tower is no longer available.

Myth Number 20

You don't need to use nutritional supplements to be really healthy.

This is absolutely true…if you happen to be what I call a "biological freak"…having been born with all the physical requirements for optimal health (see Chapter 15). If this is the case, then you probably don't need to do anything extra to stay healthy and you will probably live to be 100…**no matter what you do.** And if you are that lucky, you will undoubtedly win the lottery sometime soon too, so you might as well quit your job right now, sit back, and wait for the big bucks to come rolling in. The question now is: Do you really feel that lucky?

The rest of us are certain that we are not that lucky, so we will keep our jobs and, yes, we do need some extra help to **strengthen** our immune systems and our bodies, and to **keep** them strong (see Chapter 12). For us it is the difference between being **not too sick**…and being **truly healthy.**

I refuse to argue with people anymore about the necessity and benefits of **basic** nutritional supplements. The scientific and medical evidence proving the necessity and/or benefits of the **basic** nutritional supplements that I recommend is so overwhelming that arguing about it is like arguing whether you need to eat healthy, nutritious foods or not. Yes, you can survive by eating only fast-food, but for how long? And take a good look at the people who do. Is that something you want to aspire to in your life? How good is your health insurance?

And remember, according to some "experts," if you eat a **balanced diet,** you won't need nutritional supplements anyway (read Myth #16 again).

Myth Number 21

Nutritional supplements are dangerous.

I also refuse to argue with people about the safety of **basic** nutritional supplements anymore. The scientific and medical evidence proving the safety of the **basic** nutritional supplements that I recommend is so overwhelming that arguing about it is like arguing about whether flying is dangerous or not.

Every so often an airplane falls out of the sky and the people who are afraid of flying immediately scream, "See…flying **is** dangerous!" while completely ignoring the thousands of completely uneventful flights that take place every day, all over the world. There were 428 deaths out of eighteen billion passengers (world-wide) who flew in 2004. In spite of these facts, you will never convince someone who is afraid of flying that it is safer than driving a car, even though car accidents kill and maim millions world-wide.

I often encounter this same kind of illogical reasoning when discussing the safety of **basic** nutritional supplements. These are people who refuse to let facts interfere with their opinions!

Every now and then, one of the millions of people who regularly use nutritional supplements has a negative experience, and the cry goes out in the media, "Nutritional supplement kills athlete!" or something similar. Many times the article will neglect to mention that the person was doing something like attempting to lose weight by running in hot weather, in a plastic sweat-suit, without drinking any water, and also just happened to be taking some type of nutritional supplement as well. Yup, that nasty nutritional supplement did him in for sure. "Ban them! This proves they are dangerous." Of course some infomercial can continue to sell plastic sweat-suits as a safe, quick and effective way to lose weight…but that is OK because it was the supplement that was completely responsible for the athlete's death, not dehydration and heat stroke, right?

If you really want to be afraid of something, find out how many people die each year from OTC (over the counter) drugs that you can buy in any supermarket. In one five-year period there was **one death** from vitamins in a country (America) which has the most users of vitamins in the world. This death was the result of using a single vitamin (it was actually a mineral). In Chapter 12, I emphatically discourage the use of single vitamins, minerals, etc. In contrast, during the same five years there were **more than 2,250 deaths from OTCs,** including 640 deaths from "harmless" drugs such as simple aspirin. Prescription drugs kill another estimated 150,000 Americans every year. See also Chapter 15.

You won't find anyone trying to get these everyday drugs banned, and they shouldn't be banned. They do a lot of good for a lot of people, just as **basic** nutritional supplements do.

If I am deathly allergic to peanuts, why should *you* not be allowed to eat them. Or maybe we should only be able to buy peanut butter with a prescription. We need to be better informed and use more common sense about these things, and to stop reacting ignorantly with panic decisions.

It's like asking some guy sitting at a bar with a cigarette hanging out of his mouth if he takes vitamins. The answer you get will probably sound something like, "Nah, I don't take vitamins. I'm afraid of an overdose. Barkeep…another shot and a beer chaser here, please." Ah yes…another "expert" handing out free advice. Now there is someone whose opinion you should trust, especially about things concerning your health. Which "well-informed experts" do you rely on for your information?

Myth Number 22

You don't need nutritional supplements to realize good results from an exercise program.

This is also absolutely true. However, you do need nutritional supplements to realize **optimal** results from your exercise program. You also need nutritional supplements to realize these optimal results as quickly and as efficiently as possible. The nutritional supplements you really need are **basic** and inexpensive. There are others which are not really necessary, but which are just so darned convenient, inexpensive, and time-saving that I also recommend them. See Chapter 12 for more information.

Good, effective nutritional supplements can take your body a step beyond what it is normally capable of achieving, and do it faster and more efficiently.

Would you consider getting rid of your computer or calculator? Why not? We used typewriters and pencil and paper for many more years than we have had personal computers and calculators, and that worked just fine, so we obviously don't **need** these unnecessary gadgets either…do we? Nope, not if you are satisfied with the pace of working with manual typewriters, typing and sending each letter individually by snail-mail (yup, we don't **need** e-mail either)…and so on… and so on…and so on!

Of course this is ridiculous, just as ridiculous as **not** using **basic** nutritional supplements, both to enhance your exercise results, as well as to make building and maintaining your health faster, easier, more effective and more efficient. It is called progress, people. Hey…it is the 21st century, you know.

"But my doctor says that nutritional supplements don't work anyway." Then gently remind your doctor that it took *The Physician's Desk Reference* (which is a doctors' encyclopedia of the most commonly used drugs) **a couple of decades** to admit that anabolic steroids increase strength and muscle mass. Apparently, someone forgot to tell the athletes. So, not knowing any better, they just kept getting bigger and stronger during those many years, without the doctors' permission. How disrespectful was that? Read Myth #16 above again…same story…different subject.

After that you can ask him how many nutrition courses he took during his four years (or more) of medical school. You might be very surprised at his answer. Many medical schools still do not even offer courses in nutrition. Why not? Because nutrition is **not** what doctors study in medical school. They are too busy studying about diseases and injuries. Health-building nutrition is a completely different (but very closely related) subject.

I, along with millions of other athletes, have been safely and successfully using **basic** nutritional supplements for many decades. So, after you are finished arguing with us as to whether the **basic** nutritional supplements are safe and effective or not, we can argue as to whether the world is flat...or not. There are still people who believe that as well, and I'll bet that they are also afraid of flying.

In Conclusion

For those of you who began reading the book with this last chapter, now go to the front and read the entire book.

For those of you who have completed reading the entire book, **congratulations!** I admire your courage, persistence and self-discipline. Now go back to the front and begin **studying** the entire book as it pertains to your personal situation and goals.

Much health and happiness to all of you!

INDEX

(YOU WISH)

Nope…there is no index to this book. And you thought you were going to be able to just flip back here, look up the subject(s) that you are interested in, and then quickly read what I have to say about them. Sorry, this book doesn't work that way. If you want to know why, then go to the front of the book and read: **How to Read this Book**.

I do, however, highly recommend that you make your own personal index. As you read this book (from front to back), simply make notes of the page numbers and information which are relevant to your particular situation. This will not only provide you with a much more concise and "personalized" index for future reference, but will also serve as a tremendous learning aid. You will not only learn the information faster and better, but you will also retain the information much longer. I warned you that this is a book for serious exercisers!

Tell Me What You Think

My main reason for writing this book was to provide logical, practical, time-saving, efficient, effective and useful information to serious exercisers. I hope that I have, in the process, also been able to debunk many of the myths and old-wives' tales concerning exercise, nutrition and controlling body fat. I also hope that I have inspired you and caused you to **think** more about **what** you are doing…and **why** you are doing it…where these subjects are concerned.

If any of the information in this book is still not completely clear and understandable to you, please tell me about it. If I have missed any points which you, as a serious exerciser, feel are important and should have also been dealt with in this book, please tell me what they are. This will greatly help your fellow exercisers by making the information in further editions of this book even better, more complete and more comprehensible. It will also enable me to better cater future publications in the CTTC series to your needs.

Please direct any questions, comments or criticisms (nauseating compliments are also welcome) to our website at:

www.CTTChealthpublishing.com

I do care what you think and I would love to hear from you!

Workshops, Seminars, and Personal Training

To contact me regarding workshops, seminars or personal training, please go to our website.